W9-CFT-818

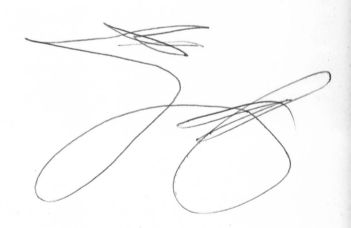

Clinical Evaluation

of the

Critically Injured

By

E. TRUMAN MAYS, M.D.
Associate Professor of Surgery
Associate Dean for Clinical Affairs
Director of the Price Institute of
Surgical Research
University of Louisville
School of Medicine
Health Sciences Center
Louisville, Kentucky

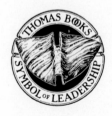

CHARLES C THOMAS · PUBLISHER
Springfield · Illinois · U.S.A.

Published and Distributed Throughout the World by
CHARLES C THOMAS • PUBLISHER
Bannerstone House
301-327 East Lawrence Avenue, Springfield, Illinois, U.S.A.

© *1975, by* CHARLES C THOMAS • PUBLISHER
ISBN 0-398-03351-X
Library of Congress Catalog Card Number: 74-23211

Printed in the United States of America
W-2

Library of Congress Cataloging in Publication Data

Mays, E. Truman, 1931-
    Clinical evaluation of the critically injured.

    Bibliography: p.
    Includes index.
    1. Medical emergencies. 2. Diagnosis. I. Title.
[DNLM: 1. Diagnosis. 2. Emergencies. 3. Hospital
emergency services. 4. Wounds and injuries.   WO700
M47c]
RC87.M387   617'.1   74-23211
ISBN 0-398-03351-X

This book is dedicated to patients who have died or suffered irretrievable impairment because of undetected, misdiagnosed or under-estimated injuries.

PREFACE

Physical injury is the leading cause of death between the ages of one and thirty-seven. United States Public Health Service and National Safety Council figures indicate about fifty million Americans each year suffer accidental injury. Eleven million of which are disabling to some degree and over 118,000 of which prove fatal. Injured patients take up twenty-two million hospital bed days a year, more than all heart patients or obstetrical patients and four times those needed by cancer patients.

The cost to this nation is estimated to be well in excess of eighteen billion dollars annually. Few comprehend the tragic and far-reaching aftermath of such critical injuries. It is impossible to estimate the irretrievable losses to individuals, families, nations or to society at large.

Quality of life as well as survival is dependent upon swift and accurate assessment of bodily damage. While consultation is obtained from all necessary specialty services, the responsibility rests with one physician who is capable of evaluating the patient's overall problem and establishing priorities. Training programs in every discipline of medicine prepare individuals for sophisticated care of specific and isolated injuries. This book deals not with the definitive treatment of an isolated injury, but the injured patient. Treatment is discussed only when it is related to immediate death, thereby becoming a first priority, e.g. airway obstruction, exsanguination, or pneumothorax. The management of individual lesions falls within the realm of numerous medical specialties and textbooks are available which cover these in detail.

High speed expressways continue to envelope every major city and intertwine states in an ever increasing network. Vehicular accidents on these high velocity roadways produce victims who have not one system injured, but many.

The recurring theme of this text is establishing priorities and accurate assessment of the patient with multiple injuries. A patient may have a horrendous scalp laceration beautifully repaired with the very latest plastic surgery technics, but if he exsanguinates from a ruptured liver or spleen while the scalp laceration is being sutured, he can never exhibit the "hardly visible hair-line scar" to the public. Better that he live with a nasty scar on the face or scalp that can be revised a year later. A man admitted to the hospital with a fractured femoral shaft after being crushed by an overturned refrigerator had his skeletal injury immediately reduced and stabilized, but he died during the night of undetected tension pneumothorax.

A recent study in Philadelphia emphasizes the problem; 950 deaths from injuries were reviewed. All but two of fifty-one salvageable cases died because of errors made at the hospital. Chief among these were: *errors in diagnosis,* failure to maintain an adequate blood volume and failure to provide specialized care early enough. These errors were all in the area of evaluation and early detection of injuries. Avoiding such errors requires emphasis on priorities, methodical assessment of bodily damage and meticulous search for concealed blood loss.

Physicians alert to these problems are urgently needed for what the National Academy of Science has termed "the neglected disease of modern society." Where are such men to care for critically injured patients to be enlisted? The solution is continued medical education—for physicians and nurses and emergency medical technicians who first encounter such patients.

The reader will be disturbed by repetition of concepts and material throughout the text. But the author feels apology for such repetition is unwarranted while injured patients continue to die or suffer brain necrosis from hypoxia, concealed or underestimated hemorrhage, and overlooked injuries.

Triage has become a popular concept. It is avoided in this text because it had its origin in military medicine. A basic assumption in triage is that there are certain patients who because of the nature of their injuries may be assigned a concrete prognosis depending upon duress, pressure and extent of facilities available. In civilian practice these basic assumptions of triage are unjustified. In the ideal emergency medical systems every injured patient should receive ultimate care for each of his injuries without prognosticating a fatal outcome. Also with proper communications, transportation and categorization of hospitals, no facility should be overtaxed.

The concept of priorities is more appropriate for civilian injuries. This concept compares one injury to another injury in the same patient, whereas triage compares the severity of one patient's injury with those of several other simultaneously injured patients and selects patients who have the best chance for surviving their injury. Establishing priorities takes into account a single patient and his various injuries. Every injury is assessed and placed into proper perspective for attention and restoration of the patient's health. After detection and evaluation, each injury is given precise skilled care consistent with the patient's survival and least possible residual impairment.

E.T.M.

CONTENTS

CLINICAL EVALUATION OF THE CRITICALLY INJURED

INTRODUCTION

The weakest spot in the whole system of care of accidents is in that uncertain period of time between arrival in the institution and definitive care in the operating room. We must accept more responsibility for what goes on in this twilight period, sometimes lasting several hours, if we hope to diminish the shocking rate of death.

Dr. R. H. Kennedy[1]

AMERICAN TECHNOLOGY, modern society and human nature have concatenated to produce injuries of a kind never before presented to the medical profession. Increasingly these critically injured patients have become a challenge. As industrial and automotive accidents spiral toward record heights, the medical profession and responsible hospital authorities must be prepared to receive and treat these patients in a competent manner.

It is now obvious that if critically injured patients are to be properly cared for attention must be directed to two areas: Phase I, initial emergency care and transportation (pre-hospital) and Phase II, in-hospital evaluation. That there have been deficiencies in both Phase I and Phase II can be confirmed by two recent accident studies. Regarding Phase I, Frey, Huelke and Gikas[2] reported 159 deaths from automobile accidents in Michigan. Twenty-eight of these were considered salvageable if adequate airway, intravenous fluids and chest tubes had been a part of the initial resuscitation and transportation. Phase II deficiencies were noted by Fitts, Lehr and Bitner[3] who analyzed 950 deaths from injuries and classified fifty-one as salvageable.

3

All but two died of errors made at the hospital. These were errors in diagnosis, failure to maintain an adequate blood volume, and failure to provide specialized care early enough.

It is impressive that in both pre-hospital and hospital mortalities proper appraisal priorities could have prevented death in many of these critically injured victims. Hence, it is imperative that early evaluation of critically injured patients become a first priority in any effective emergency medical services system. It is awesome that unlike cancer, stroke, and heart disease, no new basic scientific discovery is necessary to lower mortality rates, only the day to day application of scientific knowledge already extant. The early assessment of the severely injured patient and institution of priorities increasingly depends upon factors operative in both Phase I and Phase II.

Phase I

Properly trained and highly skilled personnel to staff adequate emergency vehicles are essential. This is evolving into the responsibility of city, county, state and federal government in the same sense that police and fire protection are basic to any organized society. It is an extremely expensive obligation. The physician must see his role in the development of Phase I as twofold: (1) instructor and teacher for emergency medical technicians who staff emergency vehicles, and (2) a catalyst to interact between government and public to create the reaction necessary to institute such expensive health care in already critically strained budgets. That such an organized effort can be effective in Phase I care is amply demonstrated by Captain Waters[4] and his now widely recognized System of Emergency Care and Transportation in Jacksonville, Florida.

Physicians must recognize their responsibilities in this area and aggressively working through county medical societies and governmental systems bring direction to the chaos that seems to be universally present in Phase I.

Phase II

Two factors are essential for improving hospital evaluation of the seriously injured:

(1) Physicians with broad backgrounds of medical training inspired with the concept of the "whole man."

(2) A geographic area within the hospital equipped and staffed on twenty-four hour basis.

Continued narrowing of fields of medical disciplines with greater degrees of specialization and sub-specialization has resulted in excellent treatment and reduced morbidity and mortality for isolated organ or system injury. But a combination of these specific lesions in a single patient often throws what otherwise is an excellent system of medical care into turmoil. While consultation is obtained from all necessary specialty services responsibility must rest with one physician who is able to evaluate the patient's overall problem and assign priorities with the "whole man" concept motivating his approach.

Infractions of this concept are so universal that it is superfluous to enumerate examples. The professional team approach is the logical answer to this dilemma. In every team there must be a "team captain." Each specialist consulted is a cooperating member of the team. He must be aware of the problems confronting his associates as well as his own problems. Of utmost importance is the fact, that upon direction of the "team captain," there is sometimes a need for varying or delaying one kind of treatment because of other associated injuries.

Finding such physicians is becoming an increasing problem. Stephenson,[5] after studying the teaching of emergency medical care in the United States and Canada, concluded, "Unfortunately, the teaching of emergency medical care of the acutely ill and injured patient too often has been given an insignificant role in undergraduate medical curricula in the United States and Canada . . . Trauma is seldom presented in its proper perspective as a disease."

Traditionally, it has been the general surgeon or orthopedic surgeon who assumed the role of primary physician in patients with multiple system injury, relying heavily upon consultation from his colleagues. His background and training in basic physiology of vital organ functions as well as technical capability of controlling hemorrhage seemed to cast him in this role. As universities are establishing residency programs in emergency medical care and as the general surgeon is gradually limiting his availability, a new physician highly trained in evaluation of patients with serious injuries to multiple systems may evolve into this primary role.

Next in importance of evaluating critically injured patients is the geographic area within the hospital where this should be done. For many years and by traditional assignment the emergency room was unquestionably the site. The "emergency room" is no longer a room but an "emergency department." "From a simple room with one or two treatment tables, a few intravenous stands and perhaps a cabinet of drugs, the 'emergency room' has now expanded into a many chambered area with facilities for many types of examination and treatment."[6]

Such a department is flooded with a diversity of patients from the critically injured individual in a state of hypovolemic shock to the individual with a viral pharyngitis or low back pain of six months duration. There are increasing numbers of nonemergency patients presenting themselves to the emergency department for health care.[7] This burgeoning utilization of the emergency departments of hospitals makes it obvious that this is not the geographic area to undertake evaluation of critically injured patients.

Many emergency departments now function as twenty-four hour walk-in clinics. As physicians in urban areas sign out to the emergency room, patients with minor ailments are learning that there is quick access to M.D.'s without long waiting periods. Traffic in the area, attendant confusion, types of illnesses being treated, distractions imposed upon medical personnel concatenate to make the emergency department the least ideal environment to evaluate critically injured patients.

A second and even more impelling reason not to utilize the emergency department is that surgical procedures such as venesections, airways, intercostal thoracotomies, and even laparotomy, craniotomy or thoracotomy become an integral part of evaluating seriously injured patients.

Efforts in the past to establish "secondary operating suites" within the emergency department have proved futile because of the now widely recognized inefficiency and high costs of duplication. Personnel staffing of such a secondary operating room on a twenty-four hour, seven day a week basis reaches impossible limitations.

Noer[6] urges the utilization of the intensive care unit or the operating room for the initial resuscitation and evaluation of critically injured patients. His proposed plan has many advantages, the greatest being immediate removal of the seriously injured individual from the mass of medical, pediatric and nonemergent patients who crowd the modern emergency department. Perry[8] adopted this system at the University of Minnesota Medical School and transfers without delay the critically injured patient to a special room in the operating suite maintained in readiness for that purpose.

The operating room is always equipped with sterile packs for venous cutdowns, central venous pressure, tracheotomy, chest tube placement, catheterization of urinary bladder, peritoneal lavage, laparotomy, thoracotomy, and craniotomy. Equipment for general anesthesia and assisted ventilation is in readiness. A special cart contains cardioscope, defibrillator, intravenous fluids, emergency drugs, etc. These supplies are not removed from this area—central supply must provide for the remainder of the hospital. This is axiomatic and if broken the entire plan for evaluation of critically injured patients may break down.

The patient is placed on a wheeled litter (with spine board as indicated) at the hospital entrance and transferred directly to the operating table—thus requiring only one move between ambulance and definitive care minimizing further trauma and preventing shuffling back and forth to X-ray (another twilight zone) and the various rooms within the emergency department.

The operating table is modified to accommodate a Bucky X-ray unit so that roentographic evaluation can proceed smoothly before, during or after an operation. In the surgical suite everything necessary for evaluation, resuscitation and definitive care is available. The nursing personnel and attendants are permanent, not rotating, and hence become extremely familiar and competent to meet the needs of the critically injured patient.

Such a system has been in effect in the University of Louisville's major teaching institution for many years. It has been extremely effective in this busy city-county hospital. The plan first evolved under the direction of Dr. R. Arnold Griswold because of his interest in salvaging penetrating wounds of the heart. The results in heart wounds proved so beneficial that over the years the plan has enlarged to include all critically injured patients brought to this regional trauma center.

In hospitals without twenty-four hour staffing of the surgical suite, the intensive care unit is the next most likely area to be utilized for initial evaluation and resuscitation, at least until the OR personnel can be called in. Most intensive care units have the basic equipment for monitoring and resuscitating while assessment of bodily injury progresses.

In the ideal emergency health services system the EMT will have established an adequate airway as first priority before transportation to the hospital, but once within the confines of the hospital the adequacy of the airway must be re-evaluated and steps taken to ensure that the airway is patent while preparations are made for thorough evaluation.

It may be that the emergency airway established at the scene of the accident has been dislodged, occluded or perhaps overlooked completely. A rapid check of the mouth and pharynx often reveals a dislodged dental plate or a "hunk" of aspirated meat or vegetable fiber occluding the hypopharynx and larynx. An index finger is the most efficient and available instrument for cleaning the hypopharynx of obstructions. The insertion of the index finger into the throat is such a simple maneuver that it is often forgotten or not done because of its simplicity. Blood, fluids and emesis should be aspirated with suction and an oropharyngeal airway or endotracheal tube inserted as indicated to ensure adequate ventilation while additional preparations are made.

Immediately upon arriving at the hospital a blood specimen should be obtained for typing, crossmatching and blood gases. At the same time a durable intravenous route must be established with a large bore needle or polyethylene catheter in the largest available vein nearest the right atrium. Venous cutdowns on the saphenous or cephalic veins are often necessary to establish a venous route in patients with reduced peripheral blood flow. The subclavian vein is a constant and convenient site for percutaneous catheterization of the superior vena cava.[9] This method avoids surgical cutdowns, saves time in critical situations, and can be accomplished from either the supraclavicular area utilizing the junction of the internal jugular vein with the subclavian vein or by an infraclavicular approach. A large bore catheter in the superior vena cava (SVC) is convenient for monitoring central venous pressure as well as giving large volumes of fluid and blood rapidly.

The pitfall that must always be avoided concerns injuries to the inferior vena cava (IVC) and SVC. If there is a possibility of injury to the IVC the saphenofemoral system of veins is contra-indicated as a venous route. More than once physicians have been caught vigorously pumping blood into an ankle vein cutdown only to find their patient deteriorate and develop cardiac standstill because the blood was running out a large hole in the IVC faster than it could be pumped in. To err in the opposite direction is just as tragic. In recent years the sterile pre-packed polyethylene catheter sets for percutaneous insertion have become so ubiq-uitous that few physicians pause to consider whether the upper torso veins or superior vena cava are injured prior to inserting an upper extremity or subclavian vein catheter. As in the lower extremities, it is futile to try to replenish blood volume by this route if the SVC has a hole in it.

The kind of fluid to be used in resuscitation has long been controversial. If blood has been lost, it should be replaced volume for volume. Recently harvested whole blood warmed during administration to near body temperature is unquestionably the ideal resuscitation fluid in situations of hemorrhage. Shires[10] demonstrated extracellular fluid deficits in hemorrhagic shock. While waiting for blood to become available extracellular fluid losses can be replaced. The large amount of data accumulated in the laboratory does not warrant the conclusion that lactated Ringer's is superior to physiologic saline nor that synthetic colloids are superior to saline solution. Of utmost importance is the recognition that extracellular fluid deficits are present in hemor-rhagic shock and partial replacement can be started while waiting for blood to become available. Hepatitis free plasma and other plasma volume expanders are indicated when an unreasonable delay in obtaining properly crossmatched whole blood is anticipated. Thus, the initial resuscitation fluid should contain both sodium and an energy substrate.[11-13]

After the patient is placed on the operating table (or other specific area for evaluation, I.C.U., etc.) clothing is cut away with large heavy bandage scissors. It is extremely important that all clothing is cut away. Numerous errors in diagnosis or failure to detect significant injury can be traced to good intentions of some kindly aide or orderly leaving underclothing intact to preserve the patient's dignity or modesty. Much more important physiologic functions need preserving in these critically injured people. A small barely detectable but physiologically highly significant penetrating wound of the thorax may be completely occluded from the examiner's eyes by items of underclothing.

The clothing must be cut away in a manner to reduce further trauma to a minimum. Never try to undress a seriously injured patient in order to keep intact an expensive sport jacket or dinner gown. Even such minimal motion as undressing has been sufficient to convert a closed fracture into an open fracture. Efforts to remove intact a pair of trousers or dinner gown can produce permanent quadriplegia in a patient with an unstable cervical spine fracture. A sharp broken rib can be pushed into the lung with sufficient force during "undressing a patient" to produce a hemopneumothorax.

After the patient is entirely nude a rapid survey of the total body surface is quickly done, taking into account areas of contusion, discoloration, penetrations, deformity, avulsion, and lacerations. It is important that this inspection include both anterior and posterior aspects of the patient. Every neophyte examiner seems to get caught offguard by obvious injuries on the ventral surface of patients failing to turn the patient over to detect a more significant wound of the back. The overall perusal of the patient must include meticulous observation of mucous membranes and nail beds for cyanosis and capillary filling, skin temperature and moisture and conjunctivae for perfusion and/or paleness. One of the earliest manifestations of hypoxia is a restless patient, thrashing around and requiring physical restraints.

As careful scrutiny of the patient continues his level of consciousness should be observed. Does he respond to verbal command? Does he move purposefully and do all extremities move equally well?

A rapid assessment of the patient's ability to give appropriate answers to questioning is exceedingly valuable at this point. Does he know or remember how he was injured? The method of injury, if it can be ascertained early, may influence the remainder of the evaluation, treatment to be instituted or a specific test to be done.

Did the patient have his seat restraints fastened? A patient thrown against the dashboard of a speeding automobile must be evaluated for deceleration injuries to the root of the aorta, the bronchus, the liver and the gallbladder. A patient thrown from the moving vehicle must certainly have a careful evaluation of the central nervous system. If seat belts were fastened, suspicion is turned to tears of the root of the mesentery and hollow viscus injury.

After this rapid general survey of the completely nude patient is completed a warm blanket is draped over the patient to prevent undue heat loss from modern air conditioning. The remainder of the examination will proceed much more efficiently if the patient is kept from chilling and made comfortable. Analgesics should be used sparingly and only for very definitive purposes; they may obscure the patient's response to pain, mask an area of localized tenderness, or cloud the consciousness.

A nasogastric tube is inserted into the stomach and the gastric contents aspirated. This is an evaluating maneuver as well as therapeutic. The presence of significant amounts of bright red blood in the aspirate lend suspicion to a major injury of the stomach. Old, dark blood may have been swallowed after injury to the nose, mouth or hypopharynx. The stomach should be as completely emptied of its contents as possible to prevent aspiration during the course of evaluation, during induction of anesthesia and in the postoperative period.

If by history, the patient has just recently taken food or liquid, it is wise to protect the airway with a cuffed endotracheal tube before gastric intubation. This obviates aspiration should the patient vomit.

Next a Foley catheter is inserted into the urinary bladder and a collection of hourly urine begun. Failure to pass urethral catheter with ease may indicate a ruptured urethra or separation of the urethra from the bladder neck. The catheter should never be forcefully inserted since this produces false passages and additional trauma! Gross blood obtained upon insertion of the catheter may indicate a torn urethra, disrupted bladder or renal contusion. The urine output should be recorded hourly as kidney perfusion is one of the chief criteria of adequate blood volume replacement. These concepts will be discussed in greater detail.

At this point the patient has been prepared for a systematic and meticulous assessment of bodily injury. An airway is ensured, a durable intravenous route is present, blood is in the laboratory for typing and crossmatching, gastric intubation has been done and a Foley catheter inserted into the urinary bladder.

REFERENCES

1. Kennedy, R. H.: Our fashionable killer. Oration on trauma. *Bull Am Coll of Surgeons, 40*:73-81, 1955.
2. Frey, C. F.; Huelke, D. F., and Gikas, P. W.: Resuscitation and survival in motor vehicle accidents, 9:292, 1969.
3. Fitts, W. T., Jr.; Lehr, H. B.; Bitner, R. L., et al.: An analysis of 950 fatal injuries. *Surgery, 56*:663, 1964.
4. Waters, J. M.: A synopsis of emergency medical services for a large city. *J Trauma, 12*:95, 1972.
5. Stephenson, H. E.: The teaching of emergency medical care in medical schools in the U.S. and Canada. *Bull Am Coll Surgeons, 56*:9, April, 1971.
6. Noer, R. J.: Emergency care of critically injured. *J Trauma. 3*:331, 1963.
7. Mays, E. T.; Mosley, D.; Rumage, W. T.; Setliffe, C.: Health care for an urban population: The emergency sector. *J Ky Med Assoc, 70*:687-693, 1972.
8. Perry, J. F., Jr.: Blunt and penetrating abdominal injuries. *Current Problems in Surgery,* May, 1970.
9. Weakley, S. D., and Mays, E. T.: Percutaneous catheterization of the subclavian vein in various clinical situations. *JKMA, 67*:902, 1969.
10. Shires, T.; Brown, F. T.; Canizaro, P. X., et al.: Distributinal changes in extracellular fluid during acute hemorrhagic shock. *Surg Forum, 11*:115, 1960.

11. Newton, W. T.; Rease, H. D., and Butcher, H. R.: Sodium and sulfate distribution in dogs after hemorrhagic shock. *Surg Forum, 20*:1, 1969.
12. Moffat, J. G.; King, J. A. C., and Drucker, W. R.: Tolerance to prolonged hypovolemic shock: Effect of infusion of an energy substrate. *Surg Forum, 19*:5, 1968.
13. Moss, G. S.; Proctor, H. J.; Homer, I. D., et al.: A comparison of asanguinous fluids and whole blood in the treatment of hemorrhagic shock. *Surg Gynecol Obstet, 129*:1247, 1969.
14. Kennedy, R. H.: The multiple injury patient. *Md State Med J, 12*:94-100, 1963.

WOUNDING FORCES

───

$\mathbf{B}$EFORE UNDERTAKING AN appraisal of injury sustained by patients, the assessor should be thoroughly familiar with kinds of wounding forces and the effects of such energy on human tissue. Violence has become ubiquitous in American society. The complexity of wounding forces and possibility of injury are accelerated yearly.

The mechanics and forces involved in wounding mankind change with changing times. It is a comment, not only on the violence inherent within man, but upon his imagination and ability to construct materials, which can make his life more comfortable or violently rip his flesh from his bones.

The development of gunpowder and the combustion engine changed wounding forces from wild animal bites, spear and rock wounds and falls from cliffs to blasting, penetrating and crushing forces involving acceleration, deceleration, impact, velocity, mass and numerous other parameters of delivering disruptive energy to human tissue. This change in wounding forces has made it mandatory for physicians to acquaint themselves with the physical as well as the biologic sciences. It is beyond reason to expect all physicians to understand completely the complex mathematics involved in deriving formulae governing all physical forces. Indeed it is beyond the scope of this text to even begin. But it is reasonable that most physicians gain at least a conceptual appreciation of a few of the formulae underlying the forces producing some of the more common injuries.

The nature of wounding forces change not only with the

physical sciences but also with the living habits and affluency of a society. The common household "ice pick," ubiquitous to the American home for four decades proved to be an easily accessible weapon. Ice pick wounds of the head, chest and abdomen were frequent in those years. As modern refrigeration displaced the "ice box" the ice pick wounds began to disappear until today they have been delegated a position with smallpox and poliomyelitis in the archives of man's afflictions.

Even stab wounds which represented a large percentage of penetrating wounds in earlier years have now decreased remarkably. They have been replaced with penetrating injuries by "Saturday night specials." The sale of small hand guns has spiraled to new heights. In our affluent society, it is a rare individual who does not possess a pistol. Many consider America an "armed camp." Following World War II it was the rare person who could not acquire an inexpensive imported handgun. Most of these imports were of .25 caliber variety. The effectiveness of these inexpensive small caliber handguns and ammunition was directly proportional to the cost. When the market flourished it was not unusual to evaluate a patient shot in the head to find with surprise that the missile lacked force to penetrate the cranium. After removing the missile from the subcutaneous tissue of the scalp the patient could be discharged and followed in the outpatient clinic.

As the gross national product increased, the buying power of the consumer paralleled it, and larger caliber weapons with greater muzzle velocity and more sophisticated ammunition became available. Magnum handguns have not only become the subject for violent movies, but are daily becoming available for an affluent populace. The physicians of the next decades will be called upon to evaluate penetrating injuries produced by weapons of increasing force.

The changing construction of automobiles influences the nature and kinds of wounding forces. Windshield construction is a prime example. Injuries sustained on pre-1966 model cars consisted of large, superiorly based avulsion flaps and deep lacerations of the eyelids, brow and forehead. Lacerations of the chin usually extended into the mouth. Such injuries usually had beveled edges or complete avulsion of tissue.[1] In 1966 an interlayer of plastic between the laminated glass was thickened to 0.030 inch and the band between the plastic and glass loosened slightly to allow some movement and slippage between the two plates of glass. This permits a degree of ballooning of the windshield. Prior to 1966 the head commonly penetrated the windshield and the sharp edges were perfect instruments for destruction of soft tissues. With the advent of the thicker plastic interlayer in the windshield there are few penetrations of the head. Soft tissue facial injuries are less frequent and of a different nature. Injuries now are small superficial lacerations, small triangular flaps and tiny avulsions.

The installation of the short stick gear shift popularized as "four-on-the-floor" has also influenced the nature of wounding capacities. I recently had a patient thrown violently onto this short gear shift ripping a large defect in the ischiorectal fossa and pararectal space.

The wearing of seat belts has remarkably decreased lethal injuries, but improper usage of such belts concentrates forces to certain organ areas and ruptures bladder, colon, small bowel and produces lumbar spine injuries.[2]

BLUNT FORCES

The destruction and tearing of tissues by blunt forces vary with the anatomical location of the impact, the contour of the impactor, and time force is applied. Trollope and colleagues[3] found the peak force and pulse duration had a high level of correlation with the estimated severity of injury (ESI) and found that when the locations of impact and mass of the subject were taken into account, the composite function:

$$\text{ESI} \; a \; \text{Log} \; \frac{f \, \tau^2}{m \sqrt[2]{a}}$$

where   f = force of impact
τ = duration of impact
m = mass of the animal
a = contact area

TABLE 2-I

ESTIMATED SEVERITY OF INJURY (ESI)

1+ Minor Trauma: Retroperitoneal hematoma, mesenteric abrasion, subcapsular hematoma of liver.

2+ Mild Trauma: Splenic hematoma, intestinal hematoma, small nonbleeding liver laceration or capsular hematoma.

3+ Moderate Trauma: Splenectomy or liver injury requiring repair.

4+ Major Trauma: Hepatic resection pancreatic fracture; survival only with maximum surgical care.

5+ Massive Trauma: Complete maceration of the liver, spleen or pancreas. Presumably lethal at scene of accident.

related well to the degree of injury produced in abdominal impacts (Fig. 2-1). They also found that the injury produced by a given blunt force, if applied over a long period of time is much more severe than if that same force is applied briefly.

The location of impact greatly influences the injury produced. Relatively small blunt forces are required to produce severe injuries of solid abdominal viscera when the point of impact is in the upper abdomen. In the lower abdomen much greater forces are needed to produce comparatively severe injuries.

Intestinal injuries occur when the intestine is crushed or impigned between the blunt forces compressing the abdominal wall and the spine.[4, 5]

When sudden severe forces are applied to fluid-filled sinusoidal, encapsulated masses, such as liver and spleen, the force is dissipated as hydrokinetic energy. It is governed by Pascal's principle and transmitted in all directions acting with the same force on all equal surfaces. A turgid organ such as the liver responds by bursting with explosive violence disrupting the internal architecture, and producing stellate and linear crevasses in Glisson's capsule. The turgidity of the organ is a definite factor in the degree of injury sustained from a given force. I studied the internal architecture of the liver by subjecting flaccid cadaver livers to blunt trauma and comparing the extent of injury to cadaver livers whose turgid state had been restored by perfusion with saline.[6] The flaccid livers showed no internal disruption after measured trauma whereas the turgid organs showed tears in Glisson's capsule and the hepatic parenchyma after similar trauma.

Energy exists in a variety of forms. Variants in which the

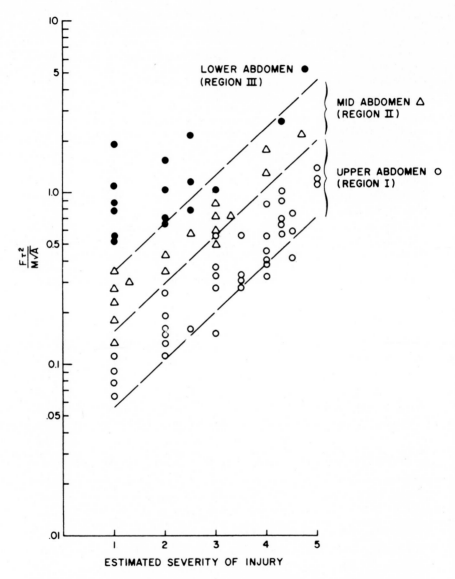

Figure 2-1.   Correlation of blunt forces to ESI. (Reproduced with permission Trollope, et al., *Journal of Trauma, 13*:962, 1973.)

energy is not dependent upon mechanical motion are referred to as potential energy. Kinetic energy is associated with bodies in motion and governed by:

$$E = \frac{m\ v^2}{2}$$

where   m = mass of body
               v = velocity

This equation is accurate in the field of trauma because the velocities we ordinarily encounter in medicine are much less than the speed of light. It is only when velocity exceeds the speed of light that the above equation becomes inaccurate involving theories of relativity and requiring correction to be made. In the English system the unit of energy is the foot-pound.

Power is the rate at which work is performed. The average power accomplished by an agent during a given period of time is equal to the total work (in trauma, destruction of tissue) performed by the agent during the period, divided by the length of time interval. The instantaneous power can then be expressed simply:

$$P = \frac{d\ w}{d\ t}$$

Applying these principles I studied forces involved in hepatic trauma. When energy in the range of twenty-seven to thirty-four ft.-lb. was transmitted to the cadaver liver it produced tears and lacerations of Glisson's capsule but intrahepatic injury involving vascular and biliary elements was absent. Increasing the energy 106 to 134 ft.-lb. disclosed crevassing of the liver externally but only an occasional disruption of a tertiary branches of bile ducts and hepatic arteries. There was no injury to major vascular and biliary structures. A further increase in energy (285 to 360 ft.-lb.) caused extensive derangement of the internal architecture of the liver, with major disruption of the tertiary dursions of the portal vein, hepatic artery and bile ducts. These injuries were similar to those seen in patients involved in high speed vehicular accidents.

Trollope and associates also studied blunt forces involved in hepatic trauma. In an animal investigation they concluded that only a small percent of the force applied to animals (and presumably to man in automobile accidents) was actually received by the liver. They found 350 lbs. were needed to produce nonbleeding liver lacerations or capsular hematomas in intact animals, whereas only 150 lbs. were needed to produce similar injuries in the exposed liver subjected to direct trauma.

Obviously rigid mathematical formulae cannot be applied directly to man because much of the energy of applied blunt forces are dampened by the protective abdominal parietes and thoracic cage. They permit some understanding of the ways various tissues respond and the amount of energy required to produce certain kinds of energy.

All tissues do not respond to blunt energy to the same degree. In the exposed rabbit colon I delivered blunt force just short of perforation and avulsion.[7] The energy was distributed by a striking weight over a 3 cm area to the terminal colon of thirty rabbits. Five animals were sacrificed at twenty-four hours, seventy-two hours and one week. Fifteen rabbits were sacrificed at one month. Hematoxylin and Eosin staining showed the muscularis to be the most susceptible layer of the rabbit colon with the mucosa and muscularis mucosa showing the greatest resistance. A force of 239 gms falling from 53 cms completely lysed the muscular layer but the mucosa and muscularis mucosa remained intact. Increasing the force ruptured the serosa and muscularis mucosa, yet the mucosa remained intact and herniated through the defect in the disrupted layers.

The serosa and mesentery of the colon respond with proliferative fibroblastic activity culminating in thickening of these structures.

Surprisingly, the vascular elements tolerate blunt forces quite well, this is likely due to the elastic elements in their structure. However, vascular elements were extremely sensitive to shearing and twisting forces. Because trauma is frequently associated with ischemia and devascularization the same model was studied after interrupting arterial flow. Here the resistance of tissue was just reversed from that found in blunt non-shearing forces. The mucosa was most sensitive to ischemia and dissolved completely and rapidly whereas the muscular layer remained intact for several days until secondary bacterial invasion dissolved the muscular layer.

Thus far we have been concerned chiefly with forces of impact resulting in avulsion, compression, crushing, and bursting of various tissues. There is another kind of force associated with blunt trauma that is often forgotten and seldom discussed. Hass[8] studied these forces in aircraft accidents and stated, "whenever one part of the body is decelerated at a rate which is different from that of another part, the connection between the two parts is placed under stress." With increased emphasis on speed and rapid transit this promises to be one of the most common wounding forces both now and in the future. The tissue injury caused by deceleration is already making itself known in frighteningly obvious ways. Our trauma team was recently impressed with the destruction discovered in the right chest of a thirty-nine-year-old man. He was brought to the hospital after his Volkswagen was struck head on at a metropolitan intersection. His chest was opened immediately because of the advanced degree of hypovolemic shock. The right lung had been torn from the hilum avulsing with it portions of the superior vena cava azygos vein and right atrium. The lung was floating free in a massive hemothorax and the right main stem bronchus could be inspected through its open end. The patient died. Such lethal tissue damage within the protected boundaries of an intact thoracic cage cannot be explained by impact. Rapid deceleration is the only force than can produce such an injury and physicians will be exposed to more and more patients who sustain these decelerative injuries. Later under cardiothoracic evaluation we will discuss a second example of such injury in tearing of the thoracic aorta at the relatively fixed region of the ligamentum arteriosum.

The amount of tissue avulsion in deceleration injuries depends not so much upon the displacement as upon gravity units. Forces of deceleration are best understood in terms of gravity units (G's). These forces increase as the square of the speed and as the stopping distance decreases.

$$G = \frac{(MPH)^2 \times 0.034}{\text{stopping distance in feet}} = \frac{(MPH)^2}{30x \text{ stopping distance in feet}}$$

As an example of the forces involved in deceleration, a moving body coming to a stop from thirty miles per hour in a distance of two inches sustains a 180 G force. A moving body suddenly stopping in two inches from a sixty mph velocity sustains 720 G and from a ninety mph velocity 1620 G. At these forces it is not necessary that organs or tissues move over great distances to avulse them from surrounding organs or tissues that are relatively fixed. Other forces of deceleration are illustrated in Table 2-II.

TABLE 2-II

FORCES OF DECELERATION

Speed of vehicle M.P.H.	Stopping Distance Feet	G's
30	2	15
30	4	7.5
60	2	60
60	4	30
90	3	90

There are many organs in the human which in relation to surrounding structures are relatively free as compared to contiguous tissue supported by heavy ligaments.[9] The lungs relationship to the mediastinal structures as described in the preceding paragraphs is only one example. The gallbladder is another. The liver is relatively well restrained by its supporting ligaments whereas the gallbladder is free. A common injury in automobile accidents is avulsion of an intact gallbladder from its hepatic fossa. Likewise the liver in relation to the inferior vena cava is relatively free and we are encountering more and more instances of avulsion of the hepatic veins from the vena cava and in some instances tearing the anterior wall of the vena cava which in relation to the posterior wall of the vena cava is relatively free.

The forces of rapid acceleration also damage tissue particularly the skeletal system. Such injuries of rapid acceleration are seen in young pilots who eject themselves from supersonic jet aircraft. Because such injuries are seldom encountered in civilian practice medicine they will not be discussed in any more detail.

PENETRATING FORCES

The degree of tissue damage produced by stab wounds is usually related only to the penetration of structures in the path of the wounding instrument. When evaluating these injuries the major concern is the number of organs penetrated and the degree of hemorrhage. But the evaluation of missile injuries is much more complicated involving velocity and mass of the missile.

Some common errors made in assessing penetrating wounds must be discussed first. The neophyte assessor usually assumes that the penetrating instrument moved through the tissues in a straight line. This assumption is usually incorrect when dealing with human subjects. Remember the injured victim does not assume the normal anatomical position portrayed in textbooks of anatomy awaiting the assault of his enemy. Rather the human body assumes a multiplicity of anatomical positions, some preparing to defend themselves, others fleeing from their assailants and others even unaware that they are about to be assaulted. Many in this latter instance will be involved in all the thousands of various manipulations the human anatomy does in carrying out hundreds of everyday common tasks. In all these anatomical positions some muscle groups are tense while others are relaxed, some ligaments are taut while others are loose, and the structural architecture of bone, cartilage, fat and muscle represents a non-homogenously laminated zone through which the penetrating instrument must move. While the wounding instrument is moving through the tissue the various tissues are also moving and gliding one over the other.

This dynamic non-homogenous anatomical system deflects penetrating objects into random patterns. When the injured patient finally comes to rest on the operating room table in a supine position, all the pierced tissue take on different relationships to each other. These factors preclude success in trying to follow the tract of a wounding instrument with either another instrument, soft catheters or pressure injection of contrast materials. This is why we condemn probing traumatic wound tracts to determine whether they penetrate certain cavities or organs.

Missiles fired from bored chambers characteristically have an axial rotation as well as forward motion. Such a spiralling mass can be deflecting in many different directions by the previously described dynamic anatomy. The inexperienced find it difficult to believe that anything but bone or metal can deflect a bullet into sharp curves and angles. But the differences presented to spiraling rapidly moving missiles by muscles, fascia and ligaments can change the course of bullets several times after they enter the body. The common error is to locate the wound of entrance on the surface anatomy and the position of the bullet on an X-ray and draw a straight line between the two, with the idea that anything in the path must be injured. Low velocity bullets do not travel in straight lines after entering human tissue. They can enter the chest, deflect to the abdomen and return to the opposite chest without ever crossing the mediastinum. The extremely high velocity missiles fired from military rifles are an exception to this rule.

Bullets also embolize. They can enter an extremity vessel and go to the right heart or enter the heart or great vessels and go to the leg. Figure 2-2a shows the chest X-ray of a thirty-year-old man shot in the chest in the xyphoid region. But the chest X-ray showed no sign of the missile. Fluoroscopy of the heart and mediastinum was equally disappointing. The patient had no complaints on examination. The right foot was cooler than the left. The poplitial pulse was palpable bilaterally but on the right the dorsalis pedis and posterior tibial pulses were absent. A roentgenogram displayed the mysteriously missing missile behind the right knee (Fig. 2-2b). Under general anesthesia an anteriotomy was done on the posterior tibial artery removing a .22 caliber bullet. A subsequent thoracotomy disclosed a three mm hole in the posterior wall of the aorta where the missile had been deflected off the vertibral bodies and entered the thoracic aorta then embolizing to the leg vessel. The adventia had effectively tamponaded the aorta and prevented the patient from exsanguinating.

As a general rule the exit wound of missile injuries is usually larger and more irregularly jagged than the wound of entry. For most bullet wounds encountered in civilian experience this is a

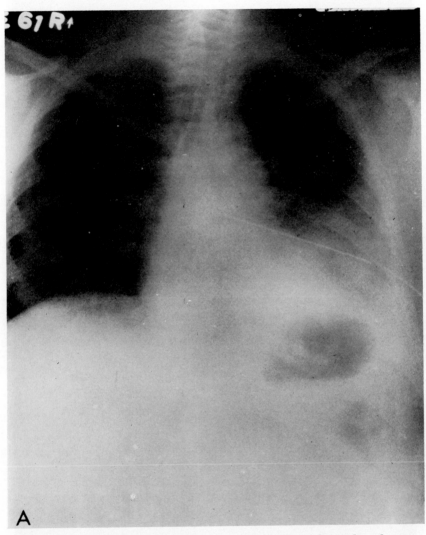

A

Figure 2-2. Chest x-ray of thirty-two-year-old man admitted with gun-shot wound of chest—but no evidence of an exit wound and no evidence of the missile (a) Roentgenogram of same victims leg showing missile embolized to popliteal artery. (b) Thoractomy disclosed the injured thoracic aorta which was repaired.

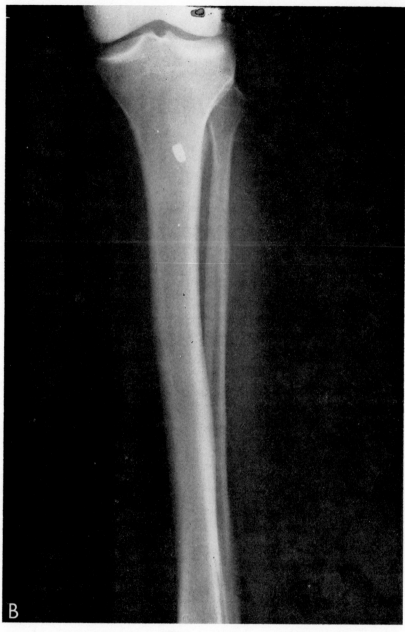

Figure 2-2b.

reliable axiom. In most instances it is an important aspect of assessment to differentiate the wound of entry and the exit wound if there be an exit wound. This is critical when examining hollow organs at the time of surgical exploration. There is a phenomenon of "splashing" which becomes operative at high velocities and may be the source of confusion. In wounds caused by extremely high velocity missiles the entrance wound may be as large or larger than the wound of exit. This is due to a retrograde jet of energy very much like the upperward jet of water when an object is dropped from a great height onto a smooth surface of water. This same effect on tissue may result in a large wound at the site of entry. Admittedly this is a rare situation, but confusion about which is entry and which exit wounds in extremely high velocity missile wounds does occur. The best illustration of this was the confusion arising over the wounds in President Kennedy.

When evaluating penetrating wounds there are often paradoxical findings that may confuse the examiner, unless he appreciates the importance of anatomical structure and relative densities of various tissues. Daniel[10] found the damaging effect of moving bullets increases with increase in specific gravity of the tissue traversed. Every clinic has encountered patients who have severe lung injury after a missile strikes the thoracic cage at a tangent and other patients who have relatively minor injuries to lung after the missile goes straight through. The effect of missiles on tissue is most evident in dense bone and least in lung. The correlation of tissue density to severity of wound is shown in Table 2-III.

TABLE 2-III

RELATIONSHIP OF SPECIFIC GRAVITY TO WOUNDING CAPACITY

Tissue	Specific Gravity	Severity of Wound
Lung	0.4—0.5	Minumum
Fat	0.8	Moderate
Liver	1.01—1.02	Marked
Skin	1.09	Marked
Muscle	1.02—1.04	Marked
Bone	1.11	Extreme

Reproduced with permission, DeMuth, W. E., *Journal of Trauma*, vol. 6, 1966, p. 226.

The evaluation of bullet wounds involves not only the tissue through which the missile passes as is true of stab or stiletto wounds. Such an oversimplification will lead to improper assessment of the injured victim. There are three major theories about the wounding capacity of bullets:

1. *Kinetic Energy Theory.* This theory explains most of the problems involved in evaluating bullet wounds and is the leading theory at this time. This theory gives greater importance to velocity according to the following:

$$\text{Kinetic Energy} = \frac{\text{Mass x Velocity}^2}{2}$$

It is obvious from this equation that if you double the velocity the Kinetic energy is quadrupled. As mentioned previously missiles possess not only forward velocity but rotation on their axis as a result of the spin imparted by the bore of the firing instrument. Therefore the kinetic energy developed through forward motion is augmented by the energy of rotation. This is calculated:

$$E = \frac{IW^2}{2G}$$

where   I = rotary inertia
         W = angular velocity in radians/sec

Rotary inertia is calculated:

$$I = \frac{Mr^2}{2}$$

where   M = weight of bullet in pounds
where   r = radius of cross section of bullet in feet

Angular velocity is calculated:

$$W = \text{rotations per sec x 2 g}$$

The spin imparted to missiles is used to stabilize the projectile in flight and increase accuracy.

2. *Momentum Theory.* This theory accepts mass as being equally important to velocity.

$$M = \text{Mass x Velocity}$$

If one accepts this theory then increasing the weight of the bullet results in greater wounding force.

3. *Power Theory.* This theory emphasizes the importance of velocity as in the Kinetic Theory.

$$\text{Power} = \text{Mass x Velocity}^3$$

Small increases in velocity result in tremendous increases in wounding potential.

In all these theories velocity is a chief determinant of wounding capacity. Once the propelling force stops velocity begins to fall. Hence, muzzle velocity, impact velocity and residual velocity are all factors that require additional delineation. Muzzle velocity is the initial velocity of the missile as it leaves the muzzle. It is limited by the weight of the projectile and size of charge. Chamber pressures should not exceed 70,000 lbs per square inch. This limit is rapidly reached as bullet weight and size of charge increase. Recoil of the firing instrument is also a limiting factor. Impact velocity is that velocity which the missile has at the instant of striking. Residual velocity is the velocity remaining as tissue is penetrated. Bullet velocity is classified in Table 2-IV.

The wounding energy actually imparted to tissue is a function of the difference between impact velocity and residual velocity.[11, 12, 13] Obviously bullets designed to remain in the organism increase the severity of wounding if bullet weight and velocity are identical. Hunting bullets are designed to expand to several times their original caliber, produce a wide wound tract and remain within the target.

Although wounding capacity seems primarily related to velocity, Demuth reports bullet design and composition are nearly equally as important[12] (Table 2-V). There are two major designs:

TABLE 2-IV

BULLET VELOCITY

Common Nomenclature	*Velocity ft/sec.*
Low	<1000
Medium	1000 to 2500
High	>2500

TABLE 2-V

CORRELATION OF WOUND VOLUME IN DOG THORAX
TO BULLET DESIGN

150 grain, 30 cal., 2,900 ft/sec

Bullet Type	Diameter Entry Wound	Diameter Exit Wound	Wound Volume
Military (full jacket)	0.75 cm	2 cm	23.5 cm^3
Sporting (expanding)	0.75 cm	12.5 cm	917 cm^3

Reproduced with permission, DeMuth, W. E., *Journal of Trauma*, vol. 6, 1966, p. 230.

1) Jacketed. Because most bullets are lead alloys, heat is a limiting factor. Lead has a low melting point. In most civilian injuries involving low velocity missiles there is no problem with distortion by barrel friction. Commercial lead bullets are rarely designed to exceed 1,500 feet/sec or they will soften and deform the barrel. Softening of lead precludes holding the barrel rifling. Above 2000 feet/sec the basic lead missile must be covered with a jacket of metal that has a higher melting point. Copper and soft steel are frequently used to jacket that portion of lead missiles in contact with the barrel. Geneva Convention rules require military bullets to be full jacketed and non-expanding. 2) Expanding bullets. These are soft nose missiles used in sporting and game hunting. This missile mushrooms after perforating the target expanding to several times its original caliber and establishing a wide wound tract. Unfortunately, most hunting accidents and home accidents involve both of the most damaging properties of missiles—high velocity and a widely expanding wound tract. The human body mass is not great enough to stop neither the full jacketed military missile nor the expanding type.

Demuth[12, 14] further states that sectional density of a missile influences how well bullet velocity is maintained and thus its wounding capacity upon perforating the target. Sectional density is the ratio of mass to cross sectional area:

$$\text{S.D.} = \frac{W}{7000\ D^2}$$

where   W = weight of bullet in grains
           D = bullet diameter in inches
           7000 = number of grains/pound

Bullets of about the same length and shape will have similar sectional densities irrespective of weight.

The impact velocity of any given missile depends not only upon muzzle velocity but also upon how effectively a bullet overcomes air resistance while in flight. The ballistic coefficient is the chief factor involved in determining how well a specific bullet remains its original muzzle velocity, or energy imparted by the charge.

$$\text{Ballistic Coefficient} = \frac{SD}{I}$$

where   SD = sectional density
           I = is a form factor (Fig. 2-3)

Ogive is the radius of bullet curve in lateral projection and is expressed as multiples of bore caliber. This means that a bullet with an ogive value of 8 would have a ballistic coefficient twice that of a bullet with an ogive value of 0.5.

Other ballistic considerations are trajectory; yaw, drag, co-efficient, and barrel design. These are not discussed here because they are not particularly applicable to clinical evaluation of wounded patients. The interested reader can pursue these in background reading by Beyer.[15] Wounding forces of some common pistols and rifles are shown in Table 2-VI.

Shot Guns

When evaluating penetrating injuries those produced by shot guns must be considered separately. The wounding capacity of shot guns differs from pistols and rifles in many aspects.[16] The shot charge consists not of one missile but a large number of small spheres. Chamber pressure and muzzle velocity are about that of a pistol (850 feet/sec). The effective wounding range of the shot gun is short. The muzzle velocity falls off much more rapidly than does that of a pistol or rifle. The pellets string out along the axis of the line of flight and dispense perpendicular

OGIVE I VALUE

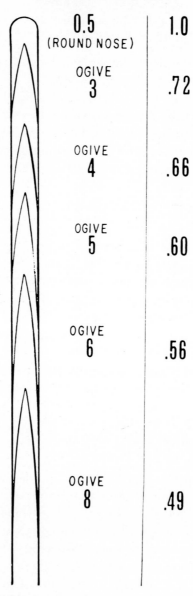

0.5 (ROUND NOSE)	**1.0**
OGIVE **3**	**.72**
OGIVE **4**	**.66**
OGIVE **5**	**.60**
OGIVE **6**	**.56**
OGIVE **8**	**.49**

Figure 2-3. Ogive values reflect the radius of bullet curve in the lateral projection and determine the Ballistic Coefficient along with the sectional density of the missile. (Reproduced with permission from Demuth, *Journal of Trauma*, 927-938, 1969.)

TABLE 2-VI

	Bullet wt. (grains)	Muzzle Vel. ft/sec	Wounding Energy ft/lbs
PISTOLS			
.25 Automatic	50	820	75
.30 Luger	93	1,250	323
.38 Automatic	95	970	199
.45 Automatic	230	850	370
.44 Smith and Wesson Russian	246	770	324
.455 Webley Mark II British	265	600	210
.38 Special hi speed	158	1,090	425
.45 Colt	250	860	410
.357 Magnum	158	1,410-1,550	695-845
.41 Magnum	210	1,050-1,500	515-1,050
.44 Magnum	240	1,470	1,150
HUNTING RIFLES			
.22 Remington	40	1,180	124
.22 Hornet	45	2,650	715
.220 Swift	45	4,140	1,825
6 mm 243 Winchester			
244 Remington	75	3,500	2,037
7 mm Mauser	175	2,460	2,350
.270 Winchester	130	3,140	2,850
300 Savage	180	2,380	2,265
30-30 Winchester	170	2,200	1,830
30-'06 Springfield	180	2,710	2,940
30-40 Krag	180	2,480	2,460
.300 H & L Magnum	180	3,030	3,670
.303 British	215	2,160	2,230
8 mm Mauser	170	2,530	2,415
.375 H & H Magnum	270	2,720	4,440
.378 Weatherby	270	3,180	6,051
.460 Weatherby	500	2,700	8,095
MILITARY RIFLES			
6.5 mm Arisaka (Jap)	139	2,428	1,880
7.7 mm Type 99 (Jap)	180	2,493	2,484
7.62 m Czech Mod 52	131	2,440	1,550
7.55 mm French M, 1949	139	2,690	2,208
7.62 mm Chinese Type 56	190	2,410	2,449
5.56 mm M-16 U.S.A.	55	3,250	1,289
8 mm German Mauser	236	2,100	2,310
7.65 mm Argentine Mauser	150	2,920	2,841
7.62 mm U.S. M-14	180	2,610	2,720
7.92 mm German Kar 98K	198	2,476	2,680
7.62 mm Russian	150	2,810	2,635
.303 British	180	2,540	2,579

Modified from DeMuth, W. E., *Journal of Trauma*, vol. 9, 1969, pp. 27-38; vol. 6, 1966, pp. 226-233, 744-755; vol. 14, 1974, pp. 227-229.

to this axis. The pellets do not all hit the target at the same time. This fact must be emphasized in light of the previous discussion about variations in anatomical positions of the victim. The first pellets may strike a person in one position and the last pellets strike the victim after he has changed from his earlier position.

Most shot gun barrels are twenty-six to thirty inches in length. The "sawed off" shot gun is approximately twenty inches and makes a particularly lethal wound at close range. It is used by some law enforcement groups and occasionally by criminals. The terminology applied to shot gun and shot gun ammunition developed over many years often in a nonsystematic and unplanned fashion. Some of the terms are not logical to individuals trained in the metric system and become somewhat confusing to physicians who are trying to understand the wounding capacity of this instrument.

Gauge

This is an archaic term designating bore caliber. It is interesting to note how the gauge of shot guns was determined originally. After the barrel was completed a single shot was poured to a size approximating the muzzle of the gun. This single round shot was calibrated so that it was just able to enter the bore of the gun. The number of such round shot required to make a pound then became the gauge of that particular shot gun. A 12 gauge shot gun could be fitted with a round ball of such size and weight that 12 of them weighed a pound. The 410 gauge shot gun is an exception to this archaic principle, in that a lead sphere approxi-

TABLE 2-VII

SHOTGUNS IN COMMON USAGE

Gauge (Archaic Term)	Bore Caliber (Inches)
10	0.775
12	0.730
16	0.670
20	0.615
28	0.550
410	0.410

Reproduced with permission, DeMuth, W. E., *Journal of Trauma*, vol. 11, 1971, pp. 219-229.

mately the bore of the 410 number 67.5 to the pound. The 410 designation refers to the bore of the muzzle which is .410 inch in diameter.

Powder Charge

Low chamber pressures are necessary because of the underlying design of the shot gun. A mixture of charcoal, saltpeter and sulfur produced "black powder." The unit of measurement was the dram. Modern "smokeless" powder replaced the original mixture, but the term "dram equivalent" persisted. A 3-dram equivalent charge is the quantity of modern smokeless powder producing the same shot velocity as 3 drams of original black powder. Shot gun powder is fast burning for use only in shot guns.

Shot Pattern

As the small lead spheres emerge from the muzzle they develop a particular pattern of flight. It forms a conical circle and ideally the spheres should be evenly distributed throughout a circle pattern when all the pellets strike their target. Because shot guns are used for small game birds and animals the effective range is twenty to forty yards. The pellets form such a dense pattern at less than twenty yards they destroy the animal to such an extent that it is no longer desirable as game. It is in this range (twenty yards) that injuries to patients are so totally destructible. Beyond forty yards the pellets take on such a sparse pattern that they lose their killing or imobilizing power for small game animals and in humans produce wounds of lesser significance.

Shot

The individual buckshot are referred to as pellets but the collective projectile mass made up of all the individual spheres is referred to as shot. At one time the individual spheres were pure lead, now they are made from an alloy of lead and antimony. For preparing magnum loads the pellets are coated with a copper zinc alloy. For larger animals larger pellets called buckshot and BB are made.

Shotgun Shell

This is a paper or plastic casing fitted into a metal cup containing the primer and "shot cap." The powder charge lies in contact with the primer. Wads made of various materials are placed between the powder and shot charge. These wads leave the barrel along with the shot when the gun is fired. In human injuries at close range this wadding is often projected into the depths of the wound. This wadding gives an added dimension to shot gun wounds about which physicians must be knowledgeable. The individual pellets can often be incorporated by fibrous tissue reaction and produce minimal foreign body problems. Many individuals have carried hundreds of pellets in their tissues for years but the wadding always acts as a foreign body particularly in the devitalized tissues produced by close range shot gun blasts. Until recently this wadding was fabricated from animal hair and as such had a significant number of tetanus spores. Once carried into the depths of the wound, this foreign body and accompanying tetanus spores produced a high incidence of clinical tetanus in patients surviving the initial blast. Now that most wadding is made of plastics, the threat of tetanus that once accompanied shot gun wounds has been reduced.

Choke

The shot pattern is largely determined by a constriction built into the muzzle end of the barrel, this constriction is termed choke and controls the shot pattern in the same way that changing the size of the nozzle on a garden hose changes the pattern of the stream of water. At the ranges where most human wounds are produced, choke is relatively insignificant in determining wounding capacity. A full choke barrel delivers 70 percent of the pellets into a thirty inch circle at forty yards. Modified choke delivers approximately 60 percent and cylinder bore (no constriction) 40 percent of the pellets into a thirty inch circle at forty yards. Since clinically troublesome injuries in patients occur at fifteen yards or less it is obvious that choke plays very little role in determining amount of tissue damage.

The tissue damage inflicted by shot guns has distinctive features depending on range. Most serious injuries to patients occur at distances of fifteen to twenty yards. At distances greater than twenty yards the wounding potential of the shot gun takes on different dimensions. The assessment of the injured patient will differ depending upon whether they have a close range injury or a long range injury.

The close range injury usually produces a skin wound with a diameter of fifteen cm or less. The real problem in these injuries is beneath the skin. Muscle, viscera, bone, fascia are pulverized to the point of devitalization. The wounding energy delivered to tissues by close range shot gun wounds is excessive (2,247 ft-lbs). The blast effect of the total mass of the shot and the wadding add further to the destruction of tissue. Clothing and other foreign particles are "sucked" into the wound by the vacuum effect. These patients are in severe hypovolemic shock and require massive volumes of extracellular fluids and blood as a first priority. Sepsis and toxicity from the dead and dying tissues is the next serious obstacle and extensive operative debridement is a major priority. These devitalized tissues serve as an excellent culture medium for anerobic organism. Tetanus prophylaxis is the third priority. The gas forming organisms find these wounds particularly habitable and appropriate antibiotic therapy is the fourth priority.

The long range shot gun injury is such a different situation that evaluation of these wounds takes on entirely different aspects. The twelve gauge shot gun loaded with 1 to 1⅛ ounces of No. 6 shot discharge 225 to 425 pellets. At forty yards approximately 200 to 300 pellets hit in a circle thirty inches in diameter. On a man six feet tall weighing 160 lbs this thirty inch circle reaches from mid thigh to the shoulders.[17] If the shot were equally distributed they would strike every two inches and about 100 to 200 pellets actually hit the patient. However, few people will get struck by the center of the shot and as previously pointed out the string of shot and the victims changing anatomical positions will also influence the number of pellets which actually penetrate the victim. These long range shot gun wounds are evaluated entirely different. They are seldom in shock from blood loss. The most serious tissue injury is usually to an organ of special sense such as the loss of an eye. The wounding energy in

TABLE 2-VIII

LONG RANGE SHOTGUN WOUNDS

Energy imparted by Individual Pellets
(Muzzle velocity 1.295 ft/sec)

| Shot Size | Energy ft/lb Per Pellet | |
	20 Yds.	40 Yds.
2	11.29	7.71
4	7.04	4.62
5	5.38	3.45
6	3.88	2.44
7½	2.31	1.37

Modified from Demuth, W. E., *Journal of Trauma*, vol. 11, 1971, p. 225.

these injuries is related to the kinetic energy of each individual pellet (Table 2-VIII). This is ordinarily quite small, the major capacity for tissue damage lies in the fact of penetration of bowel, liver, heart, aorta, emphagus, etc. The small diameter of the shot produces a wound of very small dimensions (Table 2-IX). After evaluating these patients for ventilatory defects, hemorrhage and shock these patients are managed expectantly and reassessed at frequent intervals for specific organ complications. Immediate thoracotomy and laparotomy are not indicated as they are in close range shot gun blasts. Bunch[18] observed that in long range wounds, perforations of the intestines were "mere slits in the gut. There was no pouting of mucosa, no eversion of the wound edges, no apparent leakage soiling or odor." He concluded that when the shot are scattered (as they are in injuries beyond 20 yds) the perforations of the gut are small and numerous without eversion of the intestinal mucosa conservative treatment gives the patient his best chance for survival. Paradoxically the overly anxious physician who decides to evaluate this kind of injury with exploration probably does more harm than good. Willis[19] evaluated twenty-three patients and did some animal experiments before

TABLE 2-IX

DIMENSIONS OF SHOTGUN PELLETS

| | Shot Size | | | | | | |
	9	8	7½	6	5	4	2
Pellet diameter (inches)	.08	.09	.95	.11	.12	.13	.15
No. pellets per ounce	585	410	350	225	170	135	90

concluding "If every bird shot enters the abdomen and penetrates the intestine, these perforations may be legion. Since the intestines with small wounds, unlike bullet wounds, show no pouting of mucosa there is danger of milking the germs through them and inducing peritonitis by handling. One cannot find every perforation without doing serious damage while looking for the shot." Drye and Schuster[20] confirmed the spontaneous sealing of shot gun pellet injuries after long range injury and emphasized the havoc produced by handling such an injured bowel.

Shot guns are occasionally loaded with single projectiles. From the standpoint of wounding energy these slugs compare favorably with high velocity rifles at ranges of 100 yards or less (Table 2-X).

TABLE 2-X

WOUNDING ENERGY FOR RIFLED SLUGS
FIRED FROM SHOTGUNS

Gauge	Slug Wt. Grains	Velocity ft/sec	Energy ft/lbs
12	437	1600	2485
16	383	1600	2175
20	273	1600	1565
410	87.5	1825	650

I recently spent the greater part of one night operating on a patient shot through both thighs with a shot gun loaded with a "deer slug." The single missile entered the middle third of the left lateral thigh passing behind the femur, ripping out a 4 cm segment of the femoral vein, exiting from the medial left thigh, then entered the medial right thigh and exiting from the lateral right thigh. The wounding energy of this slug was evident in the left thigh which was struck first. The slug created a large cavity in the mid-thigh leaving the muscles torn and considerably devitalized. But after expending its kinetic energy in the left thigh it produced only a through-and-through wound of the right thigh with very little surrounding devitalization of tissue. The amount of devitalization of tissue was clearly reflected in early healing of this wound compared to the more extensive wound of the left thigh. This once more points out the importance of velocity and weight of missile in disrupting human tissue.

Missiles penetrating skeletal muscle at high velocities produce temporary cavities as was evident in the patient described above. Such wound cavities reach maximum size in less than a millisecond and the volume of the cavity is proportional to the energy delivered by the missile. Coagulation necrosis of surrounding muscle occurs and gross appearance of the muscle is often misleading. This is why such wounds sometimes require sequential debridement rather than a single operation. Fascial planes provide excellent routes for dissipation of energy. Muscles adjacent to these planes are injured even though they are considerable distance from the missile tract.

Connective tissue, lung and skin resist the development of large permanent missile tracts. Cancellous bones struck by low velocity missiles may have the "fearless fosdick" or "drill hole" effect without serious comminution. The Colt .45 bullet produces such a wound. High velocity missiles striking cancellous bone produce severe comminution.

Electrical Energy

The degree of tissue damage in electrical injuries is proportional to the intensity of current which passes through the victim. Stated in Ohm's Law this is:

$$\text{Amperage (intensity)} = \frac{\text{Voltage (tension or potential)}}{\text{Resistance}}$$

In most injuries the voltage (tension or potential) remains constant. The wounding effect of the electric current depends upon the amperage (intensity of the current), the type of current, the resistance at the point of contact, the path the current takes through the tissues of the body, the duration of contact and the individuals susceptibility. Other variables also influence the degree of injury, such as humidity of the air, shape and nature of electrodes (Table 2-XI).

Electric current of 1000 volts or less is considered low tension current and above 1000 volts high tension current. High tension

TABLE 2-XI

WOUNDING FORCE OF ELECTRIC CURRENT
IS DEPENDENT UPON

1. Voltage
2. Amperage
3. Type of current
4. Resistance at point of contact
5. Path of current through tissue
6. Duration of contact
7. Individual's susceptibility

Modified from Sturim, H. S., *Journal of Trauma,* vol. 11, 1971, p. 960.

TABLE 2-XII

MANIFESTATIONS OF INJURY FROM DOMESTIC
60 CYCLE ALTERNATING CURRENT

1. Cardiorespiratory Arrest
2. Cutaneous Burns
3. Coagulation Necrosis
4. Fracture of Bones*
5. Dislocation of Joints*

* Violent uncoordinated muscle contraction.

TABLE 2-XIII

RESISTANCE OF SKIN TO ELECTRIC FLOW

Condition	Resistance (ohms)
Palm of Hand (calloused)	1,000,000
Normal Skin	5,000
Moist Skin	1,000

wires usually carry alternating current of high voltage and amperage. Alternating current has greater wounding capacity than direct current of similar intensity. As the number of cycles increase in alternating current, the wounding potential decreases. Muscle and nerves are less sensitive to high frequencies. Domestic 60 cycle alternating current is very dangerous to the heart and respiratory center (Table 2-XII). This explains the high incidence of fatal household accidents.[21]

The resistance of normal skin averages about 5000 Ohms; moist skin offers resistance of as little as 1000 Ohms (Table 2-XIII). After the current has successfully penetrated the skin it has little resistance to flow and passes quickly along blood vessels and tissue fluids.

The tissue heat may be excessive. In some instances it can momentarily approach the levels of an electric arc (2500 to 3000 C°). The heat developed is proportional to the square of the current flow. Once inside human tissues the current dissipates along paths of least resistance (Table 2-XIV). The current becomes most concentrated at the points of entrance and exit. It is these same areas where tissue coagulation is most apparent.[22]

TABLE 2-XIV

RESISTANCE OF BODY TISSUES TO FLOW
OF ELECTRIC CURRENT
(in order of decreasing magnitude)

1. Bone
2. Fat
3. Tendon
4. Skin
5. Muscles
6. Blood vessels
7. Nerves

The tissue injury produced by electric current may be the result of one or a combination of the following mechanisms:

1. electric heating elements causing thermal burns
2. electric current passing from an outside source into the body
3. electric arcs between an energized conductor and the body. In high voltage current, arcing can superimpose thermal burns onto the electric burn producing severe charring.

Tissue destruction may occur anywhere along the route the current takes through the body.[23] This path actually has more influence on survival than any other factor. Currents passing through either the heart or brain stem can cause immediate death due to ventricular fibrillation or respiratory failure. Central nervous system injury is manifested by loss of consciousness or convulsions.

Blood vessels, particularly small nutrient vessels, are extremely susceptible to electrical energy. Thrombosis of these vessels with resultant ischemic necrosis of the tissue supplied by such vessels multiplies the capability of electrical energy to destroy tissue far beyond the degree of thermal injury. High voltage current can completely necrosis the cranium and scalp requiring excision down to the meninges (Fig. 2-4). Bone can be destroyed by thrombosis of the small nutrient vessels or by destroying the periosteum and overlying soft tissue leaving exposed bone to be lost through the process of seguestration over the following months.

Intra-abdominal lesions caused by electrical energy are curlings ulcer, pancreatitis, transient ileus, perforation of hollow viscera and necrosis and perforation of the gallbladder.

High voltage electrical energy produces a peculiar two-zone phenomenon. A central zone is present at the site of contact with the conductor. Basically this is a thermoelectric injury. It has the same charred appearance as that produced by thermal energy. The adjacent tissue is coagulated and indurated. The outer zone is a band or region of ischemic injury. The ischemic tissue is pale and cold on the extremities. The degree of ischemia is difficult to evaluate and sometimes requires repeated debridement or amputations before a viable region is finally reached.

REFERENCES

1. Schultz, R. C.: The changing character and management of soft tissue windshield injuries. *J Trauma, 12*:24-33, 1972.
2. Ritchie, W. P.; Ersey, R. A., and Bunch, W. L.: Combined visceral and vertebral injuries from lap type seat belts. *Surgery Gynec Obstet, 131*:431-435, 1970.
3. Trollope, M. L.; Stalmaker, R. L.; EmElhaney, J. H., and Frey, C. F.: The mechanism of injury in blunt abdominal trauma. *J Trauma, 13*:962-969, 1973.
4. Baxter, C. F., and Williams, R. D.: Blunt abdominal trauma. *J Trauma, 1*:241-247, 1961.
5. Williams, R. D., and Sargent, F. T.: The mechanism of intestinal injury in trauma. *J Trauma, 3*:288-294, 1963.
6. Mays, E. T.: Bursting injuries of the liver. *Arch Surg, 93*:92-106, 1966.
7. Mays, E. T., and Noer, R. J.: Colonic stenosis after trauma. *J Trauma, 6*:316-329, 1966.
8. Hass, G. H.: Types of internal injuries of personnel involved in aircraft accidents. *J Aviation Med, 15*:77-84, 1944.
9. Moffat, R. C.; Roberts, V. L., and Berkas, E. M.: Blunt trauma to the thorax development of pseudoaneurysms in the dog. *J Trauma, 6*:666-680, 1966.

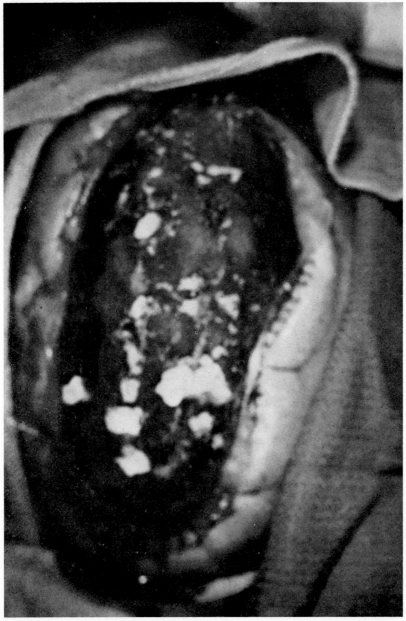

Figure 2-4. Full thickness electrical burn in workman who raised up suddenly encountering a high tension wire with his head. The wound required debridement down to the dura mater.

10. Daniel, R. A., Jr.: Bullet wounds of the lungs an experimental study. *Surgery, 15*:774-782, 1944.
11. DeMuth, W. E.: Bullet velocity as applied to military rifle wounding capacity. *J Trauma, 9*:27-38, 1969.
12. DeMuth, W. E.: Bullet velocity and design as determinants of wounding capacity: An experimental study. *J Trauma, 6*:222-232, 1966.
13. DeMuth, W. E., and Smith, J. M.: High velocity bullet wounds of muscle and bone: The basis of rational early treatment. *J Trauma, 6*:744-755, 1966.
14. DeMuth, W. E.: Ballistic characteristics of magnum side arm bullets. *J Trauma, 14*:227-229, 1974.
15. Beyer, J. C.: Wound ballistics, office of the surgeon general. *Department of the Army*, Washington, D.C., 1962.
16. DeMuth, W. E.: The mechanism of shotgun wounds. *J Trauma, 11*:219-229, 1971.
17. Bell, M. J.: The management of shotgun wounds. *J Trauma, 11*:522-527, 1971.
18. Bunch, G. H.: Shotgun wounds of the abdomen. Trans. *South Surg Assoc, 41*:38-47, 1928.
19. Willis, B. C.: Shotgun wounds of the abdomen. *Am J Surg, 28*:407-427, 1935.
20. Drye, J. C., and Schuster, G.: Shotgun wounds. *Am J Surg. 85*:438-443, 1953.
21. Dalziel, C. F.: The effects of electric in man. *IRE Trans Med Electron, 5*:44-62, 1956.
22. Sturim, H. S.: The treatment of electrical injuries. *J Trauma, 11*:959-965, 1971.
23. Baldridge, R. R.: Electrical Burns: report of a case. *N Eng J Med, 250*:46-49, 1954.

PHYSIOLOGIC CONCOMITANTS
OF INJURY

In EVALUATING CRITICALLY injured patients it is important to detect anatomic lesions and the greater part of this book is given to that purpose. But there must be an understanding on the part of the examining physician of the basic physiologic consequences of severe injury. The effects of the wounding forces, described in the preceeding chapter on the "internal milieu" must be anticipated in order that the total patient may be properly assessed. Violent forces applied to the body can have many different consequences. Every physician has encountered patients with horrendous destruction of tissue obviously incompatible with life. But there are also patients with minor local trauma sometimes of a very inconspicuous nature who mysteriously die. Yet another group suffer violence, of greater degree, spend many days in various life threatening situations and finally recover, while others develop multiple and progressive organ failure which slowly leads to death. These many different responses to trauma reflect underlying physiologic changes that influence the final outcome often to an even greater degree that the anatomic abnormality. Hans Selye[7] devoted himself to understanding these many different responses to stress. He stated, "there is an integrated syndrome of closely interrelated adaptive reactions to nonspecific stress." These adaptive responses he called the General-Adaptation Syndrome. He delineated three stages in response to stress: (1) alarm reaction (2) stage of resistance and (3) stage of exhaustion. Most of the characteristic manifestations of the Alarm Reaction (tissue catabolism, hypo-glycemia, gastrointestinal erosion, discharge of secretory granules from the adrenal cortex, hemoconcentration) disappear or actually reverse during the stage of resistance but later reappear in the stage of exhaustion. He concluded that "adaptation energy" (the ability of the living organism to adapt to severe trauma) is a finite quantity, which appears to depend largely upon genetic factors.

HEMODYNAMIC CONCOMITANTS

Wounding forces produce "shock." This is probably the most visible and obvious consequence of injury. The term "shock" though wholly undefined is a universally understood term. La Dran first used the word "choc" in 1743 but he designated an act of collision rather than the resulting functional damage. During the ensuing two centuries many have tried to adequately define the term shock. There are volumes written and one can find as many definitions as there are authors. The term itself defies an all encompassing definition and it would be ludicrous to think I could improve on previous definitions. The common denominator in all forms of shock seems to be inadequate tissue perfusion. This low flow state in vital organs reduces cellular function below a level compatible with life. Blalocks[2] 1934 etiologic classification seems to have withstood the test of time. He proposed the following categories: (1) hematogenic; char-acterized by oligemia (2) vasogenic; characterized by decreased vascular resistance and increased vascular capacity. (3) cardio-genic; characterized either by primary pump failure or a dimin-ished cardiac output resulting from numerous miscellaneous conditions. (4) neurogenic; caused by nerve reflex influence.

The symptom complex has been well described by Wiggers[3] and is shown in Table 3-I. It must be pointed out that not all the signs and symptoms appear in every patient, nor are the same ones always equally prominent. Their presence and dominance depends on the event or condition inducing the shock state. Individual patients will show various combinations of these many

TABLE 3-I

CLINICAL MANIFESTATIONS OF SHOCK

General appearance and reactions	Skin and mucous membranes	Circulation and blood	Respiration and metabolism
Mental state	*Skin*	*Superficial veins*	*Respiration*
Apathy	Pale, livid, ashen	Collapsed and	Variable but not
Delayed responses	gray	invisible	dyspneic
Depressed	Slightly cyanotic	Failure to fill	Usually increased
cerebration	Moist, clammy	on compression	rate
Weak voice	Mottling of	or massage	Variable depth
Listlessness or	dependent parts	Inconspicuous	Occasional deep
restlessness	Loose, dry,	jugular	sighs
	inelastic, cold	pulsations	Sometimes irregular
Countenance			or phasic
Drawn-anxious	*Mucous membranes*	*Heart*	
Lusterless eyes	Pale, livid,	Apex sounds feeble	*Temperature*
Sunken eyeballs	slightly cyanotic	Rate usually	Subnormal, normal
Ptosis of upper		rapid	supernormal
lids (slight)	*Conjunctiva*		
Upward rotation of	Glazed, lusterless	*Radial pulse*	*Basal metabolic*
eyeballs (slight)		Usually rapid	*rate*
	Tongue	Small volume	Reduced(?)
Neuromuscular	Dry, pale,	"feeble,"	
state	parched, shriveled	"thready"	
Hypotonia			
Muscular weakness		*Brachial blood*	
Tremors and		*pressures*	
twitchings		Lowered	
Involuntary		Pulse pressure	
muscular		small	
movements			
Difficulty in		*Retinal vessels*	
swallowing		Narrowed	
Neuromuscular	.	*Blood volume*	
tests		Reduced	
Depressed tendon			
reflexes		*Blood Chemistry*	
Depressed		Hemoconcentration	
sensibilities		or hemodilution	
Depressed visual		Venous O_2	
and auditory		decreased	
reflexes		A-VO_2 difference	
		increased	
		Arterial CO_2	
General but		reduced	
variable symptoms		Alkali reserve	
Thirst		reduced	
Vomiting			
Diarrhea			
Oliguria			
Visible or occult			
blood in vomitus,			
and stools			

Reproduced with permission Wiggers, C. J.: *Physiology of Shock.* New York, Copyright Commonwealth Fund, 1950.

components and some may disclose few or none of those listed in Table 3-I.

Most critically injured patients will have some reduction in blood volume. Reduction in blood volume is one initial step in the development of shock. Thirty-five to 40 percent reductions in blood volumes usually result in severe shock and 20 to 30 percent reductions in blood volume produce moderate shock.[3] Clinical methods of evaluating the degree of shock are illustrated in Table 3-II.

The reduction in blood volume is associated with an increased heart rate. The pulse rate is an extremely reliable method of evaluating consequences of severe trauma. As vascular volume is reduced systolic and diastolic blood pressures are decreased. Pulse pressure is reduced significantly. The small pulse pressure is due partly to reduction in stroke volume resulting from decreased venous return and partly to the acceleration of the heart. Blood pressure is not a reliable technique for evaluating the amount of volume loss nor degree of shock.

Wiggers[3] has divided the hemodynamic changes into three stages. In Stage I in addition to the above named changes in blood pressure and heart rate there is a declined portal venous pressure and a marked diminution of effective venous pressure, inferior vena cava flow and cardiac output.[3] The reduced cardiac output is predominantly responsible for the decline of arterial pressure. Such a conclusion is supported by the small pulse pressure abbreviation of systolic ejection and the configuration of arterial pressure pulses reported by Wiggers. Coronary flow is reduced.

These hydraulic components of trauma and hemorrhage are accompanied by marked contraction of the spleen and increased resistance to flow in vessels of the limbs. A high resistance develops most rapidly in vessels of the limbs and gastrointestinal tract and more gradually in the kidneys.[3] Resistance in the coronary circuit is rapidly reduced. Total peripheral resistance has less constant flux. In general however it increases until these early changes have been corrected.

As the low-flow state and decreased cellular perfusion pro-

TABLE 3-II

EVALUATION OF THE DEGREE OF SHOCK

Degree of Shock	Blood Pressure (approx.)	Pulse quality	Skin		Circulation (response to pressure blanching)	Thirst	Mental state
			Temperature	Color			
None	Normal	Normal	Normal	Normal	Normal	Normal	Clear and distressed
Slight	To 20% increase	Normal	Cool	Pale	Definite slowing	Normal	Clear and distressed
Moderate	Decreased 20 to 40%	Definite decrease in volume	Cool	Pale	Definite slowing	Definite	Clear and some apathy unless stimulated
Severe	Decreased 40% to nonrecordable	Weak to imperceptible	Cold	Ashen to cyanotic (mottling)	Very sluggish	Severe	Apathetic to comatose, little distress except thirst

Reproduced with permission, Beecher H. K., Simeone, F. A.; Burnett, C. H.; Shapiro, S. L.; Sullivan, E. R., and Mallory, T. B., Surgery, vol. 22, 1947, p. 672.

gresses to Stage II, the heart accelerates to a second maximum and arterial pressures and pulse pressure slowly decline. If volume is not replaced or if the patient continues to lose volume or has a secondary hemorrhage they decrease to serious levels and renal perfusion is interrupted. These advanced hemodynamic concomitants can be detected by failure of the patient to make urine. Coronary flow, effective venous pressure, inferior vena cava flow, cardiac output and portal pressure remain low. Vascular resistance increases progressively in the limbs and kidneys. Resistance continues to decrease in the coronary system. Total peripheral resistance may be increased, unchanged or decreased.

The critical stage III can be detected by the severe cardiac deceleration (sometimes a very marked bradycardia), very low arterial pressures, small pulse pressure and failure of the kidneys to produce urine. The pressure pulse has a very simple rounded systolic contour and a flat diastolic limb. There are further reductions in venous return atrial pressure, and cardiac output. Increased regional vascular resistance persists in the limbs and kidneys, while mesenteric vascular resistance undergoes a second increase. Coronary resistance strangely enough continues to decrease. If the total peripheral resistance has been previously increased it now shows a tendency to decline.

The importance of total peripheral vascular resistance and whether the net effect of constriction is salubrious or detrimental is contentious and has not been fully answered. Alternate opinions have been advanced by Blalock[5] and Harkins.[6] Shires[4] gives the marked increase in peripheral resistance credit for providing a life-saving diversion of the cardiac output to the brain and heart. He points out that in hemorrhagic shock the heart may receive 25 percent of the total cardiac output as opposed to the normal 5 to 8 percent and the brain as much as 80 percent of the total cardiac output instead of the normal 15 to 20 percent. Wiggers favors the concept that the net effect is harmful and that the transition from impending to irreversible shock can be retarded or prevented by abrogating sympathogenic vasoconstriction. He presented evidence that generalized vasoconstriction has only a negligible effect in sustaining arterial pressure and exerts an essentially unfavorable action by seriously throttling blood flow in states of marked hypotension. He further advocates drugs such as dibenamine and tetraethyl ammonium to block vaso-constriction of blood vessels, suggesting this prevents hemo-dynamic changes from progressing to an irreversible stage.

Diminished venous return occurs when blood volume is reduced. Evidence has accumulated that stagnation and pooling of blood in minute vessels is a dominant factor in reducing venous return. Some have suggested there is an invisible trapping of red cells in all organs of the body. The actual quantity of red cells trapped constitutes only a small fraction of total blood volume, but it represents a 20 to 40 percent reduction in capillary flow.[3] Berman and associates[7] reported intravascular microaggre-gation occurred in a high percentage of percussion type trauma and proposed a mechanical basis secondary to release of vaso-active substances from trapped and disintegrating platelets. A marked degree of platelet trapping after trauma has been reported.[8, 9] Trauma also resulted in a moderate decrease of venous endothelial activator and a complete loss of arterial endothelial activator which converts plasminogen to plasmin, and reduction of fibrinlytic activity of traumatized blood vessels.[1, 10]

Venous pressure measurements must be interpreted with great caution. The measurement of central venous pressure by catheters in the superior vena cava is not completely reliable. Artifacts due to temporary occlusion of the catheter, shifts in it or the patients position and impacts of the beating heart are not easy to avoid. It is nearly impossible to damp manometers to exclude respiratory fluctuations. The variations in pressure are as apt to reflect changes in respiration rather than cardiovascular func-tion. Such respiratory variations become deep and rapid during hemorrhage and shock. The superior vena cava is under sub-atmospheric pressure during expiration and this is even more reduced during inspiration. Many investigators feel there is no proof that the decrease in average right atrial pressure reported by some observers in human shock is not due largely to reductions in intrathoracic pressure that results from reduction of blood content within the thorax. The use of central venous pressure monitoring will again be discussed in later chapters.

Acute blood volume measurements are not a reliable method

of evaluating hemorrhagic shock. The anatomic blood volume has little relationship to what is actually available for physiologic function. Estimates of blood volume using plasma volume alone require the hematocrit for calculation. They are no more reliable than the hemotocrit which is known to be erratic in hemorrhagic shock.

Hematocrit changes with trauma have caused considerable controversy. At the beginning of World War II it had become tradition that hemoconcentration indicated by a proportionate increase in red cells and hemoglobin as compared to plasma was an essential manifestation of clinical shock. This led to the confusing belief that hemorrhage and shock were separate entities because hemorrhage was not accompanied by hemoconcentration whereas shock was inevitably accompanied by a rise in hematocrit.

Shires[4] states, "the hematocrit is not a differentiating factor." He points out the extent of hemoconcentration depends upon the proportion of red cells and plasma lost in the traumatic episode as well as upon the compensatory adjustments of the interstitial fluid in response to the intravascular volume reduction. Wiggers[3] examined the blood in all types of shock and found two categories exist as far as concentration or dilution is concerned. He found hemoconcentration in all conditions in which a large volume of fluid is lost by seepage, drainage, excretion, vomiting or is exuded into the tissues (as in crush injuries) or into the body cavities (as in peritonitis). But in shock due to skeletal muscle trauma hemorrhage or wounds, the hematocrit readings tend to be well below normal values. Attention has also been called to the fact that evidences of hemodilution may not be discernable for several days following severe hemorrhage. Wiggers summarized his investigations by stating that, "hemoconcentration is a concomitant of shock only when the injury results in large losses of plasma from the blood stream in the region of injury."

It is now clear that the hematocrit or hemoglobin concentration after trauma is a net result of the balance between relative loss of whole blood or plasma and the gain of extravascular fluid. The mechanism of hemodilution after hemorrhage is usually based on Starlings hypothesis: A reduction in hydrostatic pressure in the capillaries due to hypotension and vasoconstriction results in a shift in pressure gradient favoring the passage of fluid from tissue spaces to the capillary bed. Any implication that generalized increase in capillary permeability occurs throughout the body or that increased blood viscosity so produced is an important factor in circulatory failure has not been supported by the clinical studies of Wiggers and others.

PULMONARY CONCOMITANTS

Thoracic and lung injury are necessarily associated with various degrees of respiratory distress. These are discussed in following chapters under cardiothoracic evaluation. There is just as significant and often more lethal pulmonary insufficiency after non-thoracic trauma. Pulmonary congestion was very early recognized as a concomitant of trauma.[12] As the hemodynamic components of trauma became better understood many patients recovered from their hemodynamic deficits only to succumb to progressive pulmonary failure (Figs. 3-1a and 3-1b).

The outstanding feature of the respiratory distress is arterial hypoxemia which frequently fails to respond to increases in inspired oxygen concentration. The basic problem has been progressively confused by a burgeoning list of terms applied to a single physiologic defect.[13] The magnitude of the problems surrounding pulmonary failure after trauma were highlighted in a national conference in Washington, D.C., 1968. The proceedings of this conference are published in volume 8 of *The Journal of Trauma*, 1968 and the reader is referred to this excellent compilation of material for background reading.

Peters[14] emphasized that work to ventilate the lungs is increased after injury even without associated generalized reactions such as shock or sepsis. The effects of various forces causing increased work and deterioration of lung mechanics are cumulative. The rapidity in which they rise to intolerable proportions depends on the severity of the wounding force and the patient's reserve. When trauma is so severe that the added energy for mechanical ventilation is not available, hypoventilation results

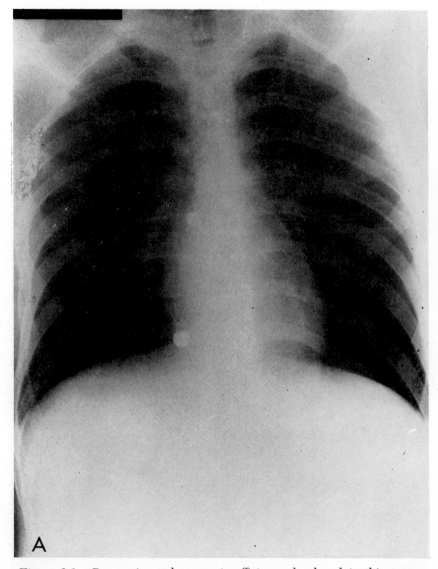

Figure 3-1. Progressive pulmonary insufficiency developed in this seventeen-year-old boy who sustained severe non-thoracic trauma. (a) chest film on admission. (b) chest film twenty-four hours after injury showing diffuse and rapidly progressing pulmonary infiltrate. Note ground glass appearance of lung.

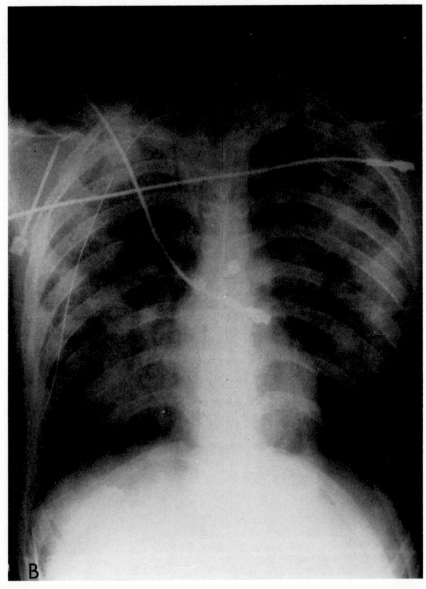

Figure 3-1b.

in respiratory as well as metabolic acidosis. In situation of less severe trauma the increased work of ventilation can be tolerated and ultimate pulmonary failure is delayed for hours or days.

But impaired mechanical ventilation due to work load is not the complete answer. Lervin and associates[15] reported patients with seriously decreased arterial PO^2 values who either had normal or reduced P_a CO_2. They felt this was good evidence that the hypoxic concomitants of trauma were not selectively due to impaired ventilation. They demonstrated functional pulmonary arteriovenous shunts. They likewise found evidence of functional peripheral arteriovenous shunting.

To evaluate the seriously injured patient physicians must be familiar with the problems caused by physiologic and anatomic shunting after trauma. The measurement and calculation of the shunt is important in assessing the injured patient. Rahn and Farhi[17] have outlined the derivation of the equation for calculating the shunt when the F_1O_2 is 0.4.

$$\frac{\dot{Q}s}{\dot{Q}_t} = \frac{Cc - Ca}{Cc - Cv}$$

where $\dot{Q}s$ = total shunt flow

$\dot{Q}_t$ = total cardiac output
Cc = Pulmonary Capillary oxygen content
Ca = Arterial oxygen content
$C\bar{v}$ = Mixed venous content

The oxygen tension in pulmonary capillaries is not measurable by present technics. The fraction of inspired oxygen, the oxygen tensions of arterial and venous samples can be determined clinically and these determinations corrected for the solubility coefficient of oxygen in plasma (0.0031) permit rewriting of the equation.

$$\frac{\dot{Q}s}{\dot{Q}_t} = \frac{(P_A - Pa)\ 0.0031}{(Ca - C\bar{v} + (P_A - Pa)\ 0.0031}$$

where P_A = alveolar oxygen tension
           P_a = arterial oxygen tension

It must be pointed out that these last equations are valid only in normal or near normal patients who are breathing 100 percent oxygen for thirty minutes. We are interested in critically injured patients and such a situation usually never exists. We have already discussed the inability of these patients to increase their arterial oxygen tension by breathing 100 percent oxygen. Most critically injured patients will have an arterial oxygen tension below 100 mm hg. Such an oxygen content and tension are in middle of the oxyhemoglobin dissociation curve where oxygen content is determined by hemoglobin saturation rather than by dissolved oxygen. Because of this the oxygen content itself must be measured or calculated and employed in the equation. Oxygen content of arterial blood can be calculated from oxygen tension and read from a monogram for the oxyhemoglobin dissociation curve.

Measuring the alveolar-arterial oxygen gradient while the patient breathes 100 percent oxygen is a good starting point. This test also allows the physician to assess the severity of pulmonary insufficiency, predicts the clinical benefit of increasing the fractions of inspired oxygen (if any) and provides objective evidence for avoiding dangerous oxygen concentrations when a lesser concentration will do for that patient or patients circulatory needs. When extremely minor increases in arterial oxygen tension occurs after the patients breathes 100 percent oxygen, there is absolutely no justification for sustaining the patient on high oxygen tension for long periods. Other means of improving pulmonary diffusion of oxygen such as positive end expiratory pressure must then be considered.

Measurement of dynamic pulmonary compliance has thrown very little light on the problem.[18, 19] Monaco and associates[17] found that in patients with reduced functional residual capacity it was impossible to interpret dynamic compliance and they reported that failure to correct a low functional residual capacity can result in an increasing shunt through non-ventilated alveoli and subsequent respiratory failure. The association of a high venous admixture with decreased functional residual capacity has been suggested as evidence that reduced functional residual capacity may be operative in controlling oxygen tension. Decreased functional residual capacity seems to accompany patients who have pulmonary insufficiency after trauma. The pathogenesis of the decreased functional residual capacity is not known.

Aveolar type II cells produce "surfactant," dipalmitoye lecithin attached to an alpha globulin.[20] The ability of type II cells to synthesize surfactant depends upon adequate pulmonary capillary blood flow. The patency of alveoli throughout the respiratory cycle depends upon adequate amounts of surfactant. After non-thoracic trauma there is an imbalance between more rapid depletion of surfactant and metabolic failure of replenishment by alveolar cells.[21]

While the characteristic physiologic concomitant of trauma is progressive arterial hypoexmia, the underlying anatomic characteristic is an increase in vascular permeability.[22] A factor carried by the blood is most likely the cause of the increased capillary permeability because studies of shock sustained while one lung is excluded from the circulation during the period of hypovolemia discloses fewer changes in the excluded lung than in the perfused lung. Also cardiopulmonary bypass divulges that exclusion of the lungs from the circulating blood protects the pulmonary vasculature from whatever blood factors cause increased vascular permeability.[23] Trauma[24] and surgery[25] cause increased plasma concentrations of free fatty acids (Fig. 3-2). Fatty acids are really not free but are under normal circumstances bound to serum albumin and as such are non-toxic. Fatty acid anions not bound to albumin are cytotoxic particularly to the lungs.[26, 27] They disrupt the capillary membrane producing increased vascular permeability.[28] After trauma and surgery serum albumin levels are decreased.[29, 30] Gutierrez and colleagues found a direct relationship between hypo-proteinemia and the development of pulmonary insufficiency in shock.[31] Ballou and associates have presented evidence of an anion-albumin association which increases with change length of the fatty acids.[32]

Although as mentioned earlier in this chapter the hemo-

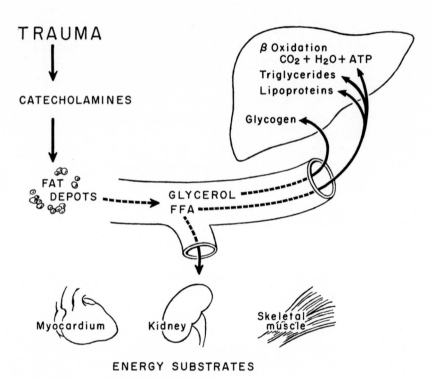

ENERGY SUBSTRATES

Figure 3-2.   Fatty acids are mobilized in response to trauma and catechol-amine stress.

dynamic concomitant of severe injury is a low flow state with lactic acidosis. Moore and associates[33] reviewed some patients whose very first findings were respiratory alkalosis compounded by some degree of metabolic alkalosis. They gave credit for the metabolic component in this mixed alkalosis to oxidation of the citrate component of transfused blood, this is accentuated by inability to excrete the sodium bicarbonate resulting from the oxidative metabolism of sodium citrate. The stimulation of the renin-angiotension-aldosterone system by injury and volume reduction produces a phase of hyperaldosteronemia which is associated with extremely high values for tubular sodium reabsorption and a persistent paradoxical aciduria despite plasma alkalosis.

The frequency and pathophysiology of post traumatic alkalosis have been discussed in greater detail by Lyons and Moore[34] and the reader is referred to their excellent work for additional information. A tabulation of the hemodynamic and pulmonary concomitants of various injuries is shown in Table 3-III.

When assessing the pulmonary sequels of severe injury the evaluator must not be deceived by chest roentgenograms. Even in the absence of radiologic lung abnormalities soon after injury there can be unbalanced ventilation-perfusion in significant segments of the lungs.[35] Determination of blood gases and calculation of shunting are much more reliable means of evaluating the pulmonary sequelae of injury.

TABLE 3-III

BLOOD CHANGES ACCOMPANYING SHOCK

	Hematocrit reading	Art. O vol. %	Art. CO_2 at 40 mm.	Art. CO_2 vol. %	pH art. blood
Controls (15 cases)	av. 45	16.6	49.5	49.1	7.42
Skeletal trauma (4 cases)	28	10.2	25.5	16.5	7.21
Hemorrhage (4 cases)	18	6.6	36.4	30.3	7.3
Burns (4 cases)	42	15.7	39.3	36.7	7.29
Abdominal injuries (3 cases)	44	12	28.4	29.0	7.17
Head injuries	39	15.4	44.9	37.7	7.38

Reproduced with permission, *Surgery*, vol. 13, 1943, p. 964.

In addition to these common pulmonary sequelae which usually accompany every severe injury there is a very rare pulmonary concomitant of head injury with which the reader should become familiar. After craniocerebral injury there sometimes develops massive pulmonary edema. This occurs even though intravenous fluids have been cautiously administered. Drucker[36] reported ten patients none of whom had received more than 500 ml of parenteral fluid by the time pulmonary edema developed. No cardiac arrhythemias were present and none of the patients responded to digitalis or positive pressure respiration. The lungs showed a uniform noncellular edema upon histologic examination. The mechanisms producing such massive edema remain obscure. Most authorities report increased intracranial pressure as the common underlying pathology.[37]

BIOCHEMICAL CONCOMITANTS

In 1877 Claude Bernard noted that hemorrhage leads to hyperglycemia. As a rule the blood sugar reaches a maximum in about thirty minutes and continues at a high plateau for three or four hours. As liver glycogen is depleted and gluconeogenesis fails to keep pace with the progressively increasing carbohydrate utilization blood sugar gradually declines until hypoglycemic levels are reached in far advanced and untreated stages.

The analysis of urinary sugars discloses significant changes in different branches of carbohydrate metabolism in injury. Regardless of the extent of glucosuria in trauma the glucose bound in oligosaccharides is consistently and significantly increased in all patients. This fraction of saccharides represents several degradation products of glycogen among them isomaltose has been determined the chief metabolite.[38]

Increased utilization of carbohydrates is associated with a shift toward anerobic metabolism. This is confirmed by a progressive increase in blood lactate and pyruvate together with an increase in the ratio of lactate to pyruvate. Acceleration of lactate production by tissues is balanced by the ability of the liver to remove lactate from the blood.[39]

After injury insulin levels are inappropriately low for the

degree of glycemia.[40] Spigelman and Ozeran found increased tolerance to irreversible shock in dogs given insulin.[41]

The insulin-glucagon ratio is usually low following injury, below the level of fasting man and in the range observed with other catabolic states.[42] Glucagon concentrations increase progressively in the twenty-four hours following trauma.[40] Glucose consumption in man increases after severe trauma.[43]

Lysosomal stability is adversely affected by tissue ischemia. Disruption of the lysosomal membranous after severe injury permits the escape of lysosomal acid hydrolases. These enzymes can digest all known biological bonds and have been shown to have damaging effects on tissues and plasma.[44] Lysosomal ezymes also have an effect on human erythrocyte membrane integrity. Concentrations of cathepsin D and Beta — glucuronidase consistent with those observed in association with trauma increase sodium ion concentrations in red cells and decrease potassium concentrations.[45]

There is severe depletion of liver, kidney and muscle adenosine triphosphate in severe shock and this is a progressive change with dephosphorylation of ATP, ADP, AMP and creatine phosphate.[46] The alterations in these compounds during shock and trauma are of considerable importance. Cellular activity is closely linked to phosphorus containing compounds. Adenosine triphospate is the most important source of high energy phosphate bonds. Other energy reservoirs such as creatine phosphate and glycogen are utilized to sustain and restore the ATP reservoir. When these mechanisms are deranged or break down, glycolytic changes begin to operate and inorganic phosphorus and lactic acid are liberated.

Protein metabolism is also significantly affected by injury. The non-protein nitrogen (NPN) is frequently elevated (Figs. 3-3a and 3-3b). There is an early rise in blood amino acid concentrations due to increased catabolism of protein and efflux of large quantities of amino acids from traumatized tissues.[47, 48] The rise of amino nitrogen in impending shock suggests the development of hepatic insufficiency. This idea of Engel and associates has been strengthened by additional observations.[3] (1) hepatic anoxia is present during shock (2) hepatic anoxia

PROTEIN METABOLISM

NORMAL

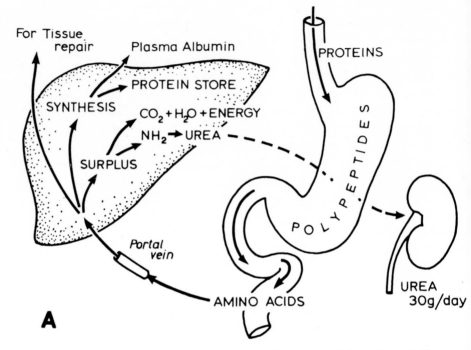

Figure 3-3. Protein metabolism in normal subjects (a) and critically injured patients (b). (Reproduced with permission Walker and Johnston. *Metabolic Basis of Surgical Care.* London, W. Heinemann Medical Books Ltd., 1971.)

causes an accumulation of amino nitrogen in the blood by impairing amino acid metabolism, (3) the rise of amino nitrogen is related inversely to the oxygen content of portal blood (4) oxygen consumption by liver slices in vitro is depressed in proportion to the rise of plasma animo nitrogen. Seligman and his associates[49] found the amino nitrogen of blood remains high or even increases in terminal stages.

Total circulating protein is diminished. The changes in concentration of serum proteins depends upon the relative amounts of fluid lost or taken in and the nature of the wounding force.

TRAUMA

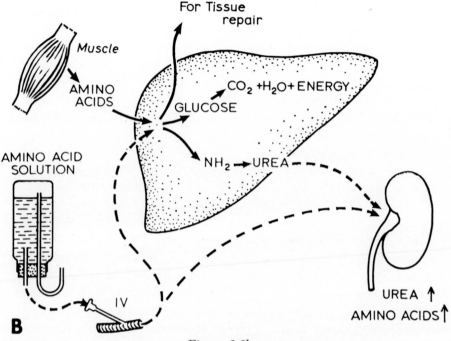

Figure 3-3b.

Although the total circulating protein may be reduced its concentration may be normal or even high when loss of extracellular fluid dominates. This reduction initially involves both albumin and globulin hence the A/G ratio is not affected. After a 30 percent hemorrhage there is continued loss of albumin from the vascular compartment. The mean decrease at one, three and six hours after hemorrhage was 13 percent, 15 percent and 29 percent, respectively, of the quantity of albumin circulating at the end of the hemorrhage.[50]

ENDOCRINE CONCOMITANTS

Injury causes an increase in adrenocorticotropic hormone concentrations in the blood.[51] Its subsequent action on the adrenal cortex produces a rise in blood cortisol concentration. More than fifty different steroids have been isolated from the adrenal cortex but the great majority of these steroids are intermediate stages with the end result that only about five classes of steroids are normally secreted into the blood stream. The glucocorticoids include cortisol and hydrocortisone. A small amount of corticosterone is secreted. The mineralocorticoids include aldosterone and 11-desoxycorticosterone. Aldosterone is the most active steroid in electrolyte control. Other active steroid hormones are androgenic and estrogenic. These are characterized by the seventeen Keto-steroids.[52]

Blood concentrations of seventeen hydroxycorticoids are acutely and significantly increased in the posttraumatic period, 70 to 80 mg per 100 ml (normal 5 to 15 mg per 100 ml).[53, 54] Although aldosterone is the most important adrenal corticoid for controlling sodium reabsorption, cortisol and cortisone also influence water metabolism and ion exchange. This elaboration of corticosteroids by the adrenal glands is dependent upon adrenal blood flow.[55] Patients in severe shock where the low flow state has existed for some time may not be perfusing their adrenal glands. This probably accounts for some investigators reporting low corticosteroids in war injuries. If adrenal blood flow is intact the peak blood levels of seventeen hydroxycorticoids are reached about six hours after trauma. It is related more to the severity of the injury than to the specific type of injury.[56] The increases in urinary nitrogen and urinary corticoids are related and parallel the degree of injury. The metabolic changes accompanying injury cannot be directly related to the absolute level of blood corticoids. This is consistent with the idea of a "conditioning action" of these hormones suggested by Hans Selye and the permissive or supporting action proposed by others.

Persisting hypovolemic shock causes an increase in plasma concentrations of epinephrine and norepinephrine.[57] The adrenal medulla produces epinephrine and norepinephrine, about 70 to 80 percent is epinephrine. These hormones mobilize free fatty acids from lipid depots and activate phosphorlase producing degradation of hepatic glycogen to glucose and increasing blood glucose concentrations. Epinephrine has a chronotropic effect on the heart, dilates bronchioles, and stimulates the central nervous system, whereas norepinephrine has a positive ionotropic effect on the heart and causes sustained arteriolar contraction. Sympathico adrenal activity has clinical signs that can be recognized if looked for. The patient is pale from vasoconstrictions and apprehensive from CNS stimulation. He is usually sweating and has a tachycardia. This produces cool moist skin to touch.

After prolonged shock there is a decline in plasma concentrations of catecholamines even though the stimuli for their release (persisting hypovolemia and increasing acidosis) is greater.[58] This suggests there is either inhibition of their biosynthesis or adrenal stores are depleted.

One of the most important hormones produced by the adrenal cortex is aldosterone. A reduction in blood volume is an extremely potent stimulus to production of aldosterone. After a bilateral nephrectomy this response is lost. Aldosterone secretion seems independent of pituitary action and will be discussed again under renal concomitants. Aldosterone has its greatest target action in the renal tubules and promotes the reabsorption of sodium and excretion of hydrogen and potassium. The increased retention of sodium and water after injury is related to production of aldosterone and the antidiuretic hormone from the posterior pituitary. After injury antidiuretic hormone is increased. This increased concentration of ADH after injury has a strong antidiuretic effect on the renal tubules by increasing reabsorption of water.

Other endocrine glands such as thyroid, parathyroids, pancreas and gonads apparently contribute in only minor ways to physiology after trauma. There is increased excretion of calcium after injury but this appears related more to the degree of immobilization than to parathyroid function. The inappropriate amounts of insulin has already been discussed. The radioactive iodine uptake and protein bound iodine have not been consistently altered in one direction or the other after injury. Gonad function appears decreased but seems to have no effect on the metabolic response to trauma.

RENAL CONCOMITANTS

The relative oligemia suffered by the kidney after injury is severe and immediate. Renal blood flow and filtration rate decrease. This is a compensatory mechanism in injured patients to divert blood flow to organs of higher priority such as the brain and heart. The development of oliguria and even in some patients anuria is a direct reflection of the severity of injury and the degree of renal ischemia.

Renal tissues removed from animals in states of shock show no significant depression in oxygen consumption. The energy reserves represented by the stores of ATP and ADP are not depleted in the renal cortex. Renal oxygen consumption decreases progressively and reaches very low levels in severe shock.[3] Contrary to most tissues renal cells appear to have the ability of reducing their oxygen consumption in proportion to that supplied.

The reduction in renal blood flow produces increases in systemic renin concentration.[59] Renin secretion is stimulated before the autoregulatory compensation of decreasing renal vascular resistance is exceeded, but much greater renin hypersecretion results from progressive hypovolemia beyond this limit.[60] The renin-angiotension system in turn cause the increased secretion of aldosterone by the adrenal cortex which was discussed in preceding paragraphs.[60, 61]

The reduction in renal blood flow also decreases the rate of glomerular filtration which in turn determines the degree of oliguria. Urea and other nitrogenous products accumulate in the blood. The excretion of potassium, inorganic phosphate and lactate is also reduced. The metabolic acidosis discussed in previous paragraphs is intensified because the increased production of acids is not compensated by their increased excretion and by the formation of ammonia to conserve base. These renal concomitants of injury hinder the recovery of the heart, brain and liver.

Renal function is additionally impaired through hemolysis, hemoglobinuria and liberation of myoglobin from damaged tissues. The acid state of the urine precipitates myoglobin and

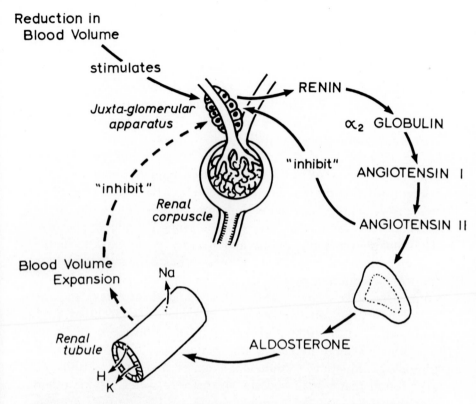

Figure 3-4. Hypovolemia stimulates the renin-angiotension-aldosterone system. (Reproduced with permission Walker and Johnson, *Metabolic Basis of Surgical Care.* London, W. Heinemann Medical Books, Ltd., 1971.)

hemoglobin in the renal tubules leading to complete blockage of many nephrons.

FLUID AND ELECTROLYTE CONCOMITANTS

Sodium and fluid retention accompany trauma. The hormonal mediators of such a response have already been discussed. After severe injury there are frequent and important changes in extracellular fluid volume. Shortly after injury extracellular fluid deficits co-exist with hemorrhagic shock. Extensive soft tissue injuries, retroperitoneal intraperitoneal and fractures may all result in significant sequestration of functional extracellular fluid. Shires and his associates[62] showed that hemorrhage was associated with a reduction in the extracellular fluid compartment as measured by tagged radio sulfate. This reduction in extracellular fluid volume could not be reversed by return of shed blood alone. They concluded that a functional defect in the extracellular fluid compartment occurred with hemorrhage and that electrolyte solution was required for replacement along with blood.

Experimental and clinical evidence has indicated that loss of water alone does not result in circulatory failure. When the salt content of the body remains unchanged and the water content is decreased, the plasma volume drops proportionately to the extracellular fluid volume and no plasma protein depletion occurs. The animals remain vigorous and healthy in contrast to those suffering from salt depletion. On the other hand salt depletion induces a reduction in plasma protein and animals so affected enter a shocklike state.[63] When extracellular electrolytes decrease water enters the cell producing a reduction in extracellular fluid and swelling of the cell with hypotoncity of both spaces.

Although fluid depletion alone does not seriously hinder physiologic function, sodium depletion is disastrous. Fulton et al.,[64] found that loss of sodium ion without water loss or other electrolyte loss caused a reduction in cardiac output, arterial pressure, urine volume, oxygen consumption and glucose utilization. They postulated that sodium deficiency may also produce derangements in cellular metabolism. Moyer[65] and his colleagues concluded that the total body sodium content was the factor most important in determining plasma volume. Moyer's group did not believe that colloid osmotic pressure was important in controlling plasma volume and pointed out that an absence of albumin in the plasma space was compatible with normal existence. They found on the other hand however, that changes in plasma volume correlated with sodium ion concentrations. As sodium is lost from the body plasma volume falls.

When quantities of sodium are lost from extracellular fluids they are replaced partly by migration of potassium into the blood stream. Ashworth and Kregel[66] concluded that a rise in blood potassium occurs only in the terminal stage of shock due to trauma or hemorrhage. Other investigators have also reported an increase in potassium concentration in the blood after injury and note that the release of potassium can occur from injured or ischemia muscle. Having entered the blood stream the concentration of potassium depends upon the state of renal blood flow and filtration rates.

CELLULAR CONCOMITANTS

Studies of ion transport across cell membranes have been done to determine the possibility of intracellular swelling in response to shock. Intracellular transmembrane potential recordings have been done with glass tips whose diameters are less than one micron. Such an electrode has been modified to record intracellular transmembrane potentials *in vivo* before during and after shock.

There is a constant and sustained fall in the normally negative intracellular transmembrane potential in skeletal muscle in acute hemorrhagic shock.[68] Other studies show that as blood pressure falls and transmembrane potential is reduced (Fig. 3-5) plasma potassium rises slowly.[69]

Surface electrometry has also shown that potassium ion activity in the extracellular fluid of skeletal muscle increases rapidly and markedly in the presence of hypovolemic hypotension, and that restoration of normal muscle surface potassium occurs when hypotension is corrected.

Studies in primates show clearly that muscle cells gain sodium, water and chloride while losing potassium. There is a decrease in resting membrane potential, a decrease in amplitude of action potential and prolongation of both replorization and depolarization time.[71] From these studies there seems little doubt that there is a change in cellular membrane transport after severe injury and shock and such changes are reversible. Are these changes due to a reduction in an electrogenic pump, sodium-potassium exchanges, or a change in cellular permeability? Authorities are leaning toward a reduction in efficiency of an electrogenic sodium pump. With a reset membrane potential extracellular fluid electrolyte concentrations are unchanged.[72] One cellular response

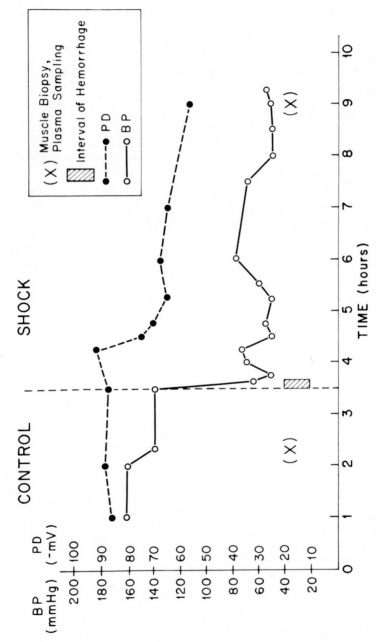

Figure 3-5.   Fall in transmembrane potential in skeletal muscle in response to shock and hypovolemia.   (Reproduced with permission Shires, G. T., *Shock*. Philadelphia, London, Toronto, W. B. Saunders, 1973, p. 29.)

to hypovolemic hypotension is a consistent change in active transport of ions.

REFERENCES

1. Selye, H.: *Stress.* First Edition. Acta, Inc. Medical Publishers, Montreal, Canada, 1950.
2. Blalock, A.: Shock: Further studies with particular reference to effects of hemorrhage. *Arch Surg, 29*:837, 1934.
3. Wigger, C. J.: *Physiology of Shock.* New York, The Commonwealth Fund, 1950.
4. Shires, T. G.: *Care of the Trauma Patient.* New York, McGraw-Hill, 1966.
5. Blalock. A.: *Principles of Surgical Care: Shock and Other Problems.* St. Louis, Mosby, 1940.
6. Harkins, H. N.: Review of shock. *Surgery, 9*:231, 447, 607, 1941.
7. Berman, I. R.; Guttierrez, V. S.; Burran, E. L., and Boatright, R. D.: Intravascular microaggregation in young men with combat injuries. *Surg Forum, 20*:14-16, 1969.
8. Peer, R. M., and Schwartz, S. I.: Prevention of pulmonary platelet trapping following trauma. *Surg Forum, 24*:5, 1973.
9. Bergentz, S. E.; Lewis, D. H.. and Ljungquist, U.: Trapping of Platelets in the lung after experimental injury. Sixth European Conference on Microcirculation Basel Karger S. 1971, pp. 35-40.
10. McGregor, F. H., and Silver, D.: Effect of trauma on the intravascular fibrinolytic activator. *Surg Forum, 20*:44-46, 1969.
11. Silver. P.: Inhibition of intravascular fibrinolytic activator by trauma. *Surg Forum, 16*:124, 1965.
12. Moon, V. H.: *Shock: Its Dynamics, Occurrence and Management.* Philadelphia, Lea and Febiger, 1942, p. 173.
13. Blaisdell, F. W., and Schlobohm, R. M.: The respiratory distress syndrome: A review. *Surg, 74*:251-262, 1973.
14. Peters, R. M.: Work of breathing following trauma. *J Trauma, 8*:915-923, 1968.
15. Leurin, I.; Weil, M. H.; Shubin, H., and Sherwin, R.: Pulmonary failure associated with clinical shock states. *J Trauma, 11*:22-35, 1971.
16. Germon, P. A.; Kazem, I., and Brady, L. W.: Shunting following trauma. *J Trauma, 8*:724-734, 1968.
17. Rahn, H., and Farhi, L. E.: Ventilation, perfusion and gas exchange—The Va/Q' concept in Field, J. (Ed.): *Handbook of Physiology,* Section 3: Respiration. Washington, D.C., American Physiological Society, Vol 1, page 735, 1964.

18. Monaco, V.; Burdge, R.; Newell, J.; Sardar, S.; Leather, R.; Powers, S. M., and Dutton, R.: Pulmonary venous admixture in injured patients. *J Trauma, 12*:15-21, 1972.
19. Powers, S. R.; Burdge, R.; Leather, R.; Monaco, V.; Newell, J.; Sardar, S., and Smith, E. J.: Studies of pulmonary insufficiency in nonthoracic trauma. *J Trauma, 12*:1-14, 1972.
20. Abrams, M. E., and Taylor, F. B.: Isolation and quantitative estimation of pulmonary surface active lipoprotein and its interaction with fibrinogen. *Physiologist, 7*:78, 1964.
21. Greenfield, L. J.; Barkett, M., and Coalson, J. J.: The role of surfactant in pulmonary response to trauma. *J Trauma, 8*:735-741, 1968.
22. Karliner, J. S.: Noncardiac forms of pulmonary edema. *Circulation, 46*:212, 1972.
23. Nahas, R. A.: Post-perfusion lung syndrome: Role of circulatory exclusion. *Lancet, 2*:251, 1965.
24. Wadstrom, L. B.: The effect of trauma on plasma lipids. *Actu Chir Scand, 115*:409-416, 1958.
25. Mays. E. T.: The effect of surgical stress on plasma free fatty acids. *J Surg Res, 10*:315-319, 1970.
26. Pomerantz, M., and Eiseman, B.: Experimental Shock Lung Model. *J Trauma, 12*:782-787, 1968.
27. Ashbaugh, D. G., and Uzawa, T.: Respiratory and hemodynamic changes after injection of free fatty acids. *J Surg Res, 8*:417, 1968.
28. Rubia, F. J., and Schulz, H.: Elektronenmikroskopische Unter suchungen des blut-Luft-weges bei der experimentellen fettenbolie der lung. *Beitz, path Anta, 128*:78-102, 1963.
29. Hoye, R. C.; Paulson, D. F., and Ketcham, A. S.: Total circulating albumin deficits occurring with extensive surgery. *Surg Gynecol Obstet, 131*:943-952, 1970.
30. Rasmussen, K. H., and Jarnum, S.: Investigations of postoperative hypoalbuninemia. *Acta Chir Scand, 122*:459-465, 1961.
31. Guiterrez, V. S.; Berman, I. R.; Soloway, H. B., and Hamit, H. F.: Relationship of hypoproteinemia and prolonged ventilation to the development of pulmonary insufficiency in shock. *Am Surg, 171*: 385-392, 1970.
32. Ballou, G. A.; Boyer, P. D., and Luck, J. M.: The electrophoretic mobility of human serum albumin as affected by lower fatty acid salts. *J Biol Chem, 159*:111-116, 1945.
33. Moore, F. D.; Lyons, J. H.; Pierce, E. C.; Morgan, A. P.; Drinker, P. A.; MacArthur, J. D., and Dammin, G. J.: *Post Traumatic Pulmonary Insufficiency.* Philadelphia, Toronto, London, W. B. Saunder, 1969.

34. Lyons, J. H., Sr., and Moore, F. D.: Post traumatic alkalosis: incidence and pathophysiology of alkalosis in surgery. *Surgery, 60*:93, 1966.

35. Cole, A. B.: Respiratory sequels to non thoracic injury. *Lancet, 1*:555-556, 1972.

36. Drucker, T. B.: Increased intracranial pressure and pulmonary edema. *J Neurosurg, 28*:112-117, 1968.

37. Cameron, G. R.: Pulmonary oldema. *Br Med J, 1*:965-972, 1948.

38. Vitek, V.; Vitek, K., and Lin, H. C.: Urinary glucose, galactose and their oligosaccharidec in trauma. *S Forum, 21*:99-101, 1970.

39. Schroder, R. K.; Eltringham, W. K.; Jenny, M. E.; Pluth, J. R.; Gumpert, J. R. W., and Zollinger, R. M.: Regional hemodynamics oyxgen consumption and lactate metabolism in a controlled reversible low flow state. *S Forum, 19*:11-13, 1968.

40. Mequid, M. M.; Brennan, M. F.; Aoki, T. T.; Ball, R. B., and Moore, F. D.: The role of insulin and glucogon in acute trauma. *S Forum, 24*:97-98, 1973.

41. Spigelman, A., and Ozeran, R. S.: The protective effect of insulin in hemorrhagic shock. *S Forum, 21*:90-92, 1970.

42. Wilmore, D. W.; Molyan, J. A.; Lindsey, C. A.; Faloona, G. R.; Unger, R. H., and Pruitt, B.: Hyperglucogonemia following thermal injury: insulin and glucogon in the posttraumatic state. *S Forum, 24*:99-100, 1973.

43. Long, C. L.; Spencer, J. L.; Kinney, J. M., et al.: Carbohydrate metabolism in man: Effect of elective operations and major injury. *J Appl Physiol, 31*:110-116, 1971.

44. Janoff, A.; Weissman, G.; Zweifach, B. W., et al.: Pathogenesis of experimental shock. IV Studies of lysosames in normal and tolerant animals subjected to lethal trauma and endotoxemia. *J Exp Med, 116*:451, 1962.

45. Starling, J. R.; Proctor, H. J., and Johnson, G.: Influences of lysosomal enzymes on human erythrocyte intracellular ion concentration. *Surg Forum, 24*:62-64, 1973.

46. Chaudry, I. H.; Sayeed, M. M., and Baue, A. E.: Alterations in adenosive nucleotides in hemorrhagic shock. *Surg Forum, 23*:1-3, 1972.

47. Engel, F. L.; Harrison, H. C., and Long, C. N. H.: Biochemical changes in shock. *J Exp Med, 79*:9, 1944.

48. Hoar, W. S., and Haist, R. E.: Amino acid nitrogen in shock. *J Biol Chem, 154*:331, 1944.

49. Seligman, A. M.; Frank, H. A., and Fine, J.: Cross circulation of the liver during shock. CHO metabolism in hemorrhagic shock. *J Clin Invest, 26*:530, 536, 1947.

50. Hoye, R. C.; Voightlander, V.; Birke, G., et al.: Changes in the total circulating albumin, plasma volume with hemorrhage and the response to cortisone. *Acta Chir Scand, 137*:299-304, 1971.

51. Moore, F .D.; Steinbreng, R. W.; Boll, M. R.; Wilson, G. M., and Myrden, J. A.: Strides in surgical endocrinology. I The urinary excretion of 17 hydroxycorticords and associated metabolic changes in cases of soft tissue trauma of varying severity and in bone trauma. *Am Surg, 141*:145, 1955.

52. Forsham, P. H.: Clinical symposium the Adrenal Gland Ciba, vol. 15, No. 1, 1963.

53. Kriegler, H.; Abbott, W. D.; Levey, S., and Holden, W. D.: Re-evaluation of the role of the adrenal and other factors in the metabolic response to injury. *Surgery, 44*:138, 1958.

54. Gold, J. J.; Singleton, E.; MacFarlane, D. A., and Moore, F. D.: Effects of adrenocorticotropsin and complex trauma in the human. *J Clin Invest, 37*:813, 1958.

55. Mack, E., and Egdahl, R.: Adrenal microcirculation in hemorrhagic shock. *Surg Gynecol Obstet, 129*:511, 1969.

56. Ingle, D. J.: Permissive action of hormones. *J Clin Endocrin Metab, 14*:1272, 1954.

57. Bauer, W. E.; Levene, R. A.; Zachwieja, A.; Lee, M. J.; Menczyk, Z., and Drucker, W. R.: The role of catecholamines in energy metabolism during prolonged hemorrhagic shock. *S Form, 20*:9-10, 1969.

58. Greever, C. J., and Watts, D. T.: Epinephrine levels in peripheral blood during irreversible hemorrhagic shock in dogs. *Circ Res, 7*:192, 1959.

59. McShane, R. H., and Stahl, W. M.: The renal response to hemorrhage in man. *S Forum, 19*:46-48, 1968.

60. Broelsch, C. E.; Chandler, J. G.; Modafferi, T.; Rosen, H., and Orloff, M. J.: Effect of acute changes in renal hemodynamics during hemorrhage on aldosterone secretion. *S Forum, 24*:23-25, 1973.

61. Modafferi, T. R.; Rosen, H.; Chandler, J. G., et al.: The role of the renin-angiotension system in aldosterone response to acute hemorrhage. *S Forum, 23*:22, 1972.

62. Shires, G. T.; Williams, J., and Brown, F. T.: A method for simultaneous measurement of plasma volume, red cell mass and extracellular fluid space in man using radioactive 1^{131} C^{35} 0_4 and Cr^{51}. *J Lab Clin Med, 55*:776, 1960.

63. Elkinton, J. R.; Danowski, T. S., and Winkler, A. W.: Salt depletion and dehydration as shock factors. *J Clin Invest, 25*:120, 1946.

64. Fulton, R. L., and Ridolpho, P.: Physiologic effects of acute sodium depletion. *Am Surg, 173*:344-356, 1971.

65. Grayson, T. L.; LoHete, J. E., and Moyer, C. A.: Oxygen consumptions; concentrations of inorganic ions in urine serum and duodenal fluids, hematocrit urinary excretion, pulse rates and blood pressure during duodenal depletion of sodium salts in normal and alcoholic man. *Am Surg, 158*:840, 1963.

66. Ashworth, C. T., and Kregel, L. A.: Partition of water and electrolytes in shock. *Arch Surg, 44*:829, 1942.

67. Carter, N. W., et al.: Measurement of intracellular pH of skeletal muscle with pH sensitive glass microelectrodes. *J Clin Invest, 46*:920, 1967.

68. Canipion, D. S., et al.: The effect of hemorrhagic shock on transmembrane potential. *Surgery, 66*:1051, 1969.

69. Cunningham, J. N.; Struis, G. T., and Wagner, Y.: Cellular transport defects in hemorrhagic shock. *Surgery, 70*:215, 1971.

70. Dmochoswki, J. R.; Deuvarert, F.; Rabelo, A., and Couch, N. P.: Muscle surface potassium ion activity in graded hemorrhage. *S Forum, 23*:12-14, 1972.

71. Trunkey, P. D.; Illner, H. M. D.; Wagner, I. Y., and Shires, G. T.: The effect of hemorrhagic shock on intracellular muscle action potential in the primate. *Surgery*, 1973.

72. Shires, G. T., and Canizaro, P. C.: Fluid resuscitation in the severely injured. *S Clin North Am, 53*:1341-1365, 1973.

MULTIPLE SYSTEM INJURIES

A s INTERSTATE EXPRESSWAYS intertwine our cities and states, as heavy industrial equipment is more frequently used, as sale of handguns spirals to new heights, the number of patients with multiple system injuries increases. The automobile is undoubtedly the most common agent in the production of multiple injuries. In an investigation of automotive crash injuries at Cornell University Medical College an analysis was made of a thousand injury-producing accidents in which 1,678 automobile occupants were injured. Multiple injuries constituted the most common pattern. Actually, over 66 percent of all injured persons suffered injuries in two or more body areas.[1]

Such seriously injured patients with multiple systems damaged require a team of physicians if they are to survive at all, and the quality of life after injury depends upon a team captain who must take complete charge of the injured patient and whose responsibility it is to determine the order of care required for the various injuries, then proceed with a concept of priorities to see that first things are done first. Kennedy[2] urged this team concept and the idea of a team captain in the care of patients with multiple injuries when he said, "Often specialists are called and each considers only the problem in his own field without sufficient co-ordination. Because of lack of authority given to one person, critical decisions may be delayed by useless bickering . . . the procedure of having a team captain to direct emergency treatment on the basis of doing first things first is the best means of giving a patient with multiple injuries a "square deal" in the use of known methods to save his life and to prevent permanent disability."

A tendency has developed in recent years to divide the patient into compartments. In patients with a single specific lesion this has provided excellent medical care. But in patients with multiple injuries a tendency to isolate injuries and ignore the "whole man" can result in tragic consequences. Many hospitals have directives that an X-ray diagnosis of fracture automatically places the patient in an orthopedic bed. A fracture, however, is one injury which rarely kills patients immediately. If the patient dies after a major fracture it is usually due to hypovolemia shock or undetected injuries.

In some instances it is routine for all rib fractures to be admitted to the chest or orthopedic service. Posterior fractures of ribs 10, 11, 12 are frequently accompanied by ruptured liver if the fractures are on the right or ruptured spleen if the fractures are on the left. Rib fractures at a higher level may penetrate the lung and cause a tension pneumothorax. The evaluation and detection of a pneumothorax and mediastinal shifts are not in the realm of the orthopedist's training, and the orthopedist should not and usually does not want the responsibility of detecting such injuries. A tragic case lingers in my memory of a young man who died during the night of a tension pneumothorax while being treated on the orthopedic service for a fracture of the femoral shaft which had been excellently reduced and immobilized with skeletal traction.

In multiple system injuries temporary arrangements are often necessary. Sometimes less than excellent results must be accepted which ordinarily would not be acceptable were that the only injury the patient had sustained. Stabilization of the vertebral column is a high priority, but temporary immobilization of a cervical vertebral fracture with a spineboard or sand bags may be necessary in a patient with respiratory embarrassment from obstructed airway, flail chest or pneumothorax. The definitive treatment of the vertebral column injury must necessarily be postponed several hours until blood gases and cardiovascular functions are optimal and permit more definitive treatment of the vertebral injury.

On the other hand, a severe injury to the vertebral column with clinical evidence of spinal cord compression in a patient with many soft tissue lacerations or fractures of the extremities should have immediate relief of the spinal cord compression in a definitive manner. The soft tissue injuries and open fractures are rapidly occluded with sterile pressure dressings delaying the definitive treatment of these wounds until spinal cord decompression has been achieved.

Severe contusions of the kidneys are impressive and obvious lesions because of the frightening gross hematuria they produce, but in a hypovolemic individual with a flail chest and hemothorax, the evaluation of the renal injury must be postponed several hours. A significant amount of time can be wasted in trying to obtain an intravenous pyelogram in a hypovolemic patient who because of the hypovolemia is not even perfusing the kidney with the injected contrast material. Blood volume repletion, aspiration of the hemothorax and stabilization of flail chests with mechanical ventilation must be done first. The hematuria is not ignored nor forgotten but evaluation by intravenous pyelography is postponed until optimal cardiorespiratory function is obtained. This may be a matter of hours or sometimes days.

Kennedy has recognized six clinical patterns of trauma and points out that the essence of treatment is organization and classification of multiple injury patients. Each type is characterized by its own particular problem although general principles remain unchanged in each. Each has a basic priority of evaluation and treatment that must be met. In each, consultants play a major role but team cooperation and effort prevails throughout.

The team captain must consider the whole man. His concept of critically injured patients must encompass the "unit concept" and at the same time the "priority concept." The team captain is usually a general surgeon orthopedist or general practitioner with the widest possible experience. However, now that several universities have residencies in emergency medicine it is logical that these individuals will also be competent to serve as team captains. Specialists have a natural bias toward their own area of concern and no criticism of highly skilled specialists is intended by the team approach.

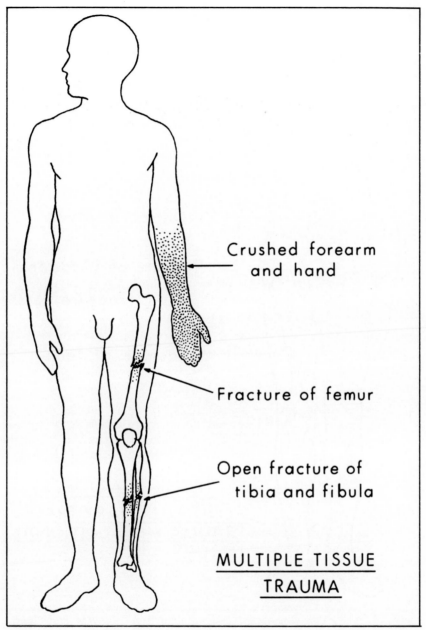

Crushed forearm
and hand

Fracture of femur

Open fracture of
tibia and fibula

MULTIPLE TISSUE
TRAUMA

Figure 4-1. *Multiple Tissue Trauma.* This type presents itself in shock, which is the chief physiologic disturbance. The essential problem, once all the sites of injury are recognized, is to determine the sequence of treatment. The orthopedist is the major consultant. The usual errors are insufficient treatment of shock, failure to recognize all the traumata, and mistakes in judgment, particularly the performance of prolonged complicated operations that could be reasonably postponed or simplified.

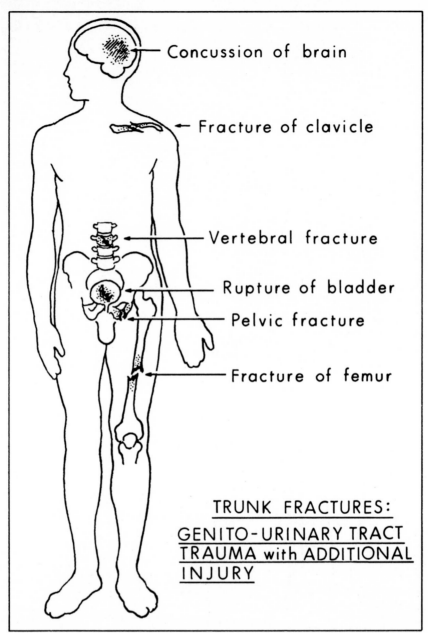

Concussion of brain

Fracture of clavicle

Vertebral fracture

Rupture of bladder

Pelvic fracture

Fracture of femur

TRUNK FRACTURES:
GENITO-URINARY TRACT
TRAUMA with ADDITIONAL
INJURY

Figure 4-2. *Trunk Fractures: Genito-urinary Tract Trauma with Additional Injury.* The presenting physiologic disturbance is shock. The essential problem is recognition of the bladder injury. While the other traumata can be identified by ordinary roentgen means, the critical bladder injury can be easily overlooked. The techniques of urinary tract investigation following trauma have been systematized in Chapter 8. The orthopedist is a close partner. He must defer treatment until the emergent urinary tract procedures have been performed. Following this, he must decide on his own regimen. The common error is to miss the bladder injury and perform extensive bone procedures.

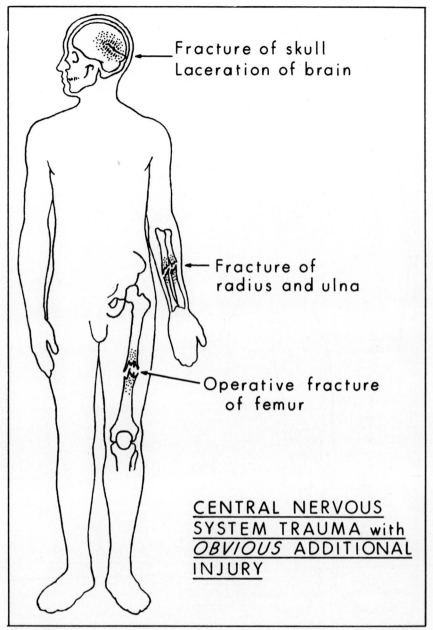

Fracture of skull
Laceration of brain

Fracture of
radius and ulna

Operative fracture
of femur

CENTRAL NERVOUS
SYSTEM TRAUMA with
OBVIOUS ADDITIONAL
INJURY

Figure 4-3. *Central Nervous System Trauma with Obvious Additional Injury.* The presenting physiologic disturbance in this type is a combination of shock and coma. The treatment of each should not interfere with the other. The presence of coma does not interdict necessary operation elsewhere as does shock. The chief consultant here is the neurosurgeon. It is important for him to cooperate with the team captain and orthopedist. Decisions as to nature and sequence of procedure must be jointly made. The common error is to place the patient on a neurosurgical service for an extended period of time with insufficient attention to the therapeutic requirements of the other injuries.

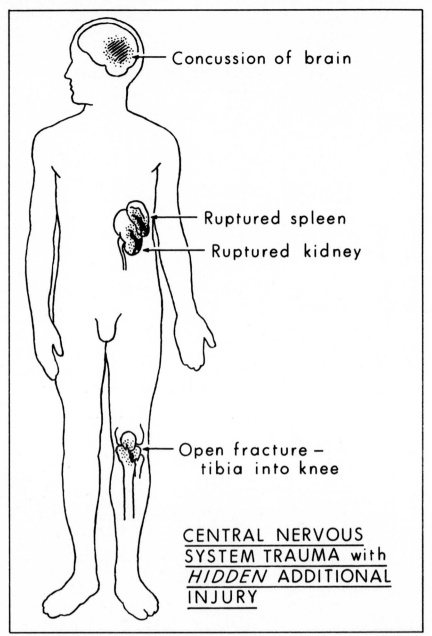

Concussion of brain

Ruptured spleen
Ruptured kidney

Open fracture —
tibia into knee

CENTRAL NERVOUS
SYSTEM TRAUMA with
HIDDEN ADDITIONAL
INJURY

Figure 4-4. *Central Nervous System Trauma with Hidden Additional Injury.* The presenting physiologic disturbance is coma. This may be transient and thereby misleading since an accurate history is unobtainable and the physical signs of bodily injuries blunted. Ultimately, the general surgeon carries the main responsibility. Shock due to internal hemorrhage may appear well after admission and the insidious nature of the clinical picture places a heavy burden on judgment as well as technical ability. The urologist and the orthopedist play important roles. The common error is to fail to recognize the severity of the intra-abdominal and retroperitoneal traumata.

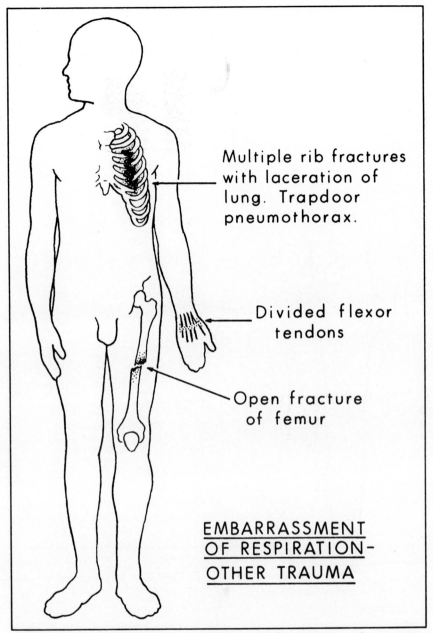

Multiple rib fractures
with laceration of
lung. Trapdoor
pneumothorax.

Divided flexor
tendons

Open fracture
of femur

EMBARRASSMENT
OF RESPIRATION—
OTHER TRAUMA

Figure 4-5. *Embarrassment of Respiration—Other Trauma.* The present-ing physiologic disturbance is asphyxia. If severe, this can be rapidly lethal. The treatment begins at the site of accident with the removal of obvious obstruction in the mouth or pharynx and the administration of oxygen. It continues as the team captain and thoracic surgeon take over. All other injuries are distinctly secondary in importance. As soon as the respiratory state is satisfactory, the other traumata can be treated according to the usual principles. The common error is to allow prolonged cyanosis to continue and to embark upon skeletal operations before a satisfactory cardiorespiratory state has been achieved.

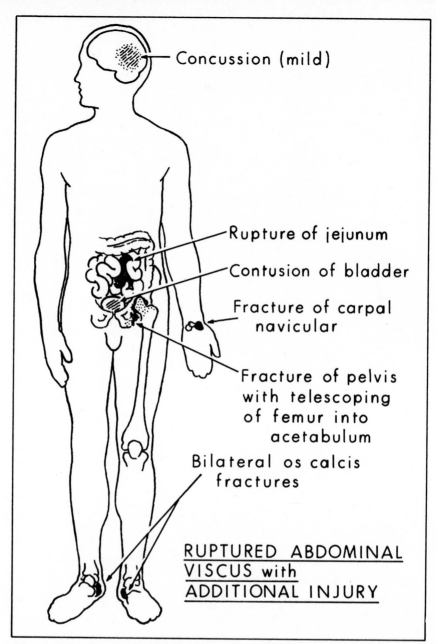

Figure 4-6. *Ruptured Abdominal Viscus with Additional Injury.* The presenting physiologic disturbance is shock. The chief problem is the decision for abdominal exploration in the presence of other obvious severe traumata. A mild concussion complicates matters. In a vigorous patient, laparotomy is indicated if the possibility of a ruptured viscus exists. In older and severely shocked patients, the surgeon's judgment is tested to the full. Abdominal roentgenograms and abdominal lavage are helpful. A laparotomy with negative findings is a preferable error to belated repair or removal of a ruptured viscus. In this type, the orthopedist's role is secondary to that of the general surgeon.

The team captain must rely heavily upon all available and indicated specialists immediately as he needs them. When operative intervention or further tests are advised by a specialist, permission must be given by the team captain. An advised operation may be required, but it may be the third or fourth procedure to be done and the team captain has that excrutiating responsibility of deciding who goes next or when the injured patient has had enough and call a moratorium on further operative procedures until the patient's condition permits.

The most important concept to be remembered is that in patients with multiple injuries it is not necessary to definitely treat and correct all his injuries within the first few hours of hospitalization. This is the most common pitfall. The American tradition of getting everything taken care of rapidly and expecting the most excellent result in every case strongly influences the management of these multiple injury patients. Quality of life after injury is important but cognizant *life* after injury is ever so much more important. Sometimes we may have to accept a little less than the best in extremity injuries or facial lacerations in order to obtain meaningful survival of the "unit."

An illustration of this point was a lovely nineteen-year-old girl who had multiple skeletal and soft tissue trauma. An impressive and obvious injury was laceration of the left arm. Hand specialists were consulted and immediately began a long and tenuous operative repair on the brachium extending from midnight into the early morning hours. Because of some technical difficulty with an arterial anastomosis the operation was prolonged. In the ninth hour the oxygen supply tank became exhausted and was unnoticed, resulting cerebral anoxia. In the postoperative period the patient never regained consciousness. Six months later she had a viable arm but no brain. She will require constant nursing home care for the rest of her life.

A seventeen-year-old boy had a laceration of the popliteal space. It was a very obvious and horrible looking injury but involved only the soft tissue and not major arteries, veins or nerves. There was no exsanguinating hemorrhage and the injury did not pose a threat to the boy's life. Because he was intoxicated and had not been fasting in preparation for his accident or operation, there was great concern on the part of the team captain whether this boy should have any repair at all of this injury. Finally the team captain gave in at the insistence of his specialist consultant and the boy was induced, intubated and turned to a prone position to facilitate operative exposure and repair of the popliteal space. While the repair was in progress the boy developed a cardiac arrest due to hypoxia. In the course of resuscitation he aspirated gastric contents. The end result: a young boy with brain necrosis requiring mechanical ventilatory assistance.

The team captain must have veto power and the strength of his convictions to use it. He must be well experienced in the amount and length of operative procedures that a critically injured individual can tolerate, or that his physician colleagues can safely provide. His judgement must be sound and founded on physiologic principles which he has mastered through the years. In definitive care cardiorespiratory resuscitation must come first; then stabilization of the vertebral column and treatment of injuries of vascular turgid organs (i.e. heart, spleen, liver, lungs). Lacerations of the hands and other soft tissue and closed fractures can wait until the patient can tolerate their operative correction and the above physiologic derangements have been corrected or compensated. Each of the lower priority systems should then receive care as decided upon by the team captain.

EVALUATING THE SEVERITY OF TISSUE DAMAGE

Most patients with multiple system involvement have been injured by excessive transfers of energy. That some method of evaluating the severity of tissue damage is needed has been agreed upon by many investigators over many years. Attempts to evaluate the severity of injuries are undoubtedly as old as is the practice of medicine. The automobile, heavy industrial equipment and ready availability of handguns has suddenly increased the number of patients with multiple system injuries by tens of thousands each year and thus emphasized the critical need for methods of assessment.

Most attempts to devise scales for measuring these phenomenon have developed in relation to automobile crashes. The National Safety Council[3] provides brief descriptions of fatal serious, minor and nonvisible injuries. It has served the National Safety Council well providing mass data, but not for research into specific injuries. The code numbers do not indicate severity but simply identify location.

For quick emergency evaluation of patients Williams and Schamadan[4] recommend a system used in air evacuation in Arizona. This scale rates the overall condition of the patient but cannot be used for rating specific injuries. A DeHaven type scale is used by the automotive crash research unit at Cornell University.[1] It provides for simple but effective identification of injuries and lists examples of injuries. Their scale covers moderate, severe, serious, critical and fatal injuries. But subjective judgement must be used to determine the severity of injuries.

The majority of these and other systems of evaluating severity of tissue damage have been designed for researchers to study and classify and evaluate multiple injuries. Kirkpatrick and Youmans[5] recommend a format to classify and evaluate multiple injuries. The advantage of their system is that it can be completed by nonphysicians and nonresearchers. It is an arbitrary number system providing a simple means of evaluating patients with multiple injuries. Their trauma index is not sensitive enough to identify small subtle differences, and is in no way a substitute for a thorough examination by a physician.

The advantage of a reliable system that can be implemented by Emergency Medical Technicians and other nonphysician personnel is pertinent. The categorization of hospitals[6, 7] under the auspices of the commission on Emergency Medical Services of the American Medical Association has thrust upon us the reality of pre-hospital decision making. In order for categorization to effectively contribute to emergency health care, individuals responsible for transporting critically injured patients must be able to select which patient needs to be taken to what category hospital. Otherwise we will enter an era of "fruitbasket turnover" in which suffering patients may be shuffled from one hospital to another because the first hospital doesn't provide for that degree of injury. There must be an initial pre-hospital decision as to

TABLE 4-I

TRAUMA INDEX

	One point	Three points	Four points	Six points
Region	skin or extremities	back	chest or abdomen	head or neck
Type of injury	laceration or contusion	stab wound	blunt	missile
CV status	external hemorrhage	BP<100 P>100	BP<80 P>140	absent pulses
CNS status	drowsy	stupor	motor or sensory loss	coma
Respiratory status	chest pain	dyspnea or hemoptysis	evidence of aspiration	apnea or cyanosis
				TOTAL

Reproduced with permission. Kirkpatrick, Jr., and Youmans, R. L., *Journal of Trauma*, vol. 11, 1971, pp. 711-714.

which patient belongs in Category I or Category IV Hospitals. Emergency Medical Technicians will be making such decisions and the Trauma Index illustrated in Table 4-I may prove useful. It has a 3 percent margin of error. The injuries producing most of the errors were: head trauma, long bone fractures and tendon lacerations.

In addition to aiding emergency medical technicians with pre-hospital decisions this Trauma Index may also be useful in smaller community hospitals staffed by nurses or paramedical personnel. A nonphysician can communicate the exact seriousness of a problem to a physician several miles away without relying on purely subjective terms. Each region of the body and each injury or each manifestation of injury are given a number value. Then the total number of points is added to achieve a total score. Kirkpatrick and Youmans found good correlation between the severity of injury and the index rating. Most patients rated between 0 to 7 have minor injuries, those rated between 8 to 18 have moderately severe injuries usually requiring hospitalization but only rarely causing death and those with scores above 18 have severe injuries with a death rate approaching 50 percent. The chief disadvantage of such evaluation is an over reliance on an arbitrary number system.

All these systems had as their prime criteria of evaluation the threat-to-life principle. The American Medical Association Committee on Medical Aspects of Automotive Safety recognized there are many criteria others than threat-to-life. They developed a new rating system in two stages. The first was called the Abbreviated Injury Scale (AIS)[8] and the second the Comprehensive Injury Scale (CIS).

With the AIS, each injury is categorized by body area (head or neck, face, chest, abdominal or pelvic contents, extremities or pelvic girdle, and general). The langauge used to describe injuries is in accordance with accepted current medical terminology except for an occasional term such as "whiplash." The AIS also categorizes each injury by severity and lists the number in the upper left hand corner of the chart, 1, minor; 2, moderate; 3, severe not life-threatening; 4, severe life-threatening, survival probable; 5, critical survival uncertain; 6 and 7 fatal within 24 hours; 8 and 9 fatal; 99 x severity unknown. 98 Z presence unknown (Table 4-II).

TABLE-4-II

ABBREVIATED INJURY SCALE

Severity Code	Severity Category/Injury Description	Police Code
0 (Zero)	No Injury	0 or D
1	Minor	C

GENERAL
   —Aches all over
   —Minor lacerations, contusions, and abrasions (first aid—simple closure)
   —All first edgree or small second degree or small third degree burns

HEAD AND NECK
   —Cerebral injury with headache; dizziness; no loss of consciousness
   —"Whiplash" complaint with no anatomical or radiological evidence
   —Abrasions and contusions of ocular apparatus (lids, conjunctiva, cornea, uveal injuries); vitreous or retinal hemorrhage

CHEST
   —Muscle ache or chest wall stiffness

ABDOMINAL
   —Muscle ache; seat belt abrasion; etc.

EXTREMITIES
   —Minor sprains and fractures and/or dislocation of digits

Severity Code	Severity Category/Injury Description	Police Code
2	Moderate	B

GENERAL
—Extensive contusions; abrasions; large lacerations; avulsions (less than 3 inches wide)
—10 to 20% body surface second or third degree burns

HEAD AND NECK
—Cerebral injury with or without skull fracture, less than 15 minutes unconsciousness; no post-traumatic amnesia
—Undisplaced skull or facial bone fractures or compound fracture of nose
—Lacerations of the eye and appendages; retinal detachment
—Disfiguring lacerations
—"Whiplash"—severe complaints with anatomical or radiological evidence

CHEST
—Simple rib or sternal fractures
—Major contusions of chest wall without hemothorax or pneumothorax or respiratory embarrassment

ABDOMINAL
—Major contusion of abdominal wall

EXTREMITIES AND/OR PELVIC GIRDLE
—Compound fractures of digits
—Undisplaced long bone or pelvic fracutres
—Major sprains of major joints

3	Severe (not life-threatening)	B

GENERAL
—Extensive contusion; abrasions; large lacerations involving more than two extremities, or large avulsions (greater than 3 inches wide)
—20 to 30% body surface second or third degree burns

HEAD AND NECK
—Cerebral injury with or without skull fracture, with unconsciousness more than 15 minutes; without severe neurological signs; brief post-traumatic amnesia (less than 3 hours)
—Displaced closed skull fractures without unconsciousness or other signs of intracranial injury
—Loss of eye, or avulsion of optic nerve
—Displaced facial bone fractures or those with antral or orbital involvement
—Cervical spine fractures without cord damage

CHEST
—Multiple rib fractures without respiratory embarrassment
—Hemathorax or pneumothorax
—Rupture of diaphragm
—Lung contusion

ABDOMINAL
—Contusion of abdominal organs
—Extraperitoneal bladder rupture
—Retroperitoneal hemorrhage
—Avulsion of ureter
—Laceration of urethra
—Thoracic or lumbar spine fractures without neurological involvement

Severity Code   Severity Category/Injury Description   Police Code

EXTREMITIES AND/OR PELVIC GIRDLE
—Displaced simple long-bone fractures, and/or multple hand and foot fractures
—Single open long-bone fractures
—Pelvic fracture with displacement
—Dislocation of major joints
—Multiple amputations of digits
—Lacerations of the major nerves or vessels of extremities

4   Severe (life-threatening, surgical probable)   B

GENERAL
—Severe lacerations and/or avulsions with dangerous hemorrhage
—30 to 50% surface second or third degree burns

HEAD AND NECK
—Cerebral injury with or without skull fracture, with unconsciousness of more than 15 minutes, with definite abnormal neurological signs; post-traumatic amnesia 3 to 12 hours
—Compound skull fracture

CHEST
—Open chest wounds; flail chest; pneumonmediastinum; myocardial contusion without circulatory embarrassment; pericardial injuries

ABDOMINAL
—Minor laceration of intra-abdominal contents (to include ruptured spleen, kidney, and injuries to tail of pancreas)
—Intraperitoneal bladder rupture
—Avulsion of the genitals
—Thoracic and/or lumbar spine fractures with paraplegia

EXTREMITIES
—Multiple closed long-bone fractures
—Amputation of limbs

5   Critical (survival uncertain)   A

GENERAL
—Over 50% body surface second or third degree burns

HEAD AND NECK
—Cerebral injury with or without skull fracture with unconsciousness of more than 24 hours; post-traumatic amnesia more than 12 hours; intracranial hemorrhage; signs of increased intracranial pressure (decreasing state of consciousness, brady-cardia under 60, progressive rise in blood pressure or progressive pupil inequality)
—Cervical spine injury with quadriplegia
—Major airway obstruction

CHEST
—Chest injuries with major respiratory embarrassment (laceration of trachea, hemomediastinum, etc.)
—Aortic laceration
—Myocardial rupture or contusion with circulatory embarrassment

ABDOMINAL
—Rupture, avulsion of severe laceration of intra-abdominal vessels or organs, except kidney, spleen or ureter

Severity Code   Severity Category/Injury Description   Police Code

EXTREMITIES
—Multiple open limb fractures
6   Fatal (within 24 hours)   K
—Fatal lesions of single region of body, plus injuries of other
body regions of Severity Code 3 or less
—Fatal from burns regardless of degree
7   Fatal (within 24 hours)   K
—Fatal lesions of single region of body, plus injuries of other
body regions of Severity Code 4 or 5
8   Fatal   K
—2 fatal lesions in 2 regions of body
9   Fatal   K
—3 or more fatal injuries
—Incineration by fire
99   X   Severity Unknown
—Injured, but severity not known
98   Z   Presence Unknown
—Presence of injury not known

The Committee on Medical Aspects of Automotive Safety readily admits that it has not been able to eliminate the subjective from the AIS but it has been able to reduce somewhat the error potential. Both scales were based primarily on the professional experience and judgment of physicians and will therefore require physician input and direction in completing the forms. Some examples of using the codes for chest and abdominal injuries in evaluating severity of various kinds of injuries are shown in Table 4-III.

TABLE 4-III

THE ABBREVIATED INJURY SCALE

Site of Injury	Terminology	AIS Code
CHEST		
Muscle ache or chest wall stiffness	Minor	1
Simple rib or sternal fracture	Moderate	2
Hemothorax or Pneumothorax	Severe	3
Flail chest or open chest wounds	Severe Life Threatening	4
Aortic laceration	Critical Survival Uncertain	5
ABDOMEN		
Muscle ache; seat belt abrasions, etc.	Minor	1
Major contusion of abdominal wall	Moderate	2
Extraperitoneal bladder rupture	Severe	3
Ruptured spleen or kidney	Severe Life Threatening	4
Rupture or avulsion of intra-abdominal organs or vessels	Critical Survival Uncertain	5

The major limitation of the AIS is that various criteria used in rating injuries cannot be readily identified and separated. Physicians are inclined to think in many other terms than threat-to-life, the length of treatment necessary for a given injury and the residual impairment after recovery, etc. are important. Researchers are also interested in the energy dissipated or the amount of force required to produce a given injury. The Comprehensive Injury Scale overcomes some of the limitations of the Abbreviated Injury Scale. Its ratings are more objective, it provides more examples of injuries, it separates the injuries by major medical specialities and it separates the criteria used to evaluate injuries into five categories, energy dissipation, threat to life, permanent impairment, treatment period and incidence (Appendix C).

Energy Dissipation

An injury can be ranked according to the wounding force and the amount of energy transferred to the patient. Another way of looking at energy dissipated is to consider the force required to produce a certain kind of injury. In automotive collisons this is the force of second impact or the energy dissipated when the occupant strikes the inside of the vehicle. This is frequently a decelerative force. Research has determined actual amounts of energy required to produce specific injuries (see Chapter 2).

Threat-to-Life

This ranking is difficult to make other than on a subjective basis. Some injuries are of such severity that death is nearly always an obvious outcome. However difficult the ranking does seem to have some validity. The long range observation of a large number of injuries of a specific nature by experienced specialists justifies some degree of objectivity. Although the ranking might well be wrong for an individual patient, its accuracy as an average is fairly reliable.

Permanent Impairment

There is considerable confusion, even among some physicians, as to the difference between impairment and disability. The

AMA Committee on Rating of Mental and Physical Impairment, which has developed guides to the evaluation of impairment for a dozen body systems, describes permanent impairment as "any anatomic or functional abnormality or loss after maximal medical rehabilitation has been achieved," whereas it describes disability as the reduction or elimination of "ability to engage in gainful activity." Impairment, therefore, is a direct relation to the severity of the injury which caused it, whereas disability reflects many other factors, such as occupation, attitude, education, and economic and social environment. A finger injury, for example, which resulted from very small forces and is of little or no consequence as a threat-to-life, might well mean total disability to a concert pianist or violinist. Actually the AMA impairment guides are based on functional loss only and have little or no basis for evaluation or rating of the injury which caused the loss. The vision guide, for instance, does not even mention specific injuries, only percentages of vision loss. In rating an injury for crash research, however, the injury itself and its cause are the prime concerns.

Investigators using the new injury severity scales must remember that they are rating specific injuries and not the "whole man." They must also remember that they are concerned only with the injury and the impairment involved, not with disability, or the man's ability to make a livelihood. An amputated leg, for instance, is obviously 100 percent impaired, but it only partly impairs the whole man. On the other hand, with certain severe injuries, such as those involving the brain or other major organs, the impairment to the whole man is often, for all intents, the same as that for the specific organs.

Treatment Period

The physician's judgment as to length of treatment is a reflection of the severity of the injury. The treatment period must not be thought of in terms of the severity of the crash which caused the injury, since a comparatively minor injury may have a longer healing period and result in a high treatment-period rating. For instance, the Comprehensive Injury Scale will show that the energy dissipation required for an amputation of a lower extremity digit is 2, a low rating, and that for an amputation above the knee it is 5, the highest rating, while both injuries have the same treatment period, 3, a moderate rating.

Incidence

A number of seemingly extraneous factors are involved in incidence, but it is important in developing data on particular injury-causing features of a vehicle. Although it could be argued that incidence is purely a statistical rating and should not contribute at all to the rating of injury severity, it is important when those injuries which cause the biggest problem in automotive safety are considered. Steering wheels and columns are a classic example in which mere incidence revealed a correctable vehicular defect. Some years ago an analysis of large numbers of chest injuries in vehicle crashes eventually led to the installation of energy-absorbing steering columns. Further studies of incidence might well lead to the elimination of other injury producers.[9]

Both the Abbreviated Injury Scale and the Comprehensive Injury Scale pertain to individual injuries. A practical reliable scale for describing multiply injured patients is not available. Everyone knows that death rates increase in the presence of injuries in a second or third body area even when the isolated injuries would not in themselves be life-threatening. This accumulative effect might be called the "Multiplicity Factor." Patients with substantial injuries to multiple body areas have higher mortality rates. Baker and associates[10] validated this multiplicity factor in a study they did to correlate Abbreviated Injury Scale ratings with mortality. Their study group included 2,128 motor vehicle occupants, pedestrians and other road users whose injuries precipitated hospitalization or caused death. They categorized injuries according to the Abbreviated Injury Scale except they left off codes 6 through 9 (see Table 4-II).

This study confirmed that a simple summation of ratings from the AIS scale did not adequately describe the patient with multiple system injuries. The death rate for persons with two injuries of AIS grades 4 and 3 was not comparable to patients with two injuries of AIS grades 5 and 2 even though the sum in both patients equal 7. This nonlinear relationship led Baker to develop the "Injury Severity Score," which they defined as the sum of the squares of the highest AIS grade in each of the three most severely injured areas. For example a patient with laceration of the aorta (AIS = 5) multiple closed long bone fractures (AIS = 4) and retroperitoneal hemorrhage (AIS = 3) would have an "Injury Severity Score" of 50 ($[5]^2 + [4]^2 + [3]^2$). By applying the concept of the "Injury Severity Score" Baker and colleagues increased the correlation between their study group as compared to the AIS grade for the most severe injury.

The "Injury Severity Score" developed by Baker and her associates is a short step in the right direction but it does not approach the overall problems of the critically injured patient who has multiple systems involved. Neither their system nor the AIS accounts for the physiologic concomitants of multiple system injuries, which frequently influence the treatment and outcome more than anatomic lesions (see Chapter 3). Neither system takes into account the priorities in patients with multiple system injuries and the effect of priorities on the survival rates. In spite of their shortcomings the concepts of evaluating injuries in all these systems are progressing in the proper direction and can be helpful until better systems are forthcoming.

PRIORITIES

What seems obvious (i.e. in patients with multiple systems injured, certain aspects of evaluation and treatment take precedence over other injuries) many times becomes obscure or at least it appears so from the everyday standpoint of what is or is not done first. For example, it is generally and widely known that the brain cannot function if deprived of oxygen two to four minutes. This is not a controversial area in which a great deal more investigation and research is necessary to establish new data, it is a well founded physiologic fact. In spite of this, it is awesome to see seriously injured patients transported many miles to hospital facilities without any preparation to maintain or ensure an airway and, hence, oxygenation of cerebral cortex. Yet this very same patient has an obvious open fracture of the femoral shaft well dressed and carefully immobilized in a Thomas splint.

It is for this reason that a chapter on establishing priorities in critically injured victims is beyond doubt the most important of this text. Yet the material and information covered is in no way unique or new. It is of such basic nature that one almost hesitates to discuss it for fear of insulting the intelligence of the reader. But if there are deficiencies in modern day methods of managing injured patients, it is in this area. Not that the information isn't widely known, but that somewhere between cognizance and application there are glaring lacunae.

The concept of priorities is discussed again in later chapters, but first it is important to establish the unmitigated role of priorities in evaluating critically injured patients.

Before any assessment of a critically injured patient begins, certain priorities must be firmly established in the physician's mind if the remainder of the evaluation is meaningful. A Steinmann pin may be inserted into the tibia and immobilization of a femoral fracture accomplished, but while this is being done if the patient exsanguinates from a ruptured liver, the well managed extremity injury has little meaning.

Cardiopulmonary Resuscitation

A functioning cardio-respiratory system is the first priority in the evaluation and care of any seriously injured patient. A cardiac arrest has occurred if:

1. the patient is not breathing
2. a pulse cannot be palpated in the neck, arm, or groin
3. heart sounds are absent
4. the pupils are dilated.

Circulation and ventilation must be restored within four to six minutes or brain death occurs. The patient should be placed supine on a firm spine board or the floor. Never attempt cardiac compression on a mattress or other soft surface. External cardiac compression is attempted first. If this fails to restore adequate brain perfusion and if the patient is in the operating room or other appropriate hospital area thoractotomy and open cardiac massage are indicated.

Cardiac compression is never effective unless simultaneous

ventilation of the lungs is also done. This is accomplished by mouth-to-mouth, mouth-to-nose or mouth-to-airway breathing until an ambu bag or a mechanical ventilating device can be obtained. In adults the lower sternum should be compressed with the heel of one hand while the other hand gives additional power. The elbows should be straight and when one attendant tires another should be ready to take over. For small children (usually under 10 years of age) only the one hand on the sternum should be employed for cardiac compression. In the newborn and infants this is further modified to using the index and middle finger over the lower sternum to achieve cardiac compression. As soon as feasible the heart action should be monitored with an electrocardiogram. Ventricular fibrillation is a major problem in these patients and electrical conversion must be done quickly. Other arrythmias are also frequent and depending upon the results of the electrocardiographic pattern intravenous atropine or lidocaine are given.

A severe metabolic acidosis accompanies cardiac standstill and sodium bicarbonate should be given intravenously until the serum pH is 7.4. Blood gases are also evaluated and corrected with appropriate ventilatory support.

Airway Obstruction

Cyanosis and forcible inspiratory efforts are signs of airway obstruction. Attention to airways must begin at the scene of the injury. Even though the physician is not present he cannot extricate himself from the responsibility of airway patency in injured patients. The physician must actively instruct EMT and other ambulance personnel in the importance of airway care.

Once the patient is under the care of a physician he must, before allowing his attention to focus on horrible-appearing injuries to bone and soft tissue, recheck and re-establish an adequate airway. First, inspection of the mouth, pharynx, and hypopharynx must be done quickly. Solid foreign bodies should be flicked out with the index finger and liquid matter removed with suction. In some patients an oropharyngeal airway is inserted and this may be all that is needed; the examiner can move on to the next priority. In more serious injuries to the face, mandible, larynx, chest wall and in serious head injuries, an endotracheal tube is required. Every physician who practices medicine should be taught this particular technic. A laryngoscope and disposable sterile endotracheal tubes must be standard equipment in any room that serves as a station for evaluating serious injuries.

At one phase in medical education students were taught that "A tracheostomy should be done when you think of it." Yet the complications of tracheostomy have proved considerable over the years until now most reputable surgeons prefer that absolute indications for tracheostomy be present.

When physicians are adequately trained in orotracheal and nasotracheal intubations the indications for emergency tracheostomy should become fewer. As EMT's are taught this technique critically injured patients who need a tracheal tube should arrive at the hospital with an endotracheal tube in place.

At one time a clinical axiom insisted that no endotracheal tube should be left *in situ* longer than forty-eight hours. Now with newer sterile disposable tubes available most endotracheal tubes can be safely left *in situ* up to seven days. Beyond this period of time if continued tracheal intubation is indicated, a tracheostomy is best done.

Once an adequate airway is established the next priority is to determine if the patient can spontaneously support the physiologic exchange of gases. If not, assisted ventilation is instituted immediately. An ambu bag can be utilized enroute to the hospital and in transit within hospitals. Mechanical ventilators can then be attached and free personnel for other duties.

If assisted mechanical ventilation does not seem indicated, the patient may be allowed to respire on his own through the airway established by the physician. In this situation frequent inspection of the nail beds and mucous membranes must be done to assess adequate ventilation. Blood gases should be drawn soon after admission and at intervals until the pattern of gas exchange is adequately evaluated.

The next priority is an intact respiratory mechanism. Multiple rib fractures cause an unstable chest and paradoxical respiration. The thoracic cage should be palpated gently and carefully, each rib is palpated to determine the stability of the thoracic cage. Rib fractures are best detected by palpation with the finger tips. Roentgenograms are notorious in failing to demonstrate rib fractures. Place a hand on each hemithorax with spread fingers and ask the patient to inspire while you exert slight pressure against the ribs. Patients with rib fractures will experience severe pain and interrupt their inspiratory movement abruptly.

The thoracic cage must be inspected front and back for penetrations. A tiny stab wound may be sufficient to produce a serious pneumothorax. The examiner should stand at the foot of the patient's bed and observe closely the movements of the thoracic wall on inspiration and expiration. If a portion of the chest wall moves inward upon inspiration and outward on expiration, this is clinical evidence of a flail chest.

The extent of outward movement of the chest wall and upward movement of the ribs should receive close scrutiny and the two hemithoraces compared with each other. The failure of one hemithorax to expand as well as the other should cause the examiner to recheck his airway and endotracheal tube to be certain the tube has not migrated to one mainstem bronchus with the inflated balloon obstructing the contralateral bronchus. This should also be evaluated by ascultation. The absence of breath sounds on the suspicious side confirms bronchial obstruction. If the endotracheal device seems properly placed, bronchial obstruction may be secondary to aspirated foreign bodies, blood, gastric contents, etc. Should catheter suctioning not immediately resolve the problem, the airway device must be removed and a bronchoscope inserted. Blood, mucous and foreign material is aspirated until breath sounds return and the involved hemithorax is inflating and deflating normally. Laryngeal, tracheal and bronchial tears or defects are searched for as the scope is passed.

If one hemithorax seems fixed in an hyperexpanded position and the patient is in severe cardiorespiratory distress, tension pneumothorax must be suspected. Deviation of the trachea is felt for in the sternal notch and ascultation of the heart determines whether the mediastinum is shifted. Patients die quickly from such mediastinal shifts and immediate relief of the tension pneumothorax is mandatory. A thoracentesis tray should be present in all evaluating centers. Needle aspiration of air from the involved side can be life-saving even though it is temporary therapy. If a syringe is not available, a finger cut off a rubber glove and tied securely to a large bore needle inserted into the pleural space can serve as a temporary one-way valve. The definitive form of therapy for tension pneumothorax is closed thoracostomy and insertion of an intercostal tube with a water seal drainage. It may be instituted later, after initial relief has been given by one of the above needle techniques.

Large defects of the chest wall produce "sucking wounds," so named because of the suctioning sound created by movement of air in and out during the patient's efforts at respiration, such defects must be occluded immediately with an airtight dressing before additional evaluation can be done.

Hypovolemia

Replacement of blood volume is also a first priority in critically injured patients. After gas exchange in the lungs there must be sufficient volume of blood to carry the oxygen to the peripheral tissues.

Evaluation of blood volume and replacement of deficits, is one of the most important aspects of evaluating critically injured patients. Some of the best clinical methods of assessing blood volume, discarded because of simplicity, should be carefully evaluated. The pulse rate, capillary filling in the nail beds, color, temperature and moisture of the skin are excellent clinical criteria of perfusion of peripheral tissues. A tachycardia associated with cold moist skin suggest hypovolemia even though the brachial blood pressure may be within normal range. The physiologic reaction to blood loss is marked peripheral vasoconstriction and increased heart rate. These compensatory mechanisms will maintain an acceptable blood pressure for varying amounts of time depending upon age of the patients and status of his vascular system. One must not be misled by normal brachial arterial pressures when there is clinical evidence of hypovolemia. When these compensatory measures become exhausted cellular changes are irreversible.

An excellent and clinically applicable means of evaluating

blood loss and degree of hypovolemia is the urine output and central venous pressure.

The kidneys are uniquely situated below other vital organs in a decreasing order in which they receive their share of the cardiac output; the brain, heart, lungs, liver all occupy higher levels of priority in demands on cardiac output. If the kidneys are making urine one can be assured that other vital organs with greater priority on the cardiac output are perfused. Exceptions to this clinical rule would be interruption of the arterial supply of these organs. If urine output is less than 5 to 10 ml/hr and the other assessments mentioned above coincide, a reduced blood volume is present. Blood and extracellular fluids must be administered in large volumes quickly.

The second means of evaluating hypovolemia in the seriously injured is monitoring the central venous pressure. A large bore polyetheylene catheter is inserted either via cutdown on an arm vein or percutaneously inserted into the subclavian vein. The catheter is connected via a three-way valve to a manometer and in this manner blood and fluids can be administered through the catheter simply by turning the three-way valve when venous pressures are not being taken.

The catheter should not be placed into the inferior vena cava as variations in intraabdominal pressure negate the reliability of venous pressures from this anatomical region.

A great amount of misconception has developed over the years regarding the value and meaning of central venous pressure (CVP) measurements. One misconception is that it can measure blood volume. The venous pressure reflects only the manner in which the heart is handling the volume replacement and whether or not an adequate amount of blood is being made available to the heart for its pumping action.

The stroke volume depends upon the extent of lengthening of myocardial fibrils and this is directly dependent upon cardiac filling during diastole. The rate and volume of filling of the cardiac chambers is in turn dependent upon duration of diastole and the venous pressure. The gradient between the SVC, IVC and the right heart and the pulmonary veins and the left heart are the major factors in filling the cardiac chambers during diastole. The generally accepted idea is that monitoring pressure in the right atrium is a fairly reliable index of pressure in the left atrium. Investigation in baboons indicate that this is an acceptable thesis for clinical application. For exceptions see Chapter 13.

The theory that as long as the cvp is within normal range or low normal the patient cannot get into any problem with "stiff lungs" or pulmonary edema from over-transfusion is unsupportable. Unfortunately, patients have been over transfused and their blood volume over expanded even though every measurement of CVP was low normal.

This pitfall can only be avoided by recognizing that CVP is not the sole criteria. A singular measurement of CVP has little meaning. It is more important to establish changes from one point in time to the next. Changes in CVP carry much greater significance than a single measurement. Central venous pressure along with urine output, ascultation of the lung fields, pulse rate, color, temperature, and moisture of the skin can help arrive at a satisfactory answer regarding adequacy of blood volume replacement. Instruments for measuring blood volume by isotope dilution techniques invaluable in animal research, have proved impractical in clinical situations.

Sequential brachial blood pressure, hemoglobin and hematocrit are unreliable when evaluating blood volume or the adequacy of replacement therapy. One must remember that hemoglobin is a test of concentration (gms solute per 100 ml solution) and in no way indicates or reflects volume. Central venous oxygen concentration can be helpful in overall evaluation of the adequacy of resuscitation but does not reflect volume.

Another important aspect of CVP is that it gives a fair estimate of cardiac function. If the overall trend is a progressive increase in CVP with scant urine, myocardial inadequacy in respect to the patients volume (irrespective of whether that volume is normal) is present. Attention must be directed toward improving cardiac function. Cardiotonic drugs (glycosides, isoproterenol, glucagon, etc.) should be given to enhance cardiac output. An important exception to this observation must be noted. When hypovolemia is profound coronary artery perfusion is reduced. Myocardial contractily is inadequate and central venous pressure is paradoxically high. It would seem from previous discussion that fluids should not be pushed in this situation. It becomes even more confusing clinically because these patients have neck vein distention and a quiet heart consistent with cardiac tamponade. A recent patient with this unique complication of severe hypovolemia had a pericardiocentesis because it so closely mimiced cardiac tamponade. Contrary to the more common circumstances volume replacement must be pushed in face of an increased CVP pressure. As volume is replenished and coronary artery perfusion improved the heart more efficiently ejects the blood in its chamber and the central venous pressure falls instead of increasing.

At this point some digression from evaluation to therapy is justified. In traditional medical practice cardiac glycosides (digitalis, digitoxin, ouabain) are rarely thought necessary in patients with normal hearts and under the age of thirty. But in critically injured patients of eighteen or nineteen years with a depleted blood volume and depleted energy stores the cardiac glycosides are not only indicated but sometimes life saving and should be utilized freely when indicated, chiefly for their metabolic effect (i.e. restoration of high energy phosphate bonds).[11] After resuscitation they can be discontinued.

Control of Hemorrhage

Control of hemorrhage in conjunction with and simultaneous to volume replacement and airway patency is essential. It is self evident that volume replacement is futile if blood is running out through a popliteal carotid or brachial artery more rapidly than it can be infused through a large bore needle or intravenous catheter.

Tourniquets and blind clamping with hemostats must be condemned. They have few indications. Although application of tourniquets to bleeding extremities have been keystones in first aid courses for years, responsible physicians should crusade against this practice. Bleeding can nearly always be controlled by finger pressure or pressure bandages. A severed carotid, brachial, femoral or popliteal artery can be better controlled and with less damage to surrounding tissues by an index finger discreetly applied. This finger pressure can be instituted at the scene of injury and maintained until the patient is anesthetized and a sterile operating field is prepared, permitting surgical dissection of the injured artery and re-established arterial flow by primary anastomosis or saphenous vein grafting.

Hemorrhage from extensive lacerations of the scalp and other soft tissue injuries are often major sources of significant blood loss in patients with multiple injuries. Severe scalp and facial lacerations are impressive and obvious sources of blood loss. The control of bleeding is a first priority but the definitive management and repair of such lacerations and avulsions is a low priority and should not be confused with the greater priority of controlling of hemorrhage. Hemostasis can usually be attained quickly in these wounds by a heavy pressure dressing. This achieves control of bleeding from sources that significantly reduce blood volume, yet time is not lost in a prolonged and careful "plastic repair" of these low priority wounds.

One of the most valuable and reliable clinical assessments in critically injured patients is the observed response to initial resuscitation efforts. Sequential observations after blood volume replacement are invaluable. After the estimated volume replacement has been given if there is a salubrious response in heart rate, CVP, urine output, skin color and temperature, and this is maintained in sequential observations, it usually indicates an optimum circulating volume.

If, on the other hand, a salubrious response is observed after reasonable volume replacement and after this initial response there is progressive deterioration in the clinical observations previously listed as indicating optimum circulating volume, one must suspect concealed blood loss. This is a classic clinical picture repeated over and over again in seriously injured patients and should not be overlooked nor misinterpreted.

Concealed Blood Loss

An initial good response after replacement therapy estimated by the physician to be adequate, followed by progressive collapse of the cardiovascular system must be given immediate priority and concealed blood loss suspected.

The regions in the body that have the capacity to conceal amounts of blood sufficient to disrupt a precarious circulating volume are limited. For that reason every physician should familiarize himself with them.

One of the most common and frequently overlooked sites are closed skeletal fractures. Because there is no obvious laceration or avulsion with visible bleeding, many examiners are misled into omitting the blood lost into fracture sites from their calculations when they add up their estimated blood losses. This failure leads to inadequate volume replacement in many injured patients and often means the difference between an optimum perfusing volume and subnormal blood volumes that retard the adequate perfusion of vital tissues slowly resulting in anaerobic metabolism and its detrimental effects on the myocardium.

A frequent site for concealed blood loss is around closed tubular bone fractures. The femoral shaft fracture is the classic example. One must calculate anywhere from 500 to 1000 ml blood loss from the circulation in these serious fractures (see Chapter 9). If there is some concern regarding this arbitrary clinical figure, a more accurate means of evaluating blood loss in extremity fractures is to measure the circumference of the injured thigh at several points and compare this with measurements of the uninjured thigh at similar points, and measure the length of the thigh. By calculating the volume of a cylinder with these dimensions from these measurements, a fairly accurate determination of extracellular fluid and blood lost from the vascular space into the tissues of the thigh can be obtained.

A second area of the skeletal system capable of concealing large volumes of blood is in pelvic fractures.[12] In some of the most extreme fractures of the pelvic girdle with displacement and rupture of pelvic venous plexuses the losses may exceed 2,000 ml. It is not only the initial losses in pelvic fractures that may influence the clinical evaluation of blood volume because often in these serious pelvic fractures there is a slow but significant continued loss as time passes. This progressive loss must be considered when summarizing the patient's response to initial resuscitation efforts.

The more minor disruptions of the pelvis lose 500 to 1,000 ml of blood and extracellular fluids but these must be kept in mind when calculating overall volume replacement.

Another region of frequent concealed blood loss is in the pleural spaces. Because a fairly large amount of blood must be present to be detected on roentogenograms of the chest or produce dullness to percussion and reduce breath sounds, suspicion is the key to uncovering concealed blood loss in this area.

The possibility of concealed blood loss in the pleural space is so great in critically injured patients that one should never hesitate to search for it with multiple needle aspirations. Needle aspiration of the pleural cavity can be done quickly and with expediency. Very little time is lost from the continuing survey of injuries and the information obtained (even a negative thoracentesis) is invaluable in so far as the overall evaluation of blood loss is concerned. The equipment needed (a blunt angled large bore needle, three-way valve adaptor and large volume syringe) and the technique are so simple that needle aspiration of the pleural space should be almost routine evaluation of critically injured patients, especially when rib fractures are detected.

The peritoneal and retroperitoneal spaces are sites of common concealed blood losses. For many years detection of hemoperitoneum was done by a four quadrant paracentesis. The abdomen is prepared in a sterile fashion as for laparotomy and after anesthetizing the skin and fascia with a local anesthetic, a long eighteen gauge spinal needle is inserted into the peritoneal space in an upper quadrant of the abdomen and attached to a syringe. If after aspiration with the syringe no blood is obtained, the remaining three quadrants of the abdomen are in turn aspirated. If no blood is obtained after this four quadrant tap the paracentesis is considered negative. If blood is aspirated, a hemoperitoneum is considered to be present and laparotomy is necessary. The incidence of negative paracentesis in the presence of a hemoperitoneum utilizing this "four quadrant tap" has been considerable (15 to 20%).[13] For many years everyone was admonished to ignore the negative abdominal paracentesis and proceed on one's clinical judgement as if a negative tap had not been done. This is mysterious advice to give a physician who is critically involved with his patient's injuries and concerned about what to do next. In fact, if a negative paracentesis is obtained, it cannot help but direct a physician's attention to the next priority at hand in his seriously ill patient. To determine the effect of a negative tap on the physician's actions Mays[14] found that in patients with ruptured livers and massive hemoperitoneums a negative abdominal paracentesis influenced the attending physician to proceed with the management of less critical injuries such as sewing up a scalp wound or inserting a Steinmann pin for traction on a femoral fracture. Several patients continued to bleed into the peritoneal space and die from cardiac arrest on the operating table. Because of the problems of the "negative tap" abdominal paracentesis as an evaluating clinical tool has now fallen into disrepute. A more accurate method of detecting concealed blood loss in the peritoneal cavity is by peritoneal lavage.

Diagnostic peritoneal lavage was introduced by Root[15] in the Saint Paul Ramsey Hospital in 1964. The simplicity and accuracy of the test are its two most important attributes and it is one of the most important techniques in evaluating concealed blood loss in the peritoneal spaces. The procedure is illustrated in the chapter on abdominal evaluation. Meticulous hemostasis is essential if false positives are avoided. A liter of normal saline or balanced salt solution is introduced into the peritoneal cavity (adults) and proportionately smaller amounts for children. In order that the lavage fluid enter all possible peritoneal spaces, the patient is turned from side to side with alternating elevation and dependency of the head and foot of the operating table.

Some advocate extensive examination of the lavage fluid for amylase, bile, bacterial and intestinal content.[16] The extent of examination of the aspirated fluid will depend upon the sophistication of the hospital's laboratory and the availability of ancillary help. For the busy physician responsible for his patient's total care, he will most likely at this point be interested chiefly in presence or absence of blood in the aspirate and chiefly concerned with whether or not blood is present in the peritoneal cavity.

In one series of 304 patients evaluated with peritoneal lavage there were nine patients (3%) with a false negative lavage and three patients (1%) with a false positive.[15] In another series of 401 patients false positive lavage was documented in only three patients 0.7 percent and false negative lavage in two patients (0.5%).[13] In 116 patients the lavage was documented positive at laparotomy and only two of these had trivial injuries from which they would have recovered without operation.[16] Hence, peritoneal lavage is a rapid simple and reliable technique for detecting concealed blood loss in peritoneal spaces.[17]

Detecting concealed blood in the retroperitoneal space is even more difficult for several liters of blood can be lost into this space without marked clinical manifestations. Sometimes a bulging in the flank area is the only physical finding present. This can be detected by careful observation of the supine patient from above so that both flank areas can be seen at the same time and compared with one another. On a plain roentogenogram of the abdomen obscured psoas shadows and enlargement or absence of renal shadows suggests concealed blood loss in the retroperitoneal space. An elevated serum amylase reflects serious injury to the pancreas and may or may not be indicative of retroperitoneal hemorrhage.[18]

After several days the extent of retroperitoneal will become obvious by the discoloration in the flank, back and lower thoracic area, but this is ordinarily a late sign and is not helpful in the early assessment of concealed blood loss. After twenty-four hours patients with retroperitoneal hemorrhage will show a progressive fall in hemoglobin and hematocrit.

Cullen has described a discoloration around the umbilicus when there is peritoneal hemorrhage but this was originally described in ruptured ectopic pregnancies and is not usually helpful in traumatic hemoperitoneum.

LESSER PRIORITY INJURIES

The order of priorities in evaluation of critically injured patients is again reviewed in Table 4-II, without apology for being repetitious, because they must become firmly fixed in the routine of every busy physician if the mortality rates in critically injured patients are to be reduced. To emphasize the importance of the first priorities, injuries of lesser priority must be outlined.

Scalp lacerations and soft tissue injuries have priority only under the category of controlling hemorrhage. Hemostasis can be achieved rapidly with sterile pressure dressings and the wounds ignored for many hours if necessary while other more important injuries are being evaluated. Before the scalp wound is dressed the cranium should be palpated with a sterile gloved finger to detect skull fractures and foreign bodies.

Although most orthopedists shudder when a surgeon states that skeletal injuries have lesser priority it is nevertheless true and must be taught and accepted. The only exception to this rule is the long bone injury associated with vascular insufficiency. This situation places the skeletal injury in a higher order of priority just beneath airway obstruction, replacement of blood volume and control of hemorrhage.

Most tubular bones can be temporarily immobilized with a quickly applied splint and do extremely well until priority injuries are cared for. This is true of even the most horrible appearing and contaminated open fractures. They should be quickly cleaned, irrigated, occluded with a sterile dressing and splinted.

Facial fractures, although producing horrible disfiguring injuries, are low priority and most physicians trained in the management of these fractures prefer to wait one to two weeks when the edema has subsided before proceeding with any definitive care. This is also true of pelvic fractures.

Hand injuries are low priority injuries and should never detract the physician from maintenance of vital physiologic functions as his first responsibiilty to the patient. These wounds can be quickly cleaned and splinted. Many surgeons even prefer secondary tenorrhapy to primary repair and while this controversy is not yet settled, a physician should never risk a patient's overall survival by diverting his attention to treating hand injuries.

At this point in the evaluation of critically injured patients, a patient airway is functioning, blood volume has been replaced, hemorrhage controlled, and a search for concealed blood loss completed. A hemodynamically stable patient perfusing vital tissues with oxygenated blood is now ready for a thorough and organized evaluation of all systems. Until these first priorities have been met, no studies, X-rays, angiograms, tests or treatment should be undertaken.

REFERENCES

1. Ryan, G. A.. and Garrett, J. W.: A quantitative scale of impact injury, publication CAL No. VT 1823-R34. Buffalo, Cornell Aeronautical Laboratory, Inc. Cornell University, Oct. 1968.
2. Kennedy, R. H.: The multiple injury patient. *Md State Med J, 12*:94, 1963.
3. Manual on classification of motor vehicle traffic accidents. Chicago Committee on Uniform Traffic Accident Statistics, Traffic Conference National Safety Council, 1962.
4. Williams, R. E., and Schamadan, J. L.: The "Simbol" rating and evaluation system. *Ariz Med, 26*:886-887, 1969.
5. Kirkpatrick, J. R., and Youmans, R. L.: Trauma index. *J Trauma, 11*:711-714, 1971.
6. Hendryson, I. E.: The revolution in emergency medical services. University Association for Emergency Medical Services. First Annual Meeting. University of Michigan, Ann Arbor, 1971.
7. Mays, E. T.; Mosely, D. H.; Rumage, W. T., and Setliffe, C.: Health care for an urban population: The emergency sector. *Ky Med Assoc, 70*:687-693, 1972.
8. Committee on Medical Aspects of Automotive Safety: Rating the severity of tissue damage. I. The abbreviated scale. *JAMA, 215*: 277-280, 1971.
9. Committee on Medical Aspects of Automotive Safety: Rating the severity of tissue damage. II. The comprehensive scale. *JAMA, 220*:717-720, 1972.
10. Baker, S. P.; O'Neill, B.; Haddon, W., and Long, W. B.: The injury seventy score: A method for describing patients with multiple injuries and evaluating emergency care. *J Trauma, 14*:187-196, 1974.

11. Best, C. H., and Taylor, N. B.: *Physiologic Basis of Medical Practice.* Eighth Ed. Baltimore, Williams and Wilkins Co., 1966.

12. Braunstein, P. W.; Skudder, P. A.; McCarroll, J. R.; Musolino, A., and Wade, P. A.: Concealed hemorrhage due to pelvic fracture. *J Trauma, 4*:832, 1964.

13. Gumbert, J. L.; Froderman, S. E., and Mercho, J. P.: Diagnostic peritoneal lavage in blunt abdominal trauma. *Ann Surg, 165*:70, 1967.

14. Mays, E. T.: Bursting injuries of the liver. *Arch Surg, 93*:92-103, 1966.

15. Root, H. D.; Hanser, C. W.; McKinley, C. R.; LaFave, J. W., and Mendiola, R. P., Jr.: Diagnostic peritoneal lavage. *Surgery, 57*: 633, 1965.

16. Divencenti, F. C.; Rives, J. D.; Laborde, E. J.; Fleming, I. D., and Cohn, I., Jr.: Blunt abdominal trauma. *J Trauma, 8*:1004, 1968.

17. Perry, J. F., and Strate, R. G.: Diagnostic peritoneal lavage in blunt abdominal trauma: Indications and results. *Surgery, 71*:898, 1972.

18. Nick, W. V.; Zollenger, R. W., and Pace, W. G.: Retroperitoneal hemorrhage after blunt abdominal trauma. *J Trauma, 7*:652, 1967.

CHAPTER 5

CARDIOTHORACIC ASSESSMENT

PRIORITIES FOR CARDIORESPIRATORY ASSESSMENT
1. Airway Patent
2. Sucking Wounds Closed
3. Chest Wall Stable
4. Lungs Expanded
5. Bleeding Controlled and Blood Volume Restored
6. Pleura Adequately Drained
7. Circulation Satisfactory
8. Blood Gases Evaluated

BECAUSE INJURIES TO the thorax and its contents interfere with ventilatory, circulatory and digestive functions, early evaluation is critical. In order of priority it is second only to cardiopulmonary resuscitation and blood volume replacement. Often it is difficult for physicians to calmly stand back and observe a person who is so seriously injured. Yet, a few minutes' inspection of the disrobed patient yields information that may well not be obtained by sophisticated laboratory studies.

Careful scrutiny of the chest, front and back, looking for penetrations or defects in the chest wall is important. If the patient is too ill to sit upright for examination of the back, he should be turned from side to side until the entire posterior surface is scrutinized. This maneuver may seem too fundamental, but the neophyte is entrapped by diverting his attention to a minor wound of the anterior chest only to find on the autopsy table that the patient had a second and much more serious wound of the posterior chest causing death while the minor anterior wound was insignificant. Thus, it is important that complete assessment be done systematically and thoroughly before giving attention to any one area. Sucking wounds of the chest wall produce havoc in ventilatory efforts and must be closed immediately with airtight pressure dressings.

FLAIL CHEST

The chest wall is observed for its symmetry and ventilatory movements and appraised to determine if the right and left hemithorax move in unison. The chest wall moves upward and outward on normal inspiration and downward and inward on expiration; the right and left hemithorax move together in synchrony.

Multiple rib fractures on one side frequently produce an unstable chest wall and paradoxical movement of the thorax. Ineffective respiration follows and the patient becomes restless, anxious and often cyanotic. Paradoxical ventilation means the chest wall moves inward instead of outward when the patient inspires. The work necessary for such ineffective movements consumes oxygen at rapid rates; requiring great effort on the part of the patient and adding to an already compromised respiratory function. Chest wall instability and paradoxical ventilation are usually detected by careful inspection and palpation of the chest (Figs. 5-1a and 5-1b).

The observer should stand at the foot of the stretcher or operating table and observe the pattern of respiration for several seconds before palpating or ascultating the chest. The movement of the chest wall should be synchronous and symmetrical. Ventilation should be easy, requiring little exertion. Expiration should be approximately equal to inspiration in length of time. A prolonged, forceful expiratory phase suggests bronchoconstriction with increased resistance in the tracheobronchial tree or loss of lung compliance. Foreign bodies in the lower airway, or retained secretions must be suspected and searched for with a bronchoscope. Difficult, forceful inspiratory movements with retraction of the sternal notch and intercostal spaces mean upper airway obstruction and is usually due to laryngeal or cervical tracheal

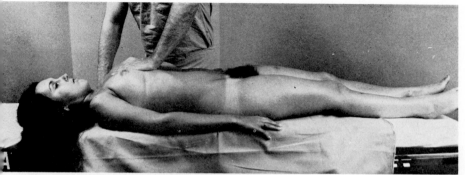

Figure 5-1. Testing for thoracic cage stability (a) anterior posterior compressions (b) lateral compression.

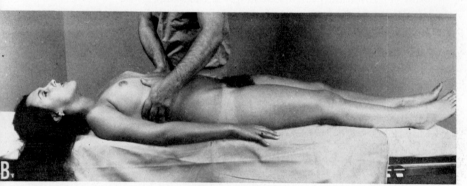

Figure 5-1b.

obstruction; severe trauma to the larynx and upper trachea can cause collapse or massive edema.

The failure of one hemithorax to move to the same extent as the opposite side must raise suspicion of a differential inflation of the lungs. This may be on the basis of two mechanisms.

(1) If one hemithorax is fixed in inspiration and remains more fully expanded than the contralateral hemithorax during expiration, a tension pneumothorax or major bronchial tear must be considered. The tension pneumothorax shifts the trachea and mediastinum toward the uninvolved side and these shifts can be detected by palpating the trachea in the sternal notch and palpating the apical heartbeat. The shifted heart can also be detected by ascultation and roentgenography.

(2) If one hemithorax is relatively fixed in a collapsed state or lags behind the other hemithorax on deep inspiration unilateral bronchial obstruction must be considered.

Once observed and suspicion is aroused, the above mentioned problems should be further evaluated with ascultation and percussion of the chest wall. If a tension pneumothorax is present the percussion note is hyperresonant and breath sounds are absent. In unilateral bronchial obstruction breath sounds are also absent but the percussion note is flat, and if the trachea or mediastinum are shifted they are shifted to the involved side instead of away from the involved side as in a tension pneumothorax. Immediate bronchoscopy is indicated.

Because of serious mediastinal shifts and death by obstruction of the afferent vessels of the heart, tension pneumothoraces are a first priority. An intercostal tube must be inserted and connected to a water seal drainage. Every physician, regardless of his area of special interest in medical practice, should be instructed in the technic of chest tube insertion. Needle aspiration is an acceptable way to temporarily manage the tension pneumothorax.

RIB FRACTURES

The most frequent mistakes in assessing the critically injured patient for rib fractures is obtaining a chest X-ray. In reality, perusal of a chest X-ray, no matter how excellent the technique may be, is the most unreliable way of finding rib fractures. The obvious displaced fractures that everyone can see on X-ray are usually no problem. It is the subtle or hard-to-visualize fracture that is most significant. The most reliable way of checking rib fractures is by careful palpation. Each rib should be palpated individually and carefully (Fig. 5-2a). When tenderness is detected the diagnosis can be confirmed by holding steady pressure on the rib (but not enough pressure to cause pain), then ask the patient to take a deep breath. If the rib is broken, as the chest wall moves outward, inspiration will be voluntarily interrupted by the patient because of pain.

Detecting rib fractures is extremely important because of implications concerning other intrathoracic organs. Sharply

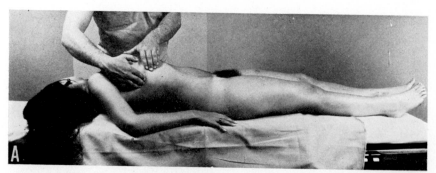

Figure 5-2. Palpating for individual rib fractures (A). Needle aspiration of pleural space for concealed hemorrhage (B).

fractured ribs often penetrate a lung. After the injuring force is removed the rib springs back into place.

Fracture of the first rib is a good example of implied information. The first rib is infrequently broken because it is protected by the clavicle and scapula. Fractures of the first rib are one exception to the usefulness of X-ray diagnosis of rib fractures. Since this rib cannot be palpated, roentgenography is the only way to detect a fracture in the first rib.

When the first rib is broken the patient has experienced unusually severe trauma and serious pulmonary or vascular injuries should be suspected. Severe pulmonary contusion, tears in major vesels, esophagus, bronchi and trachea must be assumed until proven otherwise (Fig. 5-2b).

Careful palpation is also essential to detect subtle instability of the chest wall not obvious on inspection and not causing the paradoxical movements referred to above. This palpation for areas of the chest wall that are unstable is particularly important in the stocky or obese patient and may be the only early indication of a flail chest.

Palpation of the chest wall is important also in detecting subcutaneous emphysema. The presence of subcutaneous emphysema means a break in the tracheobronchial tree. It may only be a minor rupture of a few alveoli in the periphery of the lung or a ruptured bleb that dissects back along the fascial planes of the tracheobronchial tree into the neck or supraclavicular space. On

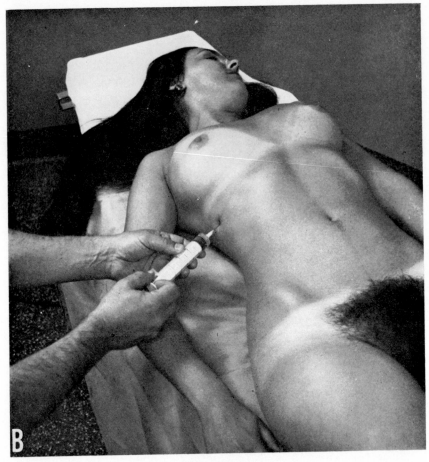

Figure 5-2b.

the other hand, massive subcutaneous emphysema progressing
rapidly means a major rupture in the trachea or one of the
bronchi. This may or may not be associated with a pneumothorax
and in some instances massive subcutaneous emphysema is the
only early indication of a major defect in the tracheobronchial
tree.

Auscultation of both hemithoraces is next done, listening for
subtle deficiencies in the ventilation of the two lungs. Are the
breath sounds equal bilaterally? Is egophony present? The non-
tension pneumothoraces or hemopneumothoraces must be de-

tected with the stethoscope and percussion. Diminished or absent breath sounds or unequal breath sounds when both hemithoraces are carefully ascultated, calls for further evaluation. If the percussion note is flat, fluid or blood are probably the source of the inadequate breath sounds.

If the percussion note is increased or nearly hyperresonant, air in the pleural space is probably the cause of the diminished breath sounds. Whether this air is nearing or exceeding atmospheric pressure must then be determined as discussed above under tension pneumothorax.

A severe pulmonary contusion will sometimes confuse the issue as breath sounds are diminished and the percussion note is flat. But here vocal fremitus is helpful. Egophony is present in pulmonary contusion but absent in a hemothorax, while tactile fremitus is increased in the hemothorax but diminished in pulmonary contusions.

THORACENTESIS

After careful inspection, palpation, percussion and auscultation of the thoracic cage, needle aspiration of the pleural space is done. Inserting a needle between the ribs into the pleural space is such a simple procedure and requires so few instruments that it is difficult to understand why physicians omit this procedure. It should always be done for the slightest suspicion of thoracic injury from either closed or penetrating trauma. The technique is shown in Figure 5-3.

The aspiration of air or blood from either pleural space dictates insertion of an intercostal tube for drainage. Some more conservative physicians may attempt to aspirate the pleural space completely and insert a chest tube only if the blood or air reaccumulate. This may be satisfactory if one is dealing with an isolated chest injury, but the critically injured with multiple systems involved prohibits this kind of sequential aspiration. Either a follow-up thoracentesis is forgotten while other injuries are being evaluated, or attention is so directed to repeated needle aspirations that co-existing injuries are ignored. In either case the hemo- or pneumothorax reaccumulates at the most em-

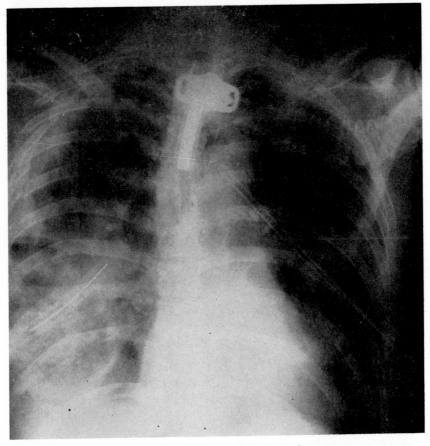

Figure 5-3. Roentgenographic evidence of first rib fracture in young man injured in an automobile collision indicates severe contusion of the lung requiring mechanical ventilation.

barassing time, e.g. while laparotomy is being done for a ruptured spleen and the patient is completely covered by sterile drapes. It is more reasonable to have the pleural space drained and the lung expanded before undertaking other corrective operative procedures.

The blood removed from the chest should be carefully measured and the collecting bottle carefully marked to determine the amount of blood loss from the chest each hour. The aspiration of 1,500 ml or more of blood per needle or intercostal tube is an indication for immediate thoracotomy. If the hourly blood loss from the chest is in excess of 400 ml/hour then thoracotomy is indicated. Other indications for thoracotomy are listed in Table 5-I.

CARDIAC CONTUSION

The chest wall is also inspected for contusions. Bluish discoloration over the anterior chest wall and vertebral column can indicate considerable myocardial contusion, and the most common is steering wheel compression injuries produced by the ever-increasing numbers of automotive vehicular accidents. Other modes of injury are blows to the chest by a fist, foot or club, a ball traveling at high speeds, kicks by animals, contact sports, blast injuries. In cases of severe trauma there was a 76 percent incidence of cardiac contusion[1] and in autopsies of patients dying in automobile accidents there is an incidence of 15 to 17 percent.[2, 3]

In addition to compression injuries, sudden extreme accelerative or decelerative motion of the chest can thrust the heart against the chest wall. The heart hangs freely and has its own inertia suspended by the great vessels and moving independently of the thoracic cage. This freedom of motion makes the heart particularly susceptible to decelerative injuries.

The examiner must not be deceived by lack of violent marks on the external chest if he suspects cardiac trauma. All the above mechanisms of injury may occur with or without actual fractures of the bones of the thoracic cage. In some cases of cardiac contusion the only external evidence is a slight bluish discoloration over the precordium, but the absence of visible external injury does not exclude heart injury.

TABLE 5-I

INDICATIONS FOR IMMEDIATE THORACOTOMY

1. Widened mediastinum with left hemothorax
2. Clotted hemothorax not relieved by intercostal tubes
3. Aspiration of 1500 ml blood per needle or intercostal tube
4. Intrathoracic bleeding greater than 500 ml per hour
5. Sudden increase in rate of intercostal tube bleeding
6. Evidence of cardiac penetration

Some cardiac contusions produce no functional disturbances and go unrecognized. At other times significant cardiac contusions are overlooked because of more obvious co-existing injuries.

Various dysrrythmias are common manifestations of cardiac contusion. Premature atrial or ventricular contractions are the most frequent but the entire gamut of atrial fibrillation, flutter, sinoatrial block, nodal rhythm, atrioventricular block, and idioventricular rhythm have all been observed.[4, 5, 6] Bradycardia and evolving changes in the ST-T segments on the electrocardiogram are the most common findings (Figs. 4a, 4b, 5a, and 5b).

Serial electrocardiograms should be done in patients suspected of cardiac contusions. Since electrical changes are not always present immediately after trauma, the changes in QRS-T complexes are similar to those seen in muscle ischemia and electrical

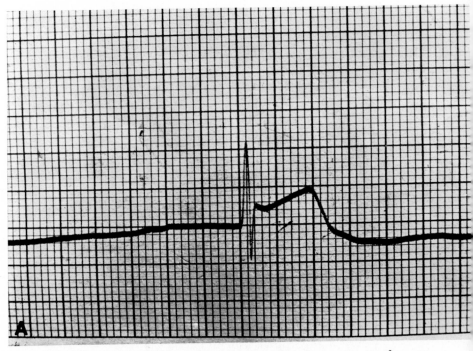

Figure 5-4.   Electrocardiographic tracing taken from a twenty-three-year-old man thrown from his motorcycle. Note (a) severe bradycardia (40 beats/min) and elevated ST segment. (b) T wave inversion in lead III.

imbalances produced by myocardial infarction due to atherosclerotic occlusive disease.

Auscultation of the heart may be normal, but occasionally the
first and second sound may be of equal intensity producing a
"tick-tick" sound. As the severity of trauma increases, rupture of
chordae tendinae produces incompetent valves with loud murmurs and progressive cardiac decompensation. Extensive traumatic heart injuries require immediate attention. Loud, harsh
blowing murmurs in critically injured patients should raise
suspicion of ruptured chordae tendinae and imcompetent heart
valves.

An example of an extreme degree of nonpenetrating cardiac
trauma has been encountered in the University of Louisville
Hospitals. The patient's case history is briefly reviewed to
illustrate the problem of blunt heart injury:

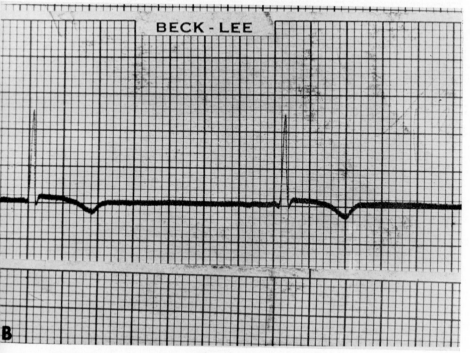

Figure 5-4b.

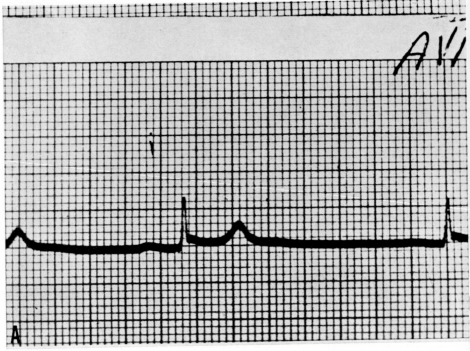

Figure 5-5. Electrocardiographic changes due to cardiac contusion in nineteen-year-old man thrown against steering wheel. Note bradycardia and ST segment elevation in leads AVF and III.

A fifty-five-year-old man was admitted to the Louisville General Hospital from the emergency department because of acute pulmonary edema. His heart rate was 150 beats per minute and he was breathing 40 times per minute with great difficulty. His brachial blood pressure was 150/90 mm Hg. A balloon-tipped flow-directed catheter was inserted into the pulmonary artery and wedged. The pressure was 30 mm Hg. His pO_2 was 60 mm Hg; pCO_2, 26; and pH 7.3.

Right and left heart catheterizations disclosed 4+ aortic insufficiency and 2+ mitral valvular insufficiency. The left ventricular end-diastolic pressure was <50 mm Hg and pulmonary wedge pressure 45 mm Hg with the free pulmonary artery pressure ranging 45 to 50 mm Hg. The coronary arteries were normal by angiography.

It was learned that the man had had a serious automobile accident one month before he became ill. He was thrown violently against the steering wheel of his car and the steering wheel broke from the force of the impact. The patient did not think himself injured and did not seek medical advice.

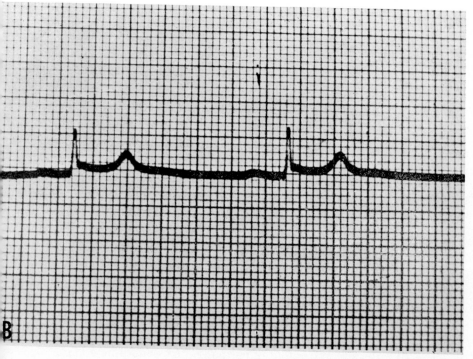

Figure 5-5b.

Because of normal coronary arteries and the strange history of trauma the patient was explored with extracorporeal assistance. At the operating table all heart chambers were enlarged. There was a tear in the commissure of the aortic valve between the right and left aortic cusps. There was soft necrotic tissue in the septum with a small ventricular septal defect. A tiny sinus tract was discovered opening from the root of the aorta and ventricle into the surrounding periaortic tissue.

Without evidence of pre-existing heart disease and because of recent severe chest trauma these pathologic cardiac findings were considered to be traumatic in origin. The patient did well after surgery and was discharged to the outpatient clinic.

PENETRATING WOUNDS OF THE HEART

Penetrating wounds of the heart have first priority over all injuries. A cardiac perforation should be suspected when the condition of the patient and the degree of shock are out of proportion to the obvious wound. The patient is usually bathed in perspiration and is delirious. Acute ethanol intoxication is frequently present. The pulse rate is usually slow unless there has been concomitant hemorrhage from other wounds super-imposing a severe hypovolemia. If acute cardiac tamponade is present the classic triad described by Beck can usually be detected. This consists of distended neck veins (or increased central venous pressure when there is time to measure it), diminuted heart sounds and reduced pulse pressure.

In many instances there is no time for evaluating test. Thoracotomy and control of the heart wound with an index finger preempt diagnostic test. This kind of patient has caused great confusion in managing heart injuries. In our institution patients are transferred rapidly from the scene of injury to the operating table. This method of immediate thoracotomy was developed by Dr. Arnold Griswold.[7] His experience caused he and his colleagues to advocate immediate thoracotomy and con-demn pericardiocentesis. His reasons for this aggressive approach were:

(1) the site and extent of cardiac injury cannot be adequately determined without exploration

(2) associated injuries to other important intrathoracic struc-tures may be overlooked unless exploration is done

(3) intra-pericardial clotting can prevent effective needle aspiration

(4) blind aspiration even by the costoxyphoid approach may be hazardous

(5) delayed hemorrhage can result from unsutured wounds of the heart (Matas referred to this in 1909)

(6) the organization of clots in the pericardial sac may be followed by pericarditis.

Others did not agree with Dr. Griswold's aggressive approach and advocated aspiration as the sole method of treating pene-trating wounds of the heart.[8, 9] Both views can be reconciled by considering time lapse from injury to hospitalization. In institu-tions where the bars and areas of injury are nearby, the patients with severe heart wounds arrive with some residual signs of life. Other institutions have a selective influence on the kind of patient they encounter. The very bad wounds are dead on arrival, if there is significant time lapse between injury and physician encounter. Some patients are seen at one hospital and referred to another. Institutions serving as a referral center or remote from regions of incidence of heart wounds are obviously encountering a selected population; the severe wounds have died before arriving at their institutions and those still alive after a significant time lapse obviously have lesser injuries and can be treated by initial pericardiocentesis and observation.

It seems wise then to assess the patient's condition and time lapse between injury and primary encounter with physicians. Those patients described by Griswold in profound shock with bradycardia and covered with perspiration should have immediate thoracotomy and few if any diagnostic evaluations. Other patients may permit additional evaluation. Needle aspiration of the pericardial sac can disclose a cardiac tamponade. This is a life-threatening injury and must be evaluated accurately. Neck vein distention, distant muffled heart sounds, and narrow pulse pressure should motivate the careful monitoring of central venous presure (CVP) with a catheter in the superior vena cava. Increasing CVP and decreasing cardiac output with a paradoxical pulse must cause great suspicion and if fluoroscopy is reasonable, the cardiac silhouette shows very minimal pulsations.

These findings should urge the examining physician to aspirate the pericardium. This is both a diagnostic and therapeutic maneuver. A needle with a short bevel is attached to an aspirating syringe via a three-way stopcock. The patient is connected to an electrocardiograph. The needle is inserted at the angle formed by the junction of the xyphoid process and the chondrosternal junction (Fig. 5-6). The tip of the needle is directed toward the left axilla and the barrel of the syringe is elevated approximately 15 degrees anterior to the midcoronal plane. In unusually obese or stocky patients the 15 degree angle is increased to a 45 degree angle with the coronal plane or the operating table. As the needle progresses, the electrocardiogram is monitored and indicates when the needle has gone too far and entered the myocardium. If this should occur, the needle is slowly withdrawn while aspirating constantly.

After an initial definitive diagnosis of cardiac tamponade any

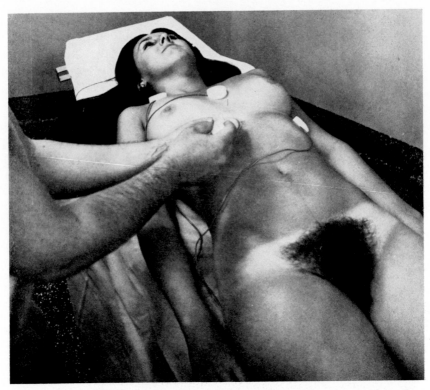

Figure 5-6. Method of pericardiocentesis. The needle is inserted at the xyphoid-costal angle and directed toward the left axilla. The barrel of the syringe is elevated 15 to 30 degrees above the coronal plane. This procedure is less hazardous if done while monitoring the electrocardiogram. One lead can be attached to the needle.

re-accumulation indicates thoracotomy and exploration of the heart and pericardium. Echocardiography offers a safe non-invasive method of detecting blood in the pericardium but is not yet widely available.

RUPTURE OF AORTA

This extremely critical injury is due to rapid deceleration and results in death from exsanguination. Early detection of such injuries is necessary for survival. Because the aorta is ensheathed in a tough layer of adventia, the extent of the rupture does not have great significance on immediate survival, as some patients may live twenty-four hours or more with a complete transection. Yet, if undetected, nearly all of these patients die within the succeeding twenty-four hours because of secondary rupture in the mediastinum and pleura.

The ligamentum arteriosum plays a rather important mechanical role in ruptures of the aorta for it acts as an anchoring site against which maximal shearing stress may develop in situations of rapid deceleration. The aorta distal to this point is relatively free to continue forward movement against the relatively fixed point of the ligamentum arteriosum and the aorta ruptures at this point most frequently. Extravasation of blood widens the mediastinal silhouette on chest films and this is the most common method of diagnosis (Figs. 5-7a and 5-7b). Sequential widening of the mediastinum after serious trauma must be considered aortic rupture until proven otherwise. Other points of relative fixation where the aorta tears less commonly are the junction with the heart and even less frequently at the junction with the innominate artery. Tangential tearing at the junction of the aorta with the heart may result in cardiac tamponade. In such instances the cardiac tamponade should be evaluated in a similar manner described in the preceding paragraphs.

In aortic ruptures there are some common pitfalls. Errors in evaluating these injuries are, strangely enough, not failures to suspect aortic rupture but the physician is often deterred from his conviction that a major intrathoracic vessel has been lacerated, simply because pulses are present distal to the point of a suspected tear. Two of the most impressive patients I have seen had complete transection of the aorta at the site of the ligamentum arteriosum, yet pulses were palpable in the femoral vessels. Likewise, a normal appearing aortogram does not preclude significant aortic injuries. Evaluation of the arterial tree by contrast roentgenography (Fig. 5-8) is usually definitive in divulging aortic rupture. Aortography will be discussed in later chapters. But tears in the thoracic aorta do not always show in the arteriogram. Strong fibrous adventia may prevent early extravasation of contrast material and give a fairly normal contour

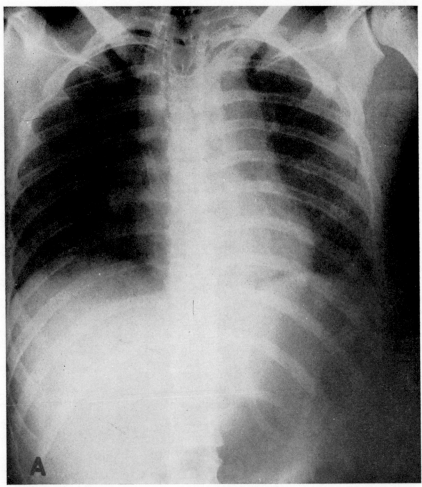

Figure 5-7. Roentgenogram of the chest showing progressive widening of mediastinum in a twenty-four-year-old man who had rupture of his aorta at the ligatmentum arteriosum in a car accident. (A) Admission (B) One hour later.

to the thoracic aorta. For these reasons, aortography is not always indicated, especially in multiple system injuries where the patient's cardiodynamics are failing and peripheral perfusion is inadequate. If the width of the mediastinum is increased in these patients, time consuming catheterizations and X-ray evaluation of the arterial tree is poor judgement. Surgical exploration should proceed simultaneously with blood volume replacement and cardiopulmonary resuscitation.

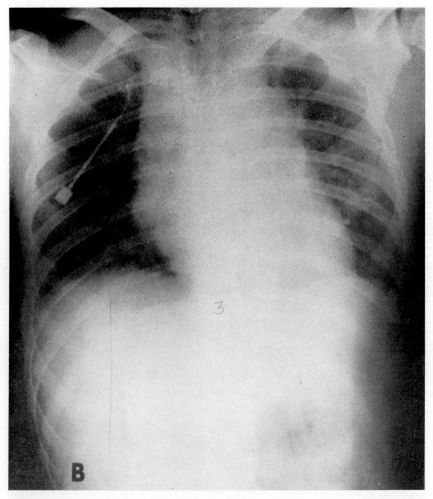

Figure 5-7b.

ESOPHAGEAL INJURIES

Any missile injury traversing the mediastinum must be suspected of injuring either the aorta, esophagus, or trachea. A roentgenogram of the chest must be scrutinized for mediastinal air. The presence of air does not differentiate between tracheobronchial or esophageal lacerations. A barium swallow is a simple, effective and reliable means of evaluating the esophagus.

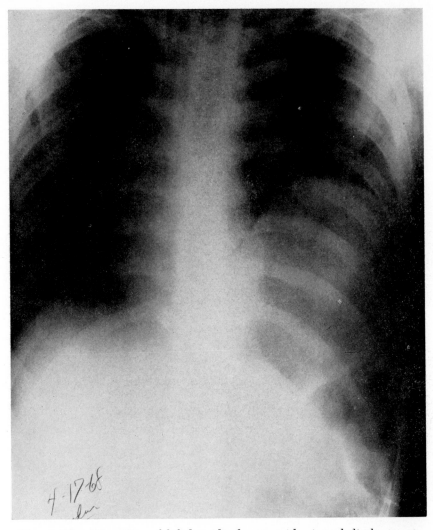

Figure 5-8.   Disruption of left hemidiaphragm with visceral displacement.
into the left chest.

Extravasation of contrast media outside the contour of the
esophagus or interruption of the normal smooth cylindrical
appearance should be interpreted as esophageal injury after
serious trauma.

Even the most insignificant esophageal defects if undetected produce mediastinitis within twenty-four hours. These patients are impressive because they present a clinical picture of being the "sickest" patients seen in the experience of medicine. They are extremely hypermetabolic with hyperpyrexia. Once a physician encounters one of these extremely ill patients he is impressed that the early detection of esophageal tears is the area of emphasis rather than the treatment of an established mediastinitis.

TRACHEOBRONCHIAL INJURY

Tracheobronchial injury is divulged by dyspnea, pneumothorax, mediastinal emphysema, and subcutaneous emphysema. When these signs are present in critically injured patients bronchoscopy and bronchography are mandatory.

Rupture of the trachea is an uncommon injury. But in spite of its rarity physicians and EMT must be aware of its seriousness. Difficulty breathing is the most characteristic early suggestion that there is an injury. This reflects back to earlier chapters pertaining to airway obstruction. In complete transections the tracheal ends retract and soft tissue intrudes into the gap. A functioning airway must be established. Whether this is done by tracheal intubation, emergency cricothyroidotomy or tracheostomy is at the discretion of the responsible physician. In the cervical trachea the recurrent laryngeal nerves are sometimes involved along with tracheal disruption. This produces abductor paralysis of the vocal cords and further increases the difficulty in breathing. Hoarseness of the voice, aphonia, difficulty swallowing and blood tinged sputum are additional signs of cervical tracheal injury. Associated laryngeal injury should also be suspected and looked for with a laryngoscope or bronchoscope.

Contusions and discolorations about the anterior neck with massive emphysema spreading rapidly and widely should alert responsible persons to tracheal disruptions in the neck. If there is complete transection of the cervical tracheal, palpation will disclose the gap between the two ends. This kind of injury is usually caused by an impact which compresses the trachea against the cervical spine while the cervical vertebrae are forcefully extended. A kick on the neck by horse or man, a handlebar of a motorcycle, a steering wheel or dashboard of a car, a tight wire, chain or rope can all produce the injury.

Disruption of the mediastinal trachea by blunt or penetrating forces usually causes massive subcutaneous and mediastinal emphysema which progresses even while the examiner is inspecting the patient. In smaller tears a pneumonomediastinum can be detected on chest roentgenography.

Almost all bronchial injuries are located in the main stem bronchi.[10] There are two major clinical problems created by bronchial injury. The first occurs immediately after the injury and is created by the open bronchus and its effect on gas exchange. Should it communicate with the pleural space a tension pneumothorax ensues resulting in mediastinal shift, occlusion of venous return to the heart, cardiac arrest and death. Should the open bronchus communicate, with the mediastinum, severe and progressive pneumomediastinum and massive subcutaneous emphysema develops.

The second clinical problem occurs two to three weeks after injury and is produced by stenosis of the bronchus at the site of the tear. Lung tissue beyond this stenotic segment is without function and often becomes infected. Both the early and late problems of ruptured bronchi are serious. Early detection of bronchial injury becomes very important.

It is clear that the key to early recognition of tracheobronchial injuries is in recognizing the defect in the tracheobronchial tree and not in any pattern of associated injuries. Pneumothorax hemoptysis and emphysema are too inconstant to prove reliable diagnostic guides.

Ninety-one percent of 167 patients with bronchial rupture had one or all the first three ribs broken.[10] Rib fractures, particularly ribs one, two and three are always associated with bronchial rupture after blunt trauma in patients over the age of thirty years. The only patients who rupture a bronchus without breaking a rib are children or young adults under the age of thirty years.

Useful signs in early detection of bronchial injuries are listed in Table 5-II. Roentgenograms of the chest are mandatory. In suspicious patients bronchoscopy and bronchography must also be done soon after injury.

RUPTURE OF THE DIAPHRAGM

Graded degrees of respiratory distress are frequently present in patients with multiple injuries and physicians cannot rely solely on this observation for selecting patients in whom diaphragmatic defects may be present.

Penetrating injuries are usually no problem because either thoracotomy or laparotomy is done for the penetrating injury and lacerations of the diaphragm are discovered incidentally at the time of exploration. Repairs of the diaphragm then become coincidental with repair of other organs.

The major problem arises in detecting diaphragmatic disruption after closed trauma. Defects in the diaphragm can cause significant derangement in gastro-intestinal and cardio-respiratory function. After blunt trauma early diagnosis and repair is critical to quality of life after survival.

Disruption of the diaphragm may occur after either thoracic or abdominal blunt trauma. It is usually a blowout kind of tear due to transmission of energy according to Pascal's principle. The fixation of the diaphragm around its circumference by strong fascial attachments lend itself well to a shearing force. Diaphragmatic rupture does not of itself threaten life nearly so much as other co-existing injuries compromising vital organs. For this reason diaphragmatic tears may go undetected unless other reasons precipitate celiotomy or thoracotomy.

Experience in evaluating injured patients stresses suspicion of diaphragmatic rupture in all critically injured patients when

TABLE 5-II

SIGNS OF BRONCHIAL INJURY

Respiratory Distress
Mediastinal Emphysema
Subcutaneous Emphysema
Pneumothorax with great tension
Fracture of ribs 1 and 2 on side of pneumothorax

initial assessment demonstrates factors that do not fit common or well known injury patterns.

Proposed methods of evaluating patients for diaphragmatic defects are: (1) auscultation of lung fields, (2) plain chest film, (3) insertion of nasogastric tube.

If bowel sounds are heard in the chest the diaphragm is ruptured until proven otherwise. Careful examination of the chest X-ray for an abnormally high diaphragmatic shadow, gas containing viscera above the level of the normal diaphragmatic apex, or unusual markings in the lower thorax such as liver or splenic shadows, confirms suspicion of a tear. A nasogastric tube that curls up above the diaphragm is clinically helpful. If the patient's general condition permits, contrast roentgenographic evaluation is a good definitive diagnostic method.

The majority of diaphragm injuries occur on the left side. The liver forms a baffle, protecting the right hemidiaphragm from transmitted forces allowing only the shearing forces to tear the right leaf of the diaphragm.

Twenty-one patients with proven disruption of the diaphragm after blunt injuries have been treated in the University of Louisville Hospitals. The right hemidiaphragm was involved in five and the left in sixteen patients. When the right diaphragm is injured the liver is almost always severely traumatized. Only two of these patients survived. Seventeen diaphragmatic injuries were due to automobile accidents and one each from a blow to the lower abdomen and a fall from twenty feet. Twenty patients had associated skeletal fractures, fourteen had intra-abdominal injury, and ten had intrathoracic injuries. Only one patient had rupture of the diaphragm with no other injury.

Defects in the diaphragm produced by penetrating wounds are usually small and discovered during thoracotomy or laparotomy done for other reasons. Such penetrating injuries are more frequent than closed injuries but present few problems in either diagnosis or surgical correction.

The real difficulties in diaphragmatic trauma occur after closed injuries. Tears and lacerations are large and detection is perplexing. Diaphragmatic tears usually are not undetected unless other reasons precipitate celiotomy or thoracotomy. Our experience stresses specific methods of evaluating critically injured patients. When a cursory clinical assessment demonstrates factors that do not fit common, well known trauma patterns, pleuro-peritoneal lavage should be done.

The operative repair of diaphragmatic rupture is done through either the chest or abdomen and is highly effective, regardless of technic of repair. Hence, the operative management is relatively unimportant compared to early diagnosis, which is the major problem in all reported series. Bernatz[11] reported the average delay in diagnosis of ruptured diaphragms secondary to blunt trauma to be three and one-half years. Epstein[12] reported an average delay of nine years in detecting ruptured right diaphragms.

While the operative repair is simple if done immediately; it is difficult when done months or years later. The reasons for early diagnosis and immediate repair are cogent. The diaphragm is a muscle. Retraction and atrophy occur quickly and tissues that could easily be approximated on the day of injury may never approximate after retraction and atrophy have taken place. Adhesions become a hazardous problem in late repairs and resulted in death in at least one patient.[12] The tissue at late repair is poor and if the edges of the defect cannot be approximated prosthetic agents must often be inserted. Marlex mesh is ideal for bridging large defects in the diaphragm,[13] but if discovered early and repaired immediately alloplasty is usually not necessary.

In addition to the physiologic and anatomic reasons for early detection and repair of ruptured diaphragms, there is the socio-economic aspect. Most litigation in multiple injury accident cases are settled within two years. When the diagnosis is missed initially, it is usually not detected within this two-year period and patients lose financial compensation from insurance companies without the right to regain their losses.

These simple but pertinent facts about rupture of the diaphragm condense the physician's chief responsibility to early diagnosis. The entire outlook of the patient, physical and socio-economic health, depends upon the initial evaluation on the day of his injury.

Detailed investigations and multiple X-ray studies are perilous in the patient with multiple injuries. Four of our patients had no blood pressure at time of admission. All had multiple problems. Priorities of airway, ventilation, and blood volume replacement must come first. Disruption of the diaphragm does not of itself threaten life nearly so much as hemorrhage, shock, or airway obstruction.

A nasogastric tube should be inserted into the stomach and contents aspirated. When the nasogastric tube is seen coiled in an intrathoracic stomach the diagnosis is established and no detailed investigation is needed. The chest should be asculted for presence of peristaltic sounds above the diaphragm.

The universal admonition for early diagnosis and repair of traumatic disruptions of the diaphragm is valid. Quality of life in survivors is reduced by missed defects in the diaphragm. However, when medical reports are perused for aids in diagnosing this injury one is confronted by the empty cliche "high index of suspicion." The young physician in training wonders how he achieves this high index of suspicion so vaguely ruminated by his mentors.

Because multiple co-existing injuries preclude sophisticated diagnostic technics, an accurate, reliable means of detecting diaphragm defects is urgently needed. To be of value it must be simple and practical. The triad described by Pomerantz[14] of mediastinal shift, dullness or tympany over left chest and bowel sounds in the thorax are present in so many severely injured patients that they are of little help.

The roentgen detection of such defects is treacherous. The keystone of roentgen diagnosis is the presence of extraneous or unusual shadows above the diaphragm. The pitfall is that herniation of abdominal viscera does not always occur immediately after injury. Carter[15] declares shifts of the heart and mediastinum, disc-like atelectasis, an arch-like shadow over the diaphragm, and extraneous shadows on chest roentgenograms are diagnostic of traumatic disruption. Yet anyone exposed to critically injured patients is aware that heart and mediastinal shifts are frequent in pneumo- and hemo-thoraces, atelectasis in thoracic cage trauma, and peculiar shadows in pulmonary contusions. The dilated intrathoracic stomach can look very much like a simple elevated diaphragm (Fig. 5-9). Roentgen findings that are supposed to point to diaphragmatic rupture are present in many patients with severe multiple system injuries and statistics show it is these patients who usually have tears in the diaphragm.

Fluroscopy for assessing movement of the diaphragm is likewise misleading. Desforges[16] reported the herniated liver in his patient moved with respiration. Gastrointestinal studies with contrast materials is not wise in these patients. The manipulative requirements to achieve technically reliable roentgenograms are often prohibitive in the patient who is in shock with multiple organ systems injured. The insertion of a tube by the nasogastric route is a simple and quick method of assessing stomach position. Instillation of contrast opaque through the tube helps delineate air and organ shadows. Such evaluation depends upon the abnormal position of the abdominal viscera. The problem has been pointed out by Ebert and associates: early herniation of abdominal organs does not always occur.[13]

Pneumoperitoneum is undependable. Deceptive shadows in the chest of severely injured patients are confusing. If the patient already has a pneumothorax upon admission to the hospital, it is futile to proceed with a pneumoperitoneum to detect a ruptured diaphragm.

This brief critical review of methods of diagnosis establishes one clear fact. Added dimensions of diagnosis are needed and not rhetorical admonitions such as "high index of suspicion." To that end we propose the modified peritoneal lavage technic. Multiple system injuries in patients with ruptured diaphragms, mandate peritoneal lavage, which has proven extremely reliable in detecting intraperitoneal injuries. Insertion of intercostal tubes in suspected cases of ruptured diaphragm, even in the absence of any obvious hemopneumothorax, is a benign procedure when compared to the complications of ruptured diaphragms. Mortality doubles and death is rapid after visceral strangulation or obstruction develops.[17, 18]

The volume of Ringer's lactate instilled into the peritoneal cavity must be sufficient to fill the large perihepatic spaces and the lateral gutters, then spill over the hole in the diaphragm into the pleural space and out through the intercostal tube. In the

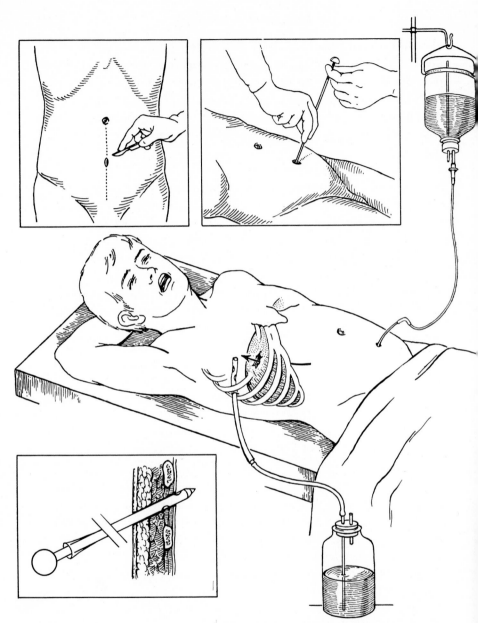

Figure 5-9. Method of detecting diaphragm defects by pleuroperitoneal lavage. A standard peritoneal dialysis catheter is inserted into peritoneal cavity (top insets) Intercostal chest tubes are placed (lower inset) A liter of Ringer Lactate is infused into the peritoneal cavity. If clear Ringer's solution returns through chest tube the diaphragm has been injured.

average size individual two or three liters are adequate. Even in the presence of a hemothorax or active intrapleural bleeding the outflow of clear Ringer's lactate in large amounts through the chest tube is noticeable. This added dimension of pleuroperitoneal lavage should lower drastically the percentage of missed diaphragmatic injuries in patients with multiple systems injured.

TRAUMATIC ASPHYXIA

In 1837 Ollivier[19] observed that patients trampled to death by crowds in Paris had a very characteristic "masque ecchymotique." In America this syndrome has been called traumatic asphyxia and is recognized by cervico-facial cyanosis, subconjunctional hemorrhages and ecchynosis of the face. It is produced by severe sudden compression of the upper chest. Williams and colleagues[20] have recognized four components necessary for the syndrome to develop: (1) deep inspiration before injury (2) closure of the glottis (3) tensing or bracing of the thoracoabdominal muscles in preparation for the impact, (4) sudden severe compression of the chest.

The major cause of traumatic asphyxia is blunt trauma acutely compressing the chest wall. Other less common injuries producing it are deep-sea diving accidents, blast compression of the chest and close range shot-gun blasts to the chest. These severe compressing forces to the anterior chest push the heart against the vertebral column suddenly ejecting blood from the right atrium into the veins of the upper thorax and neck. This sudden thrust of blood in a retrograde fashion through the valveless system of veins produces acute venous stasis of the smaller veins of the mucous membranes and skin. Tiny hemorrhages occur in the subconjunctional tissues and there is a purplish mantle over the face and neck leaving a distinct line of demarcation between the upper thorax and head (Figs. 5-10a and 5-10b). This clinical picture is frightening but unless there are concomitant interthoracic or neurologic injuries traumatic asphyxia is usually insignificant and resolves spontaneously in most instances.

Haller and Donahoo[21] observed two major complications:

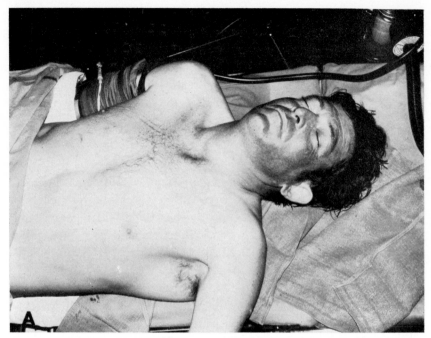

Figure 5-10.   Traumatic asphyxia in man whose chest was acutely compressed by large crane. Note (a) sharply demarcated "masque ecchymotique" and (b) subconjunctional hemorrhage.

(1) neurologic (2) pulmonary. They reported their patients were rarely semi-comatose, but most were disoriented and agitated. The neurologic symptoms were rapidly and spontaneously reversible within twenty-four hours. Pulmonary complications were much more serious. A few patients had major hemorrhage into the pulmonary parenchyma and pulmonary edema. Pneumomediastinum and pneumothorax were rare. Flail chests may also accompany these injuries. Such pulmonary and thoracic cage involvement can lead to poor gas exchange. Blood gases must be determined and deficits corrected by appropriate ventilatory support.

If co-existing neurologic and pulmonary injuries are not present traumatic asphyxia is rapidly reversible and the patient recovers uneventfully. There is usually no residual impairment.

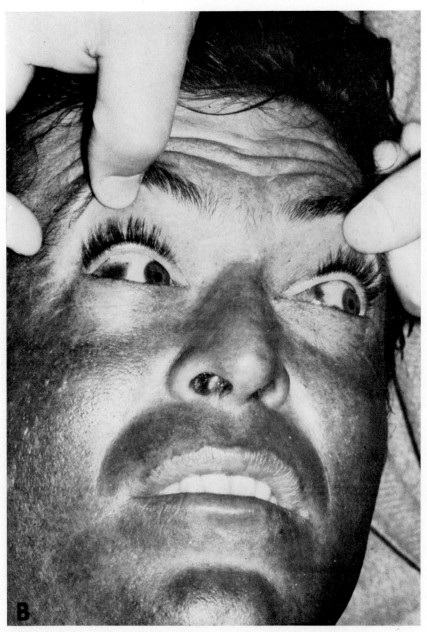

Figure 5-10b.

REFERENCES

1. Leinhoff, H. D.: Direct nonpenetrating injuries to the heart. *Ann Intern Med, 14:*653, 1940.
2. Kissane, R. W.: Traumatic heart disease. *Circulation, 6:*421, 1952.
3. Sigler, L. H.: Trauma of the heart due to nonpenetrating chest injuries. Report of cases with recovery of long survival. *JAMA, 119:*855, 1942.
4. Chapman, M. G., and McEachem, J. A.: Cardiac contusion caused by use of a jackhammer. *Am Heart J, 54:*625, 1957.
5. Harthorne, J. W.; Kantrowitz, P. A., and Sanders, C. A.: Traumatic myocardial infarction. Report of a case with normal coronary angiogram. *Ann Intern Med, 66:*341, 1967.
6. Bright, E. F., and Beck, C. S.: Nonpenetrating wounds of the heart. A clinical and experimental study. *Am Heart J, 10:*293, 1934.
7. Griswold, R. A., and Maguire, C. H.: Penetrating wounds of heart and pericardium. *Surg Gynecol Obstet, 74:*406-418, 1942.
8. Elkin, D. C., and Campbell, R. E.: Cardiac tamponade: Treatment by aspiration. *Ann Surg, 133:*623, 1951.
9. Ravitch, M. M., and Blalock, A.: Aspirations of blood from pericardium in treatment of acute cardiac tamponade after injury. *Arch Surg, 58:*463-477, 1949.
10. Burke, J. F.: Early diagnosis of traumatic rupture of the bronchus. *JAMA, 181:*682-686, 1962.
11. Bernatz, P. E.; Burnside, A. F., and Clagett, O. T.: Problems of the ruptured diaphragm. *JAMA, 168:*877-881, 1958.
12. Epstein, L. I., and Lempke, R. E.: Rupture of the right hemidiaphragm due to blunt trauma. *J Trauma, 8:*19-38, 1968.
13. Ebert, P. A.; Gaertner, R. A., and Zuidema, G. D.: Traumatic diaphragmatic hernia. *Surg Gynecol Obstet, 125:*59-65, 1967.
14. Pomerantz, M.; Rodgers, B. M., and Sabiston, D. C.: Traumatic diaphragmatic hernia. *Surgery, 64:*529-534, 1968.
15. Carter, B. N.; Guiseffi, J., and Filson, B.: Traumatic diaphragmatic hernia. *Am J Roentgenol, 65:*56-71, 1951.
16. Desforges, G.; Streider, J. W.; Lynch, J. P., and Madoff, I. M.: Traumatic rupture of the diaphragm: Clinical manifestations and surgical treatment. *J Thorac Cardiovasc Surg, 34:*779-797, 1957.
17. Hedblom, C. A.: Diaphragmatic hernia. *JAMA, 85:*947-953, 1925.
18. Sullivan, R. E.: Strangulation and obstruction in diaphragmatic hernia due to direct trauma; report of two cases and review of the English literature. *J Thorac Cardiovasc Surg, 52:*725-734, 1966.

19. Ollivier: Relation medicale des evenemens surveis an Champs-de-Mars le 14 junin 1837. *Ann Hyg, 18*:485-489, 1837.
20. Williams, J. S.; Minken, S. L., and Adams, J. T.: Traumatic asphyxia-reappraised. *Ann Surg, 167*:384-392, 1968.
21. Haller, J. A., and Donahoo, J. S.: Traumatic asphyxia in children. *J Trauma, 11*:453-457, 1971.

CHAPTER 6

EVALUATION OF THE ABDOMEN

PRIORITIES AND CHECK LIST FOR ABDOMINAL ASSESSMENT

1. Ventilation Adequate
2. Vertebral Column Stabilized
3. Blood Volume Replaced
4. Tissue Perfusion Adequate
5. Peritoneal Lavage

THE CONTENTS OF the abdominal parieties are the most difficult of all systems to evaluate rapidly and accurately. This is particularly true after blunt trauma in patients with co-existing injuries, especially head injuries. Intoxication with alcohol or other drugs is an increasing problem in evaluating these patients.

Trivial or sometimes forgotten trauma to the abdomen has the potential of producing a serious injury without producing a significant history. The index of suspicion of abdominal injuries must always be high in the examining physician's mind. Every patient involved in a serious accident must have repeated, careful examination of the abdomen even when the patient gives no complaint referable to the abdomen, and irregardless of obvious and frightening associated injuries.

Before beginning with an account of evaluating methods, there are a few clinical axioms that have been thoroughly established by universal experience, but because of their simplicity are often neglected or forgotten at the critical time. Roentgenographic assessment for abdominal injuries is not an efficient means of evaluating these patients. A few exceptions to this rule will be described later but valuable time should never be wasted in a fruitless search with multiple X-rays. Clinical findings are more reliable than either roentenograms or abdominal paracentesis. It is the missed or overlooked intra-abdominal injury that accounts for mortality in abdominal injuries. In evaluating the abdomen it is better to err on the side of laparotomy than to miss a deadly intraperitoneal lesion. In an analysis of 200 cases of abdominal injuries there were no deaths from laparotomy in whom no intra-abdominal injury was found, but three patients died from intra-abdominal hemorrhage in whom exploration was not performed.[1] Increased mortality also results from delay in laparotomy.[2, 3]

As in all other chapters of the text, the emphasis in evaluating the abdomen includes a thorough and careful recording of methods of injury and a meticulous inspection, palpation ascultation and percussion of the abdomen. This clinical evaluation, if done carefully, accurately, and repetitively, is the most reliable means of evaluating the traumatized abdomen. As has been noted by others, no laboratory or roentgenographic finding substitutes for frequent and repeated evaluation by an alert clinician.[2] Intelligent interpretation of the findings disclosed by history and physical examination is the last, but not by far the least, of this important triad of systematic evaluation.

In the conscious, alert patient, the presence of abdominal pain is extremely reliable in leading the physician to detect abdominal injuries. In some instances the injury may be to the abdominal parieties rather than intra-abdominal organs. Tears in the rectus or oblique muscles of the abdomen may cause severe pain and discomfort.

The patient who complains of pain should be listened to carefully. The pain experienced by the peritoneal response to blood or succus entericus bathing the parietal and visceral peritoneum is intense and persistent. The careful assessment of the patient's pain is important in determining whether additional evaluations and careful attention to the abdomen is justified.

The abdomen must be carefully inspected front, flanks and back. Bluish discolorations in the parieties often point to areas of impact and suggest torn viscera or rupture of solid organs.

Bluish discolorations over one or both flanks progressing anteriorly but sparing the most anterior abdomen frequently point to retroperitoneal hemorrhage when other abdominal signs are absent. Bluish discolorations localized to the umbilical area without flank or pelvic involvement suggest intraperitoneal blood, whereas bluish discolorations localized to and appearing to arise from out of the pelvis indicate extraperitoneal bleeding.

Aside from the bluish discolorations produced by blood dissecting in the various spaces and tissue planes, frank avulsions of tissue or obvious abrasions of the abdominal wall should be carefully noted as these most often indicate a shearing or tangential force of the kind producing intra-abdominal shearing of the hollow viscera.

Inspection should also be carried further to look for asymmetry between the flanks, which frequently in older persons with lax abdominal walls indicates accumulation of fluid, or blood in a lateral gutter. In younger individuals, it is probably extraperitoneal. Discrepancies in the contour of the abdomen are helpful. The normal abdomen is scaphoid in appearance. If while the evaluation is taking place the concavity from xyphoid to pubis is lost, one must suspect accumulation of blood, fluid or gas within the abdomen.

Abrasions and contusions in the area of seat belts or matching the contour of a seat strap must raise suspicion of intra-abdominal visceral injuries. A seat belt properly positioned and fastened should restrain individuals by means of anchoring the pelvic girdle and thoraco-vertebral axis. However, as with most human devices seat belts are often not worn or adjusted properly. When inspecting the critically injured patient the imprint of a seat belt across the lower abdomen or at waist level suggests improper positioning and must raise the suspicion of intraperitoneal shearing of the mesenteric vessels or perforations of hollow viscera.

Next, careful palpation of the abdomen is done. The gentleness of approach and the reassuring touch of the physician's hands are critical in collecting information to diagnose the injured abdomen. An immediate rough palpating hand in an already frightened, hurting, miserable human being may cause such exquisite additional pain that further physician approaches are invalidated.

As the examining hand carefully determines how much pressure can be applied without aggravating pains, the empathizing hand can progress gradually deeper into the abdominal wall evaluating resistance or spasm and probing for masses. Tender, painful masses are strong indications that large solid, organs (liver and spleen) have ruptured beneath their capsules but retained the blood in the shape of a mass rather than allowing it to diffuse out into the free peritoneal space. Quite often only the slightest pressure over a limited area, sometimes with only one or two fingers, gives the greatest information. This is especially true in frightened children.

Rigidity in the abdominal parieties must be evaluated as to whether it is voluntary on the part of the conscious patient, or whether it is involuntary and due to the peritoneal response to trauma. If a patient has a contusion of the gastrointestinal tract, liver or spleen he will voluntarily resist the examiner's fingers by tensing muscles to keep the physician's hand from inducing further pain by pressure palpation. But if the gastro-intestinal tract is disrupted, the urinary bladder perforated or hemorrhage develops, the response of the peritoneum is immediate and impressive. As time passes the irritation of the peritoneum is reflected in the abdominal muscles, they develop varying degrees of spasm, the most extreme of these leading to generalized spasm, commonly termed "board-like rigidity."

In the conscious patient tenderness, guarding, rigidity, and spasm are very reliable indices of intra-abdominal injuries. The palpating fingers must also be educated to search out unusual masses and determine whether they are enlarging as time progresses. Just looking at the size of the abdomen is not sufficient. The girth should be measured at its greatest diameter and recorded, with the passage of time increasing size of a palpable mass or increasing girth size are measurable indices to add to other positive evaluations.

The most common error in evaluating the abdomen by palpation is to consider the examination complete after feeling the major area between xyphoid and pubis. This is a frequent pitfall. The palpating fingers must progress from the traditional anterior xyphoid to pubic examination to include the rectum, pelvis, flanks and posterior abdomen.

A finger inserted into the rectum and returned with bright red blood mandates sigmoidoscopy. No free blood but the presence of fluctuant, boggy masses extrinsic to the rectum points to pelvic hematoma, ruptured urinary bladder and fractured pelvis.

The search by palpation is not complete until pelvic examination is done. Small intestinal injury in the pelvis with intraperitoneal bleeding limited to the cul-de-sac may show very little on standard abdominal examination; the tender mass in the cul-de-sac may be the only suggestion of injury.

Some have proposed culdocentesis as a reasonable method of detecting free intraperitoneal blood. When "four quadrant tops" were in vogue, a strong case could be made for culdocentesis before considering the four quadrant tap complete. However, with the advent of peritoneal lavage and its greater efficiency in detecting even small amounts of free blood in the peritoneal cavity, it is difficult to any longer advocate culdocentesis as an evaluating tool in most critically injured patients.

Percussion is quickly carried out, paying particular attention to loss of dullness over areas of solid organs (liver, spleen) indicating the presence of free air. The presence of dullness over normally gas containing regions indicates the presence of blood. An astute clinician can use these two findings to great advantage, but he must be familiar with normal subjects and of the normal distribution of dullness due to the configuration of the liver and spleen. Aside from those two careful observations, percussion is of no great value in the injured abdomen.

Ascultation of the abdomen involves chiefly the presence or absence of bowel sounds. Bruits in hypovolemic states do not have the same meaning as in routine examinations of the abdomen. The presence of peristaltic sounds do not help in a positive manner and should never be relied upon to the extent of relieving suspicion of abdominal injury. On the other hand, most people feel the absence of bowel sounds in the injured patient are an extremely reliable indication of intra-abdominal injury. Some even go so far as to make their decision for exploratory coeliotomy if peristaltic sounds are absent. Peristaltic sounds may be analagous to the discussion on central venous pressure monitoring. Taken alone as a single determinant and making a judgment decision without incorporating modifying factors of additional clinical information leads to pitfalls in both instances.

The effect of intra-abdominal injuries on bowel sounds must be reviewed. There is a lag period between time of injury and cessation of peristalsis. This lag period will vary in individuals and in relation to extent of spillage of feces, succus entericus, air or blood. This time factor is frequently undeterminable in critically injured patients.

The time between injury and assessment of the abdomen by a physician also varies from hospital to hospital and medical center to medical center. In the University of Louisville Affilated Hospitals, due to the rapid transit within the city of injured patients, many abdomens are ausculted within ten to fifteen minutes of injury.

In our experience we have not relied heavily upon the presence or absence of bowel sounds as a single determining factor indicating intra-abdominal injury. We assess many of our patients so quickly after injury that peristaltic sounds are present even in the face of life threatening intraperitoneal injuries.

For this reason we urge that presence or absence of peristaltic sounds be incorporated into the total clinical assessment and that if a number of other factors accumulate in favor of intra-abdominal injury, the ascultatory finding of presence or absence of bowel sounds be weighed in with the rest of the findings.

At the Louisville General Hospital in the conscious patient abdominal pain and one or more of the physical findings of tenderness, rigidity, fractured ribs, spasm, absent bowel sounds, abnormal percussion, and asymmetry of abdominal contour proved highly effective and reliable clinical evaluations denoting intra-abdominal injury and requiring laparotomy.

The unconscious patient presents a different and more difficult problem, and it is in this group that added dimensions of clinical evaluation is essential. Several years ago abdominal paracentesis was advocated as an added dimension in detecting concealed intra-abdominal injury. The single tap was rapidly refined to include a "four quadrant tap" because there were too many negative single taps in the face of serious injuries.

The false negative taps continued to plague advocates of four quadrant needle aspiration of the abdomen. They avoided the sensitive problem of false negative taps by stating that clinicians must ignore the four quadrant tap if negative and proceed on the basis of their clinical findings as if a negative needle aspiration had never been done. Psychologically this proved difficult and physicians found themselves in the position of making judgment decisions and assigning priorities of care based on "negative taps." Mays[4] reviewed four fatalities resulting from severe intra-peritoneal hemorrhage in whom it was obvious from the hospital record that negative needle aspirations of the abdomen influenced the responsible surgeons to delay laparotomy and attend other more obvious but less serious injuries.

It became obvious from this and many similar experiences that single or multiple needle aspirations of the injured abdomen were unreliable and even misleading. In 1965 Root and associates[5] refined the technique and developed the concept and practice of diagnostic peritoneal lavage. A standard peritoneal dialysis catheter is introduced into the low mid-line of the abdomen (Fig. 6-1) under local anesthesia. If gross blood is not present, 1,000 ml of Ringer's lactate solution is infused rapidly into the peritoneal cavity. In children, appropriately smaller amounts (300 to 500 ml) are used. The empty bottle is then lowered to floor level creating a siphon to return the excess fluid. The urinary bladder must always be drained with a catheter prior to this procedure and areas of old surgical incisions avoided as sites for catheter insertion. As little as 0.5 ml of free blood in the peritoneal cavity colors the perfusate a salmon pink and indicates intra-abdominal injury (Figs. 6-2a, 2b, 2c, and 2-d).

The peritoneal lavage has been further refined by some physicians to do cell counts on the returned fluid and microscopic inspection of a spun down sediment to look for intestinal content.

Peritoneal lavage has proven to be a highly reliable means of evaluating abdominal injuries. Gumbert and associates[6] reported

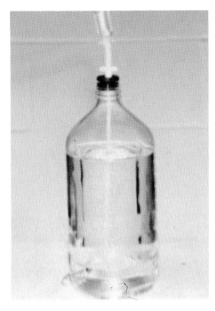

Figure 6-2a. Clear solution, negative lavage

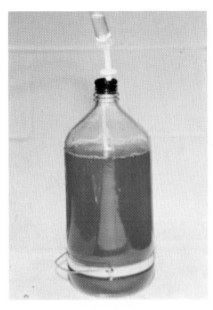

Figure 6-2b. Salmon pink produced by as little as 0.5ml whole blood

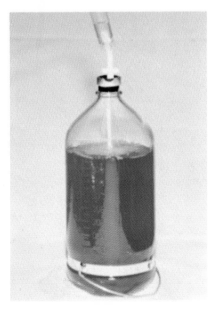

Figure 6-2c. Deeper red lavage solution produced by 1.0ml whole blood

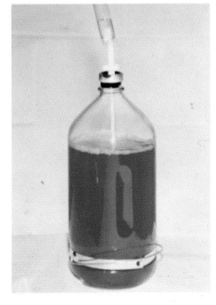

Figure 6-2d. Dark red lavage solution from ruptured spleen

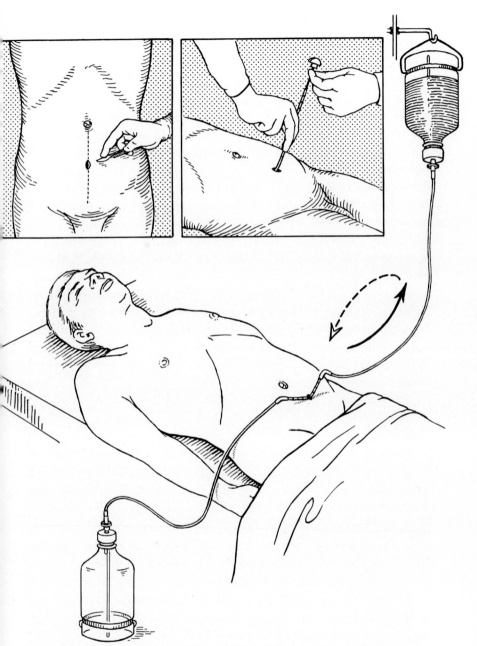

Figure 6-1. Method of lavaging the peritoneal cavity to detect intra-abdominal injuries. Upper inset: midline incision below umbilicus after emptying urinary bladder; insertion of peritoneal dialysis catheter. After infusion of a liter of balanced salt solution the flask is placed on floor for gravity drainage.

an incidence of false negative needle aspirations of the abdomen between 15 to 20 percent, but after instituting diagnostic peritoneal lavage, they increased their accuracy of diagnosis to 97 percent and had only one false positive.

The efficiency of peritoneal lavage has been so great that now the major problem in its use is injuries not requiring operative correction. Such minor or insignificant injuries from which patients spontaneously recover without operative intervention are the nemesis of peritoneal lavage in the same manner that false negatives were the pitfall of the four quadrant tap. Hence, we arrive at the conclusion that diagnostic peritoneal lavage is an extremely efficient and highly reliable means of evaluating the traumatized abdomen in unconscious patients, patients with unexplained shock and patients with confusing abdominal signs and multiple system injuries. Ahmad and Polk[7] reviewed sixty-three consecutive patients and concluded that conscious patients with obvious physical findings should undergo operation without delay, but the patient who has sustained serious cranio-cerebral injury and is not fully conscious benefits the most from peritoneal lavage.

In addition to being an extremely reliable means of detecting hemoperitoneum, Root and associates[8] have refined the technique ever further to include gastro-intestinal injuries in which bleeding is minimal. Isolated tears and perforations of hollow viscera are quite often unassociated with severe enough hemorrhage to cause hypovolemia and shock. Root and colleagues showed that the peritoneum responds to contamination with succus entericus, feces or bile by an outpouring of polymorphonuclear leukocytes and plasma into the peritoneal cavity. They used this characteristic to detect ruptured viscera in the absence of severe intraperitoneal bleeding. Of 189 patients studied, 100 had positive peritoneal lavage. Six of these patients had gastro-intestinal tract injury detectable only by the presence of peritoneal leukocytes. Again, however, there is a time lag before the appearance of peritoneal leukocytes in the range of two to three hours after injury and the assessor must take this into consideration in hospitals where patients arrive ten to twenty minutes after injury.

SPLENIC INJURIES

The spleen continues to be the most common abdominal organ injured (Table 6-I). For this reason any evaluation of the abdomen must be associated with a high index of suspicion of splenic trauma. Early diagnosis is critical not only for survival but for quality of life after survival. Accurate prompt appraisal of splenic injuries is directly related to reducing the morbidity and mortality from this injury. In a collective review by Griswold and Collier[15] which included the years 1900 to 1956, the average mortality rate was 30 percent. Other more recent series report a mortality rate of 9 percent.[16]

A review in the University of Louisville Hospitals for the years 1967 to 1972 disclosed there were no deaths in fifty-eight patients with isolated splenic injuries and splenectomy.[17] The absence of death in this series is directly attributable to careful meticulous abdominal examination by a physician, peritoneal lavage, and utilization of selective splenic arteriography in 16 percent of the patients where there was doubt about the diagnosis of splenic injury.

TABLE 6-I

ORGANS MOST COMMONLY INJURED WITH
ASSOCIATED OPERATIVE MORTALITY*

Organ	Number of Injuries	Total	Number of Deaths Intraoperative	Postoperative
Spleen	124	9	0	9
Liver	80	13	3	10
Small bowel	43	7	2	5
Kidney	35	2	1	1
Mesentery	32	7	1	6
Colon	29	7	1	6
Pancreas	27	5	0	5
Stomach	15	2	1	1
Diaphragm	15	1	0	1
Pelvic bones	14	6	1	5
Duodenum	13	2	0	2
Bladder	12	5	3	2
Aorta and branches	12	6	4	1
Vena cava and branches	8	6	5	1
Gallbladder	5	2	1	1

* Reproduced with permission from Gerald O. Strauch, M.D. and *The American Journal of Surgery,* vol. 125, p. 417, 1973.

Physical findings of abdominal tenderness, voluntary muscle guarding and/or rigidity of the abdominal parieties, associated with hypovolemia are effective and reliable signs of splenic injury. Fracture of the posterior segments of ribs 9, 10, 11, 12 in the left chest is an extremely reliable indication of trauma of the spleen. Kehr's sign (left shoulder pain) occurs only when the patient is supine or in a head-down position. A falling hematocrit and leukocytosis of more than 15,000 mm creates suspicion but is not reliable.

In questionable situations or in the unconscious patient peritoneal lavage detects hemoperitoneums but is not specific for splenic injuries. With a positive diagnostic lavage it really doesn't matter because the abdomen will be opened anyway and the spleen can be visualized directly.

Plain roentgenograms of the abdomen are not usually helpful. If the stomach or air bubble in the stomach is displaced medially, the stomach unusually dilated or the splenic flexure depressed inferiorly, one must suspect trauma to the spleen and pursue additional evaluating procedures

In approximately 16 percent of patients with splenic trauma, there is sufficient doubt to justify more sophisticated assessment. Selective splenic arteriography is an extremely reliable means of detecting injuries to the spleen.[17] Indications for selective splenic arteriography are listed in Chapter 14.

Others have found radionuclide photo images valuable in the study of possible splenic injuries. Technetium sulfur colloid 99m is perhaps the most popular and most readily accessible agent for scanning the spleen in emergency situations at night and on weekends. For spleen scanning 10 to 15 mC: of 99m Tc-S-C is given intravenously to the patient and imaging on a camera with a diverging collimotor is started immediately; 100,000 to 300,000 counts requiring about three minutes are accumulated per image. Six images can be obtained: 1. anterior, 2. posterior, 3. right lateral, 4. left lateral, 5. left anterior, and 6. right anterior oblique. The last three are highly specific for the spleen. Polaroid images are available immediately and an analysis of the findings can be made within thirty minutes after starting the procedure.

Collections of blood with the splenic parenchyma and compression of surrounding tissues show up as focal non-functioning areas and as concave defects.[18] The scintiscans are mostly valuable in detecting parenchymal and subdiaphragmatic lesions. The liver also picks up the technetium sulfur colloid and the margins of spleen and liver cannot be distinguished.

LIVER

The second most common abdominal organ injured is the liver. The mortality rate from hepatic trauma is much greater than splenic injury. Again, abdominal pain, tenderness, rigidity are the common findings. The degree of shock due to hypvolemia is usually greater than in splenic trauma and should lead the examiner to suspect hepatic rupture rather than splenic rupture. Diagnostic peritoneal lavage is again efficacious in detecting hemoperitoneum but is not specific for organ injury.

Pain is increased by deep inspiration and sometimes referred to the right shoulder. Fracture of the lower right rib cage, elevation of the right diaphragm and an enlarged or distorted liver shadow suggests liver injury in some instances. The technetium sulfur colloid scintiscan described above has also been found helpful by some in displaying space occupying lesions caused by subcapsular hematomas. This technique has merit only for the asymptomatic patient who is not in shock. It has no place in evaluating a patient with hemorrhagic hypovolemia.

I must emphasize that the most effective and safe evaluating method for liver injuries is coeliotomy. The mortality rate is too high in these patients to spend futile, wasteful moments in unfruitful diagnostic tests or evaluations. The hemogram is not helpful and if hypovolemia is present the best way to evaluate liver trauma is opening the abdomen. Once inside the abdomen after hemorrhage is controlled, operative cholangiograms and angiograms are helpful in evaluating the extent and severity of intrahepatic damage. Because hemorrhage from the liver is so life-threatening, laparotomy and control of hemorrhage must often be the primary evaluation methods.

In less serious hepatic trauma where hemorrhage is not a

threat (contusions, subcapsular hemotomas, etc.) laboratory evaluations can be productive. A falling serum albumin and prothrombin with an increase in serum bilirubin, latic dehydrogenase and serum transaminases after trauma assess the degree of hepatic injury. The return to normal of these tests is reliable evidence of healing of the injured liver. The initial improvement in hepatic function tests with a sudden reversal and deterioration of these functional tests indicates abscess formation (intrahepatic or extrahepatic) or additional hypoxia (atelectasis, pneumonia, pulmonary insufficiency) or hypovolemia.

STOMACH

A tube inserted through the nose into the stomach and aspirated is the most simple and reliable means of detecting injury to the gaster. The presence of blood in the aspiration indicates some degree of injury. This is such a simple test that it is often overlooked and not done at all. The major caution is in the unconscious patient with a full stomach in whom aspiration of gastric contents into the tracheobronchial tree can be a real threat to recovery. Contrast material can be inserted through the tube and an x-ray taken if there is suspicion of disruption of the stomach.

DUODENUM

In the early paragraphs of this chapter I mentioned that roentgenograms are not usually very helpful in evaluating the injured abdomen. This was emphasized to prevent patients from having multiple X-ray pictures made in efforts to diagnose an abdominal injury while other more effective evaluating tools are available.

However, the duodenum is an exception to this general rule. Because it is a fixed retroperitoneal organ some disruptions are retroperitoneal injuries and diagnostic peritoneal lavage and physical examination can both be negative yet there can be significant retroperitoneal disruption of the duodenum. Some of these patients are actually sent home because their findings after trauma are so minimal.

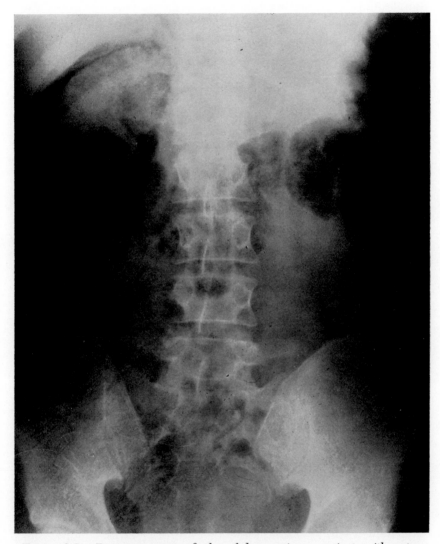

Figure 6-3. Roentgenogram of the abdomen in a patient with retroperitoneal rupture of the duodenum. The retroperiotoneal air dissecting around the right kidney causing an "air nephrogram" was the only indication in this patient of serious injury.

Since it is fairly well fixed by its peritoneal attachments, the duodenum is susceptible to shearing forces that compress the posterior wall of the duodenum against the rigid vertebral column. When there is an isolated injury to the retroperitoneal duodenum the only way to detect it immediately is with a plain X-ray of the abdomen. The diffusion of air into the retroperitoneal space gives a distinct "air nephrogram" and after blunt trauma to the epigastrum is pathognomonic of retroperitoneal rupture of the duodenum (Fig. 6-3).

If duodenal injuries are missed initially, the patient may return in extremis with oliguria and sepsis; therefore, it is extremely critical that duodenal injuries be diagnosed early.

Penetrations or disruptions of the anterior duodenum permit bile and gastric juices to bathe the peritoneum and cause the usual physical findings of rigidity and tenderness. Such duodenal injuries are usually no problem in diagnosis since the peritoneal lavage will show bile or leukocytes as described earlier in this chapter or the physical findings will be so distinct as to precipitate laparotomy.

Not all injuries of the duodenum result in complete through and through perforations or tears. Hematomas beneath the mucosa or within the wall of the duodenum is a significant variant of duodenal trauma. They occur most frequently in children. The average age of eleven patients seen over a ten-year period in the University of Louisville was nine years.

This entity is also best detected by X-ray examination. Serious nausea and vomiting with abdominal pain and epigastric tenderness should lead to a contrast study of the upper gastrointestinal tract. Occasionally a pathognomonic "coiled spring" sign can be seen as the submucosal hematoma pushes the valvulae conniventes close together and into the duodenal lumen (Fig. 6-4). The "coiled spring" roentgenogram is infrequent and more commonly duodenal obstruction, either partial or complete, is observed on the upper gastrontestinal series. Other roentgenographic pictures show edematous mucosa bulging into the lumen sometimes creating a picket fence appearance.

Unless coexisting injuries require laparotomy, the diagnosis of this particular variant of duodenal injury does not warrant

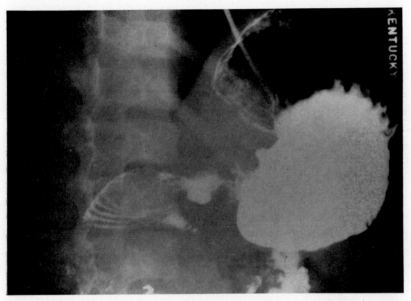

Figure 6-4.   Contrast study of stomach and duodenum after blunt trauma to the abdomen of a nine-year-old boy. Note the obstruction of the duodenum by a submucosal hematoma and "coiled spring" appearance of Valvulae conniventes.

laparotomy. Most of these patients do extremely well, with supportive nasogastric decompression and intravenous ailimentation allowing spontaneous absorption of the duodenal hematoma.

PANCREAS

The pancreas is fairly well protected and not injured as frequently as other organs. Just as the duodenum is an exception to the general axiom that X-rays are not helpful in evaluating injured abdomens, so pancreatic trauma is an exception to the axiom that laboratory studies are not usually helpful. Elevated serum amylase concentration is frequently the only indication an appraisor has that this organ has been significantly injured. Few injuries of the pancreas are isolated and more often the duodenum or stomach are also injured. A perforation of the duodenum may also allow absorption of enough extravasated pancreatic amylase by the peritoneum to elevate the serum amylase; interpretation of these laboratory findings must proceed with intelligent caution.

Olsen[19] reported a single determination of serum amylase done within a few hours after abdominal injury can neither identify nor exclude serious pancreatic injury. He suggested that in these situations hyperamylasemia may often be nonpancreatic in origin. Thirty-three percent (12 patients) with hyperamylasemia had no significant intra-abdominal injury. But he found that a rising or persistently elevated serum amylase strongly suggested pancreatic injury. Naffziger and McCorkle[20] found elevation of the serum amylase in every case of pancreatic injury in which the test was performed.

Pancreatic trauma occurs in degrees and the severe transsections or avulsions of the head or body are associated with the physical findings that normally precipitate laparotomy and the extent of pancreatic trauma is evaluated further by operative techniques.

There are no classical signs of pancreatic injury. The early clinical picture in the more severe disruptions or transections of the body across the vertebral column is hypovolemic shock with peritoneal irritation or generalized peritonitis. No other organ injury produces such agony and profound collapse in the absence of massive blood loss. Intense epigastric pain is the chief complaint of the part of the patient. Roentgenographic and other laboratory procedures are of little help except in turning up co-existing injuries. Approximately 50 percent of patients with pancreatic injuries have an associated retroperitoneal injury. Blunt trauma to the abdomen with a rising or persistently elevated serum amylase concentration is usually an indication for abdominal exploration. Diagnostic peritoneal lavage is again helpful when one is suspicious of an injured pancreas. Perry[21] states that an amylase concentration greater than 100 Somogyi units per 100 ml of lavage fluid is diagnostic of injury to pancreas or small bowel.

SMALL INTESTINE

Eighty percent of bowel injuries occur between the duodenojejunal junction and the terminal ileum. Blunt injuries produce the most difficult diagnostic situations. The abdominal wall should be carefully scrutinized for discolorations, contusions, etc., or any indication that a severe and sudden compression of the abdomen occurred. The bowel does not blow out after the fashion of a balloon rupturing but is sheared or torn between the anterior force suddenly compressing the abdominal wall and impigning the intestine against the rigid vertebral column. The response of the peritoneum to torn or penetrated jejunum can be detected as described earlier in this chapter by diagnostic peritoneal lavage.

Stephenson advocates an interesting method of detecting intestinal perforations. Sodium Diatrizoate (Hypaque®) is given orally (50 ml) and urine specimens collected. It is essentially unabsorbed by the intestinal mucosa. If there is loss of the Hypaque into the peritoneal cavity, it is rapidly absorbed by the peritoneum and excreted in the urine where it can be detected by precipitation with concentrated Hydrochloric acid (one drop). If diatrizoate is present in the urine an immediate dense chalky white precipitate is seen.[22] Free intraperitoneal air on abdominal roentgenograms is helpful in deciding for laparotomy, but if absent, is not sufficiently reliable to allow the physician to omit intestinal perforations from consideration.

After evaluating for small intestinal injury, the examining physician must be aware that even though the small bowel itself has escaped injury, long tears of the inesentery or hemorrhage into the leaf of the mesentery can cause segmental ischemia of sufficient degree to produce gangrene of the intestine. Such mesenteric tears can usually be detected by peritoneal lavage.

COLORECTAL INJURIES

Injuries to the intraperitoneal colon are detected as described for small intestine. External evidence of severe blunt trauma should be assessed. The peritoneal response to colon injury is much more intense and rapid than duodenal perforations, hence the abdominal signs of tenderness, pain, guarding are very reliable and usually all that is needed to justify laparotomy. Free air is again helpful but rarely present in injured patients.

The examination of the rectum both with a gloved finger and a sigmoidoscope is critical. Such simple evaluating procedures as inserting a finger into the rectum may be forgotten or ignored in this enlightened age of technical advances, but it still gives invaluable information. Bright red blood in the rectum or sigmoid must arouse suspicion of injury.

Penetrating wounds of the intraperitoneal colon are usually no problems in evaluation and laparotomies give a definitive and quick diagnosis. Wounds of the extraperitoneal rectum are extremely difficult to detect. Even at the operating table with the abdomen opened widely, the extraperitoneal rectum defies adequate inspection or observation. From inside the abdomen, there is just no easy means of detecting wounds of the extra-peritoneal rectum. It is for this reason that evaluation of the patient's rectum by finger examination and direct inspection with a sigmoidoscope can not be omitted.

In questionable situations a rectal and colon evaluation with an aqueous opaque media should follow the finger and sigmoido-scopic evaluations. Colorectal lesions are so lethal that such examinations should not be procrastinated to a more convenient time.

Not all colon injuries result in perforations or tears. Blunt trauma sometimes produces colonic obstruction by hematoma in the early phase or cicatrical stenosis late[23] (Figs. 6-5a, 6-5b, 6-5c). Portions of the colon with a mesentery are mobile enough to be impinged between the spine and injuring force and tear or perforate leading to peritoneal signs that dictate laparotomy and repair. The right colon and descending colon being relatively fixed in their retroperitoneal positions, cannot be sheared across the vertebral column and, hence, do not tear or rupture by blunt forces but may develop hematomas and stenoses that obstruct. These are detected by colon studies with contrast media and if suspected are really no problem in diagnosis. If physicians are not aware of this entity the diagnosis may be delayed for months or even years (Figs. 6-6a, 6-6b, 6-6c).

FEMALE REPRODUCTIVE ORGANS

Female reproductive organs are infrequently injured either by blunt or penetrating trauma. In fact rupture of the non-pregnant uterus is a medical curiosity and so rare that it is seldom mentioned. Two patients who were in the immediate postpartum period are reported by Quast and Jordan[24] as the only recorded cases of uterine rupture in the non-gravid state. In a gravid state the uterus rises from its protected position deep within the bony pelvis to become an abdominal organ, and thus equally susceptible to injury as other abdominal organs. Reproductive organs which are not enlarged were reported injured only eight times from gunshot wounds out of twenty-seven patients with gynecologic injuries (Table 6-II).

In pregnant women the presence or absence of fetal movements and fetal heart sounds should always be ascertained on initial evaluation. Evaluating gravid females after trauma involves being highly suspicious of uterine rupture. The signs and symptoms are the same as in other severe hemorrhagic hypovolemic states. Shock is severe, immediate and dominates the

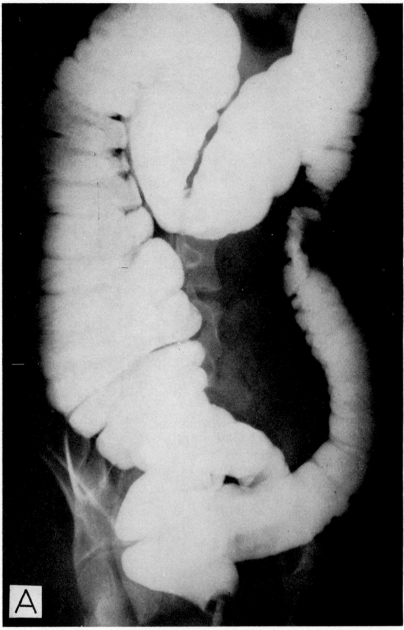

Figure 6-5. Colon study with Barium after penetrating abdominal trauma shows obstruction at splenic flexure by subserosal hematoma in descending colon. (a) absorption of hematoma and resolution of obstruction occurs spontaneously (b) two weeks (c) three months after injury. (Courtesy *J Trauma, 6*:319, 1966.)

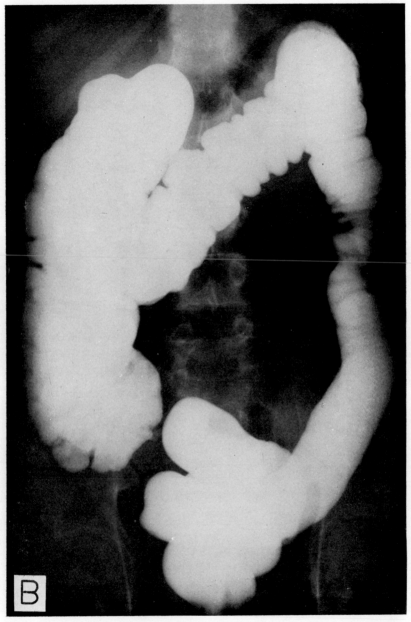

Figure 6-5b.

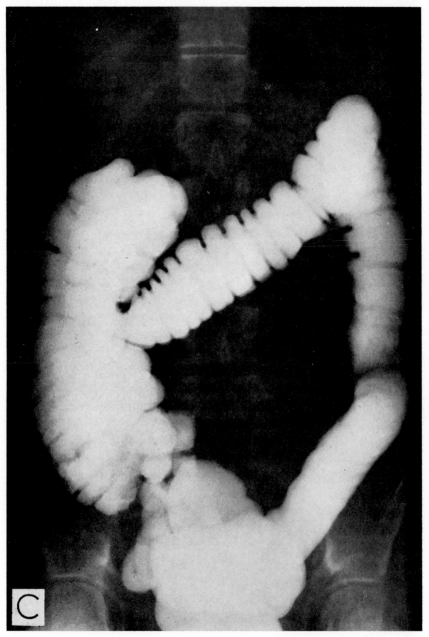

Figure 6-5c.

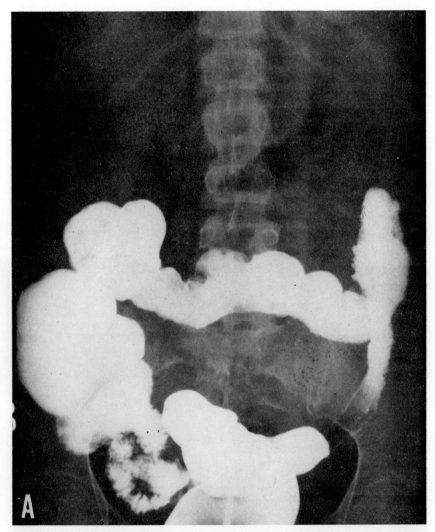

Figure 6-6. Colon study with Barium after blunt abdominal trauma showing cicatricial circular fibosis of descending colon causing obstruction. (a) Initial hospital admission.

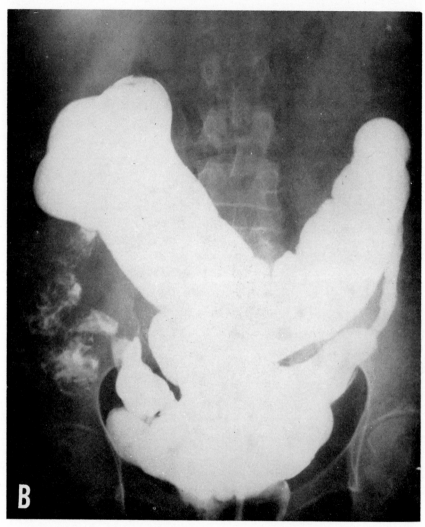

Figure 6-6b.   Two months after injury.

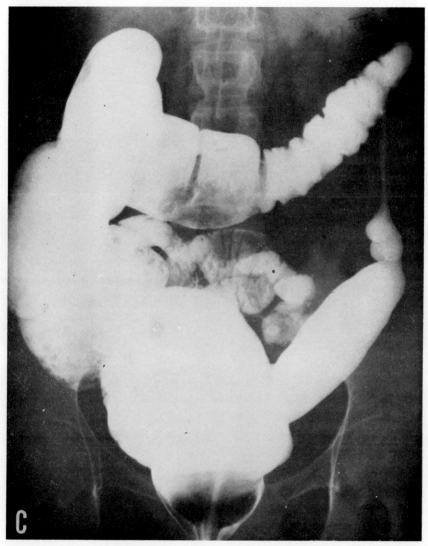

Figure 6-6c.   Eight months after injury.

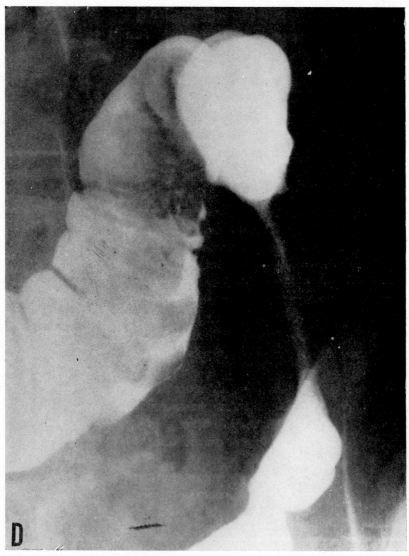

Figure 6-6d.   Close up of area shown in (c). This patient required colon resection and primary anastomosis. (Reproduced by permission, Mays, *J Trauma*, 6:320, 1966.)

TABLE 6-II

WOUNDS OF FEMALE REPRODUCTIVE ORGANS

(Site of Injury in 27 Patients)

Uterus	18
Uterus and Tube	4
Tube	2
Ovary	1
Tube and Ovary	1
Cervix	1

Reproduced with permission of Quast and Jordan and the *Journal of Trauma*, vol. 4, 1964, p. 839.

clinical picture throughout. It soon becomes obvious with oliguria, reduced central venous pressure and tachycardia that exsanguinating hemorrhage is imminent.

In addition to these findings, there is abdominal pain, tenderness, distention, ileus and absent fetal heart sounds and fetal movements.

Because of the tremendous vascularity of the gravid uterus, these patients will die of exsanguination or irreversible shock unless there is rapid replacement of blood volume and laparotomy to control hemorrhage.

RETROPERITONEAL HEMATOMA

Pelvic fractures account for nearly 60 percent of all traumatic retroperitoneal hemorrhage. Abdominal pain and back pain are frequent symptoms. Careful inspection of the abdomen will show unilateral or, in some instances, bilateral bulging of the flanks and sometimes there is discoloration present slowly progressing out of the flanks and anteriorly toward the umbilicus. This area of the flank will be very dull to percussion. Palpation may uncover a boggy mass and rectal examination may confirm this palpatory finding.

Roentgenography is valuable in two respects: 1. obliteration of the psoas shadow, 2. pelvic fractures. Progressive fall in hemoglobin and hematuria on urinanalysis in 80 percent of patients are helpful laboratory guidelines. Varying degrees of shock are present depending upon the size and volume of the hematoma. The most common pitfall in replacing blood volume is underestimating the retroperitoneal losses.

PENETRATING INJURIES

The penetration of the abdominal parieties by wounding objects must be considered separately insofar as clinical evaluation is concerned. Many feel that any patient whose abdominal parieties have been penetrated by a wounding object deserves laparotomy. We have followed this course almost consistently and still believe it to be in the best interest of the patient.

Shaftan,[9] in 1960, began to differentiate between the propulsive missile type injury and stab wounds. He pointed out that many exploratory laparotomies after stab wounds were negative and emphasized the morbidity and mortality associated with laparotomy. On this basis criteria for coeliotomy after stab wounds were used to separate patients into two groups. A review of 535 patients with penetrating trauma showed a 0.5 percent mortality in patients treated by selective conservatism as contrasted to 7.3 percent mortality in patients who had laparotomy. By using the criteria listed in Table 6-IV, Shaftan and associates explore only 28 percent of penetrating wounds of the abdomen. Others report good results with expectant management of stab wounds of the abdomen. Mason[10] noted that over a three year period at the University of Illinois Research Hospitals the exploration rate for abdominal stab wounds were reduced from 98 percent to 61 percent. All stab wounds were observed closely and celiotomy done only for specific indications. They had no

TABLE 6-III

PERITONEAL LEUKOCYTE RESPONSE IN PATIENTS
Aliquot Peritoneal Fluid Leukocytes/cu mm

	WBC Range	No. of Patients
FLUID WITHOUT GROSS BLOOD		
No abdominal visceral injury	0.50	21
With abdominal visceral injury	2,300-27,500	6
FLUID WITH GROSS BLOOD	20-3,160	8
	(Mean—1,275)	

Reproduced with permission of Root, et al., *Arch Surg*, vol. 95, 1967.

TABLE 6-IV

CRITERIA FOR CELIOTOMY IN PENETRATING
ABDOMINAL WOUNDS

1. Peritoneal Irritation
2. Positive Peritoneal Aspirate
3. Free Air on Roentgenograms
4. Persistent Unexplained Shock
5. Absent Bowel Sounds

mortality or morbidity in those patients managed nonoperatively.

As experience with conservative management of stab wounds developed, Shaftan and Mason placed great weight on the presence or absence of bowel sounds in evaluating patients with penetrating trauma leading Shaftan to comment, "The absence of peristaltic sounds is an absolute indication for exploration and presence of them is a reliable guide toward conservative management."[11] Mason also relies heavily on presence of peristaltic sounds in evaluating penetrating wounds of the abdomen. He stated "experience indicates that few errors will be made when this rule (absent bowel sounds) is followed. . . ."

Two points must be emphasized in regard to observation of penetrating wounds: (1) these experiences reflect a civilian setting, (2) the speed of transportation of the injured to the hospital influences the findings. If one places great importance on bowel sounds, you must remember that even in the presence of an injury they may not completely disappear for three hours after injury. Such a fact is critical in intelligently evaluating abdomens with penetrating wounds. Finally, the physician must be free and available for frequent and repeated examinations of his injured patient. If he is called away from the injured subject's bedside and cannot return for six to twelve hours he must make some arrangement for someone else to be briefed in the patient's care and urge him to do repeated and careful examinations.

Another problem in assaying penetrating abdominal wounds is determining whether or not the peritoneal cavity has been entered. Some wounds of the abdomen are tangential and others superficial and never enter the peritoneal cavity.

One approach to evaluating the penetrating wound of the abdomen is to prepare and drape the patient in the same manner as for a sterile surgical laparotomy. With anesthesiologists standing by, the wound is explored under local anesthesia to determine whether the peritoneum has truly been traversed. If the depths of the wound end in the abdominal muscles or go off in a tangent to the abdominal wall and do not enter the peritoneal cavity, the procedure is terminated and the patient sent to the ward or discharged as indicated.

Another method is radiographic evaluation of the wound by injecting contrast media. The area around the wound is cleaned and draped. After infiltrating the tissue with a local anesthetic, a purse string suture is placed around the penetrating wound. A 12 or 14 French rubber catheter is advanced into the wound and the purse string tightened. For very small penetrating wounds as made by an ice pick or stiletto, an intracath is substituted for the rubber catheter. Sixty to 80 ml of Hypaque 50 percent containing 1 ml methylene blue are injected through the catheter under pressure sufficient to create a slight bulge in the skin surrounding the wound. The methylene blue is added to detect leaks to the outside. After injection of contrast media, the catheter is clamped and the patient tilted on the X-ray table up and down and side to side. Roentograms are taken in the anteroposterior, lateral and oblique positions.

Such a study is considered satisfactory only if a large amount of contrast material is seen in the abdominal wall proving there was sufficient injection pressure to outline a tract had it entered the peritoneum.

A positive study shows the contrast material outlining intestinal loops or collecting around or below the spleen or liver.

Steichen and associates[12] studied 100 patients with abdominal stab wounds with this technic. Thirty-seven had positive signs of peritoneal penetration. In twenty-four there were injuries to one or several intraperitoneal organs.

Shotgun wounds of the abdomen present such unique problems that they must be considered separately. In evaluating shotgun wounds the major factor is the distance. A long range shotgun injury involves numerous small penetrating injuries of low velocity. Each pellet injures the tissue locally by its own kinetic energy which is very little for each individual pellet. These long range shotgun injuries may be treated expectantly by the same selective conservatism described previously for stab wounds. Laparotomy is done only for specific indications such as abscess formation, urine or bile extravasation. Evaluating signs are those of tenderness, rigidity and absent bowel sounds. Many of these individuals require only antibiotics, tetanus immunization and supportive care.

On a man about 6 feet tall, and weighing 160 pounds, shot at a distance of forty yards by a twelve gauge shotgun loaded with No. 6 shot, a little over 100 pellets would be distributed from mid-thigh to the shoulders. When the abdomen is involved in this scatter wound pattern, there are many visceral perforations (fifty to one hundred fifty). These perforations in almost all instances seal over and do not require laparotomy. Antibiotics, nasogastric intubation, and intravenous alimentation are usually all that are required in these scatter type wounds. Operations are reserved for specific complications such as delayed localized abscess formation. It is unusual for shotgun pellets to cause tangential wounds of the intestine in which the bowel wall is laid open for several centimeters such as is sometimes seen with pistol and rifle wounds.

The close range shotgun blast is entirely different and cannot even be considered as even the same injury though made by the same wounding instrument. The individuals pellets or wounding missile are unimportant. The kinetic energy applied to tissue by the blast effect is the most important factor. For a 12 gauge shotgun loaded with No. 6 shot discharges 275 pellets and the kinetic energy at the muzzle is ($K = \dfrac{Mv^2}{2}$) 2,300 foot pounds. The awesome destructive effect of such kinetic energy can better be appreciated if compared to the high velocity military M-16 rifle whose kinetic energy is only 1,530 foot pounds at the muzzle (see Chapter 2).

The assaying of close range shotgun blast hinges chiefly upon determining the amount of devitalized tissue and amount of blood volume lost.

LABORATORY DATA

Laboratory studies are of limited value in assessing intraabdominal injuries. The hemoglobin concentration and hematocrit have little significance in the early stages of blood loss. Many clinicians have traditionally attached importance to the leukocyte count as an indication of concealed hemorrhage. This tradition has been largely based on a report by Berman and associates[13] in which they believed they could correlate leukocytosis with internal hemorrhage in 338 patients after blunt trauma. In their opinion, a leukocyte count of 15,000 or more justified suspicion of a ruptured liver or spleen. They reported this finding of greater significance than blood pressure and serial red blood cell counts. Others have not found the leukocyte count helpful. At the Louisville General Hospital leukocyte counts of 15,000/mm³ or greater were present in only 8 percent of patients with splenic rupture.[7] Williams and Zollinger[14] urged that white blood count not be the sole criterion for laparotomy. They reported leukocyte counts greater than 20,000 mm in patients with fractures and chest injuries.

Hemoglobin and hematocrit determinations are completely unreliable in respect to estimating blood loss or blood volume in the early hours after abdominal injury. A falling hemoglobin may be useful in the late twenty-four to forty-eight hour period

TABLE 6-V

PERITONEAL LEUKOCYTE COUNT WITH
GASTROINTESTINAL INJURY

Diagnostic Peritoneal Lavage
Peritoneal Leukocytosis

Injury Site	No. of Patients	Peritoneal WBC/cu mm
Small Bowel	4	146*-27,500
Duodenum	1	4,800
Bladder	1	8,000
Gastrojejunostomy	1	2,300

* 1½ hours after injury.
Taken from Peritoneal response to injury with permission of Root, et al., *Arch Surg*, vol. 95, 1967.

to arouse suspicion of a ruptured spleen or liver and precipitate more definitive evaluations.

Serum amylase concentrations are helpful after abdominal trauma, especially if the pancreas represents the only intraperitoneal injury. An elevated serum amylase may be the only abnormal test. If there is no free air and peritoneal lavage is negative, these patients can be observed and many times treated nonoperatively.

An evaluation of lactic dehydrogenase, transaminases, serum bilirubin, albumin and prothrombin time can be very helpful in hepatic contusions. If the abdominal injury doesn't rupture Glisson's capsule and produce a hemoperitoneum, these laboratory studies are often the only indication of liver trauma. A negative peritoneal lavage is very helpful in deciding on nonoperative management of a contused liver.

REFERENCES

1. Fitzgerald, J. B.; Crawford, E., and DeBakey, M. E.: Surgical considerations of abdominal injuries: Analysis of 200 cases. *Am J Surg, 100:*22, 1966.
2. Strauch, G. O.: Major abdominal trauma in 1971. *Am J Surg, 125:*413-418, 1973.
3. Penberthy, G. C., and Reiners, C. R.: Visceral injury resulting from nonpenetrating trauma. *J Mich Med Soc, 54:*1057, 1955.
4. Mays, E. T.: Bursting injuries of the liver. *Arch Surg, 93:*92-1-6, 1966.
5. Root, H. D.; Hauser, C. W.; McKinley, C. R.; LaFane, J. W., and Mendiola, R. P.: Diagnostic peritoneal lavage. *Surgery, 57:*633, 1965.
6. Gumbert, J. L.; Froderman, S. E., and Mercho, J. P.: Diagnostic peritoneal lavage in blunt abdominal trauma. *Ann Surg, 165:*70-71, 1967.
7. Ahmad, W., and Polk, H. C., Jr.: Blunt abdominal trauma: A study of relationships between diagnosis and outcome. *S Med J, 66:*1127-1130, 1973.
8. Root, H. D.; Keizer, P. J., and Perry, J. F.: The clinical response and experimental aspects of peritoneal response of injury. *Arch Surg, 95:*531, 1967.
9. Shaftan, G. W.: Indications for exploration in abdominal trauma. *Am J Surg, 99:*657, 1960.

10. Mason, J. H.: The expectant management of abdominal stab wounds. *J Trauma.* 4:210-218, 1964.

11. Ryzoff, R. H.; Shaftan, G. W., and Herbsman, H.: Selective conservation in penetrating abdominal trauma. *Surgery, 59*:650, 1966.

12. Steichen, F. M.; Pearlstein, D. M.; Dargan, E. L.; Prommas, D. C., and Weil, P. H.: Wounds of the abdomen: Radiographic diagnosis of intraperitoneal penetration. *Am Surg, 165*:77, 1967.

13. Berman, J. K.; Habegger, E. D.; Fields, D. C., and Kilmer, W. L.: Blood studies as aid in differential diagnosis of abdominal trauma. *JAMA, 165*:1537-1541, 1957.

14. Williams, R. D., and Zollinger, R.: Diagnostic and prognostic factors in abdominal trauma. *Am J Surg, 97*:575-581, 1959.

15. Griswold, R. A., and Collier, H. S.: Blunt abdominal trauma. *Surg Gynecol Obstet, 112*:309, 1961.

16. Shirkey, A. L.; Wukasch, D. C.; Beall, A. C.; Gordon, W. B., and Debakey, M. D.: Surgical Management of splenic injuries. *Am J Surg, 108*:630, 1964.

17. Villarreal-Rios, A., and Mays, E. T.: Efficacy of clinical evaluation and selective splenic arteriography in splenic trauma. *Am J Surg, 127*:310-313, 1974.

18. Witek, J. T.; Spencer, R. P.; Pearson, H. A., and Touloukian, R. J.: Diagnostic spleen scans in occult splenic injury. *J Trauma, 14*:197-199, 1974.

19. Olsen, W. R.: The serum amylase in blunt abdominal trauma. *J Trauma, 13*:200, 1973.

20. Naffziger, H. C., and McCorkle, H. J.: Recognition and management of acute trauma to the pancreas with particular reference to use of serum amylase test. *Ann Surg, 118*:594, 1943.

21. Perry, J. F., Jr.: Blunt and penetrating abdominal injuries. *Current Problems in Surgery,* May 1972, p. 28.

22. McGraw, J.; McLeod, R.; McDonald, W., and Stephenson, H. E., Jr.: A urine precipitation test for intestinal perforation. *Arch Surg, 91*:148, 1965.

23. Mays, E. T., and Noer, R. J.: Colonic stenosis after trauma. *J Trauma, 6*:316, 1966.

24. Quast, D. C., and Jordan, G. L.: Traumatic wounds of the female reproductive organs. *J Trauma, 4*:839, 1964.

EVALUATION OF NEUROLOGIC INJURIES

PRIORITIES AND CHECK LIST FOR
NEUROLOGIC EVALUATION

1. Airway Patent
2. Stabilized Vertebral Column
3. Cerebral Circulation Intact
4. Cautious Volume Repletion
6. Fracture Dislocations Impinging on Nerve or
   Spinal Cord Reduced

H YPOXEMIA IS PRESENT immediately after cranio-cerebral injury and immediate assessment of the degree of hypoxemia is important. Blood gases should be drawn soon after admission and monitored sequentially as described in Chapter 13. Sinha and associates[1] studied arterial oxygenation in a control group and in patients wtih head and spinal cord injuries. They found one half of the head and spinal cord injuries had arterial oxygen tensions below 60 mm Hg.

This hypoxemic concomitant of head injury is aggravated by airway obstruction and shock. It is a tragic commentary on American medicine that many patients with minor head injuries, potentially salvagable, are converted to decerebrate vegetables because of the poorly understood relationship between cerebral trauma and hypoxia. The very worst environment for the injured brain is hypoxia. The simplest way to convert a minor head injury with a fully recoverable potential into permanent brain damage is failure to detect airway obstruction from whatever causes. Hypoxia causes profound cerebral edema far beyond what would be expected from minor trauma.

Profound circulatory collapse (shock) is not usually caused by head injuries but increases greatly the hypoxic environment of the brain. Campbell[2] stated "as an absolute rule the presence of shock following injury to the head is indicative of injury elsewhere until it is proved that it is not. . . . In the presence of shock, head injuries should be ignored and the patient treated precisely as if he had any other sort of injury." Youmans[3] also reported shock due to brain injury to be an unusual circumstance. He studied 654 patients and found only twenty-one (3.3%) patients with shock due to brain injury. Another way of stating the same finding is that 97 percent of patients with cranio-cerebral trauma and shock as the presenting complex have some reason for their circulatory collapse other than brain injury per se. The criteria that must be met before the circulatory collapse is considered secondary to neurologic injuries are: 1. Severe brain stem injury, 2. severe spinal cord damage at high level. Brain stem injuries can be detected by the profoundly unresponsive patient, with bilaterally dilated and fixed pupils, with decerebrate posturing and altered respirations. Before these criteria can be accepted as reliable, adequate airway, ventilation and arterial oxygen tensions with an intact cerebral circulation must be ensured. Dilation of the peripheral vascular bed due to severe spinal cord injury is usually so obvious that it usually does not present a problem in detection.

Youmans concludes his study by stating, "If a severely injured patient does not have dilated and fixed pupils bilaterally and ventilation and airway are adequate his shock is almost always on a basis other than his head injury."

It is also tragic that many critically injured patients who survive accidents without permanent paralysis or weakness develop irreversible neurologic damage in the ambulance or somewhere between hospital stretchers, X-ray or operating room tables. Stabilization of the cranioverterbral axis is critical and must begin at the scene of the accident. The most skilled neuro-surgeon in the world cannot restore a spinal tract that has experienced pressure by a displaced vertebra for several hours.

This is the reason at the beginning of this text I stressed the responsibility of medicine begins at the scene of the injury rather than at the hospital's back door. The personnel transporting these patients must be made aware of the strict need of stabilizing the cranio-vertebral axis and attaching appropriate spine boards to these patients before extrication and transportation. Otherwise, all the medical skill in the world cannot restore a lacerated spinal cord. Physicians cannot shirk responsibility simply because they take over only after the patient arrives at their office or hospital. We are charged with the responsibility of providing the public with technicians trained in the use of spine boards and extrication skills to prevent additional trauma and ultimate paralysis in these patients.

The same holds true in the hospital environment. The number of times a patient is transferred to and from various transporting elements increases the likelihood of cord damage. This is why we at the University of Louisville have advocated for many years that special operating rooms be set aside to receive these patients. All evaluating procedures and X-rays should be done in this one area, thus minimizing the number of times the patients cranio-vertebral axis must be stressed.

There are many ways of immobilizing and stabilizing the spinal column on a temporary basis to prevent the non-paralyzed patient with a cervical or thoracic vertebral fracture from permanent cord damage. Spine boards and sand bags are excellent for this purpose.

The intubation of the trachea in patients with cervical spine injuries is a difficult problem. The kinds of movement necessary for positioning the head and exposing the larynx can produce irreparable spinal cord damage in patients with unstable cervical fracture. This situation contraindicates insertion of tracheal tubes until the patient's arrival in the operating room where lighting and equipment are ideal. Until that time airway patency will have to be maintained by oropharyngeal airways and frequent pharyngeal suctioning.

Even under the most ideal circumstances the problems of getting a tube into the trachea of a patient with an unstable cervical spine fracture are many. In any event the "team captain" is responsible for reminding supporting members of the team in anesthesia, neurosurgery and orthopaedics that the problem is present and is a real threat. In critical circumstances in which the tracheal tube had to be inserted before body cavities could be opened to control exsanguinating hemorrhage it was necessary to proceed regardless of the risks to the spinal cord. Now however with the advent of fiberoptics and the new flexible bronchoscopes the intubation of the trachea can proceed quickly through either the nose or mouth with almost no movement of the head or neck. The endotracheal tube is first threaded over the flexible fiberoptic bronchoscope. The bronchoscope is inserted under direct vision into the trachea. The endotracheal tube can then be pushed into position over the bronchoscope letting the bronchoscope act as a guidewire. This part can be done blindly if the bronchoscope has been properly inserted. Then holding the endotracheal tube in position with one hand the bronchoscope is removed leaving the endotracheal tube behind in its proper position in the trachea.

It must be emphasized that although stabilization of the vertebral column is a high priority, this priority does not necessarily refer to definitive, permanent techniques of stabilization being done while hemorrhage and shock are reducing the patient to a vegetable with renal shut-down. An example of this is taking time to insert Crutchfield tongs to stabilize a C_6 or C_7 fracture in a patient with a hemoperitoneum from a ruptured liver or lacerated spleen. Any dislocation should be reduced and the cranio-cervical axis stabilized temporarily with sand bags while immediate attention is directed to stopping hemorrhage.

After stabilization the cervical vertebrae are palpated individually evaluating crepitance, false motion and tenderness. Any suspicious findings must be considered a serious vertebral fracture until confirmed or disproved by roentgen exam. Figure 7-1 shows a C-2 fracture in a sixteen-year-old boy thrown from a motorcycle. This fracture was suspected because of tenderness to palpation over the area. The boy had very wisely been placed on a spine board by EMT's at the scene of the accident and the vertebral column immobilized. Even though a cervical

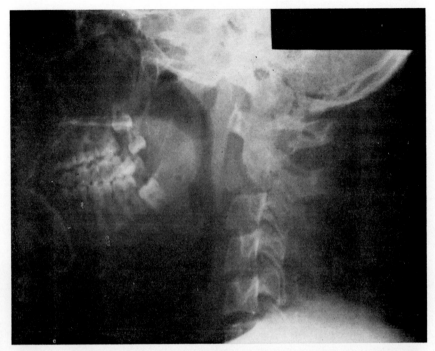

Figure 7-1. Roentgenogram of sixteen-year-old boy after a motorcycle accident shows fracture of cervical vertebrae number two.

fracture was suspected immediate x-rays were not done. The patient was exsanguinating from an extensive scalp wound which had completely scalped the boy "Indian fashion" and left the entire scalp hanging over his face attached by a pedicle.

Without being moved from the spine board the boy was taken to the operating room and hemorrhage controlled and the scalp returned to its normal position and sutured. After hemorrhage was controlled, still on the original spine board, X-rays were obtained which confirmed the suspected C-2 vertebral fracture. Crutchfield traction was then instituted and after four weeks the boy was discharged wearing a brace. Throughout this sequence he showed no paralysis and is active today with functioning spinal cord. At any point in his care, reckless abandon in transporting or failing to palpate the vertebral column in this boy could easily have resulted in permanent quadriplegia.

The thoracic and lumbar spine should also be palpated and percussed carefully but only after all question of cervical spine injury has been excluded. Strength and motion of all four extremities is tested. In the conscious patient, the fifth cervical segment can be evaluated by asking the patient to flex his elbows (biceps), then squeeze the examiners fingers (eighth cervical) and extend the elbows (seventh cervical, triceps).

The pattern of respiration is observed. Intercostal paralysis produces paradoxical movement of the chest and abdomen. Inefficient ventilatory exchange indicates the level of transection is so high that all intercostals are paralyzed and the patient will need immediate assisted ventilation.

The head is carefully inspected for scalp lacerations, local edema, and indentations. With an otoscope the external auditory canal and the nasal canals are visualized, looking for blood or cerebrospinal fluid. If blood is present in the external auditory canal and there are multiple scalp or facial wounds, some judgement must be used to determine whether the blood ran into the auditory canal from the external injuries or is present in the auditory canal because of a basilar skull fracture. The same is true of the nose. On the other hand, the presence of clear or bloody cerebrospinal fluid in either the external auditory canal or the nasal canals or blood behind the tympanic membrane usually signified a basilar skull fracture. Basilar skull fractures are rarely seen on roentgenograms of the skull.

With gloved hands and clean technique, the head is palpated for lacerations, embedded foreign bodies and depressed fractures. This is extremely important as it is surprising how large a foreign body can be hidden in a scalp laceration and the laceration sutured, leaving the foreign body behind. Palpation is the most reliable means of preventing such errors as some foreign objects are not opaque to X-ray and may not be detected.

Very little important information can be obtained by carrying this palpation further into the depths of compound wounds and it is better to apply a temporary occlusive pressure dressing and wait until X-rays are obtained and the scalp is shaved and cleaned with surgical soap before carrying this examination of the cranium further.

TABLE 7-I
EVALUATION OF HEAD INJURIES

General Principles
TRIAGE
—Rapidly assess the total patient
—Treat life-threatening injuries first
AIRWAY
—Highest priority is the airway, especially in supine unconscious patients
—Institute corrective measures immediately
—Beware of cervical spine fractures when intubating trachea
—Obtain serial arterial blood gases
—Obtain Fibrinogen Factor V, VIII concentrations, platelet count and protamine
  paracoagulation studies
Neurological examination
—Avoid terms such as stupor or semi-coma; rather describe patient's reactions
—Use simple check-off sheet as noted on opposite page
—Unilateral dilated and/or fixed pupil with contralateral hemiparesis suggests
  intracranial hemorrhage requiring immediate neurosurgical intervention
—Systolic hypertension and/or bradycardia supports this diagnosis
—Hypotension infrequently due to head injury; search for other causes
—Bleeding from auditory canal or blood behind the drumhead indicates basilar
  skull fractures rarely seen on X-ray
Neck injury in the unconscious patient (5 to 10%)
DIAGNOSTIC HINTS
—Flaccid areflexia, especially with flaccid rectal sphincter
—Diaphragmatic breathing
—Patient can flex forearms but not extend them
—Facial grimaces to pain above the clavicle but not below
—Hypotension without other evidence of shock
—Priapism is an uncommon but characteristic sign
CROSS TABLE LATERAL CERVICAL SPINE X-RAY
—Obtain in emergency department to reduce unnecessary patient movement
—Visualize all seven (7) cervical vertebral bodies, if necessary depress
  shoulders by pulling upper extremities toward feet
—Widening of posterior pharyngeal soft tissue shadow suggests spine injury
Scalp wounds
—Inspection difficult because of bleeding
—Debride, cleanse, and suture simple lacerations at a later time
—Palpate wound (sterile glove on index finger) for bone fragments
—Flaps with narrow base or poor blood supply require plastic surgery
Skull X-rays
Skull X-rays seldom contribute to the acute program. When obtained, the
following are important:
—Double density (depressed bone fragment)
—Linear fractures across major meningeal vessels, especially temporal bone
  or dural sinuses (epidural hematoma)
—Pineal shift (intracranial hematoma)
—Pneumocephalus (basal skull fracture)
—Foreign body
Special procedures
CEREBRAL ANGIOGRAPHY
—Best method to diagnose neurosurgical lesions
—Requires a trained team
ECHOENCEPHALOGRAM
A midline echo shift suggests a neurosurgical emergency
—Normal tests do not rule one out
ELECTROENCEPHALOGRAM
—Only to provide a baseline for brain death
LUMBAR PUNCTURE
—Contraindicated in obvious head injuries

Reproduced with permission, *Bulletin of the American College of Surgeons,*
vol. 59, 1974, p. 22.

The accurate assessment of cranicerebral trauma does not require unusual or sophisticated equipment. Although special tests will be mentioned briefly, the emphasis is placed on what any physician nurse or trained paramedic can observe (Table 7-I).

The most important guideline is the patients' level of consciousness. This is such a simple observation that it is often neglected. But the most important information a neurosurgeon can receive when he is finally called in consultation is "what was the patient's level of consciousness immediately after the accident?" and, "How has his level of consciousness changed in the intervening time?"

Even in obtaining such simple information, there are many pitfalls. Traditionally, vague, subjective terms such as drowsy, stuporous, semicomatose, comatose have been utilized. It becomes obvious when asking various physicians the meaning of these terms each one has his own idea and many times different meaning of these nonspecific terms. Avoid such terms in evaluating head injuries.

Objective information is always much more meaningful and helpful. This is especially true in evaluating neurological injuries because the first observer is very rarely the same individual who must make the final responsible decision in the definitive management of the neurologic system. In fact, the neurosurgeon is more frequently the tertiary or even in some cases the quaternary physician and as information is passed along the line of communication such non-objective terms such as drowsy or comatose become vague and misunderstood. As already pointed out the most valuable information the neurosurgeon can obtain is the level of consciousness of the patient prior to, and immediately after, the accident. In some instances in which the neurosurgeon does not have patient contact for several hours or days the changes in level of consciousness are most important.

For these reasons good records must be kept and communicated to others. Objective data regarding level of consciousness should be recorded accurately, objectively and concisely. If the patient appears sleeply or confused, but responds to verbal stimuli, it is more useful to others participating in the care and management of the patient to record "responds to verbal stimuli" rather than writing down "drowsy"; "unaware of time, place or person" rather than "confused" or "amnesic."

If the patient is unresponsive to verbal stimuli but responsive to pain, it is simpler and better to record this. If unresponsive to either verbal or painful stimuli, but makes purposeful movements, record this objective data instead of 'coma" or "semi-coma." Finally if the patient is unresponsive to verbal and painful stimuli and makes no purposeful movements, but has decerebrate posturing this information is more useful than terms such as "deep coma."

There also needs to be a standard means of evaluating a patient's response to painful stimuli. If the response of the patient to pain is to be meaningful as the hours elapse after injury then nearly the same degree or at least kind of stimulus should be evaluated. Again, this is especially important in these patients because often several physicians will have examined the patient over a period of time and if different kinds of painful stimuli are administered the patient's response may or may not be the same.

A standard evaluating procedure must be one which requires no special instruments and can nearly always have the same response. For this reason, it is best to determine the patient's response to pain by pricking the nasal mucosa with a pin or other sharp instrument. Safety pins are nearly always easily available and these make excellent instruments because everyone everywhere can utilize this evaluating mechanism and record the patient's response. If the patient responds with purposeful movement this should be recorded as important objective data. If the patient responds with decerebrate rigidity to this standard stimulus, this also is important objective data and should be recorded and communicated to others.

Some examiners prefer knuckle pressure over the sternum as a method of delivering a standard noxious stimulus. This is acceptable but the amount of stimulus will vary from time to time and vary with examiners. This method is usually done by rubbing the examiners knuckles firmly against the patient's sternum. Enthusiastic examiners may produce visible contusions which later under a different group of physicians might be

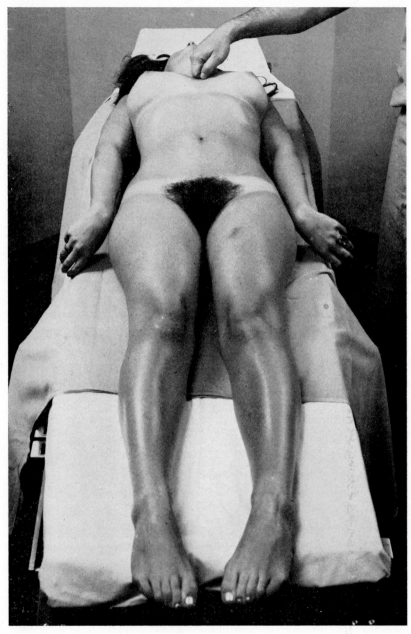

Figure 7-2. Sternal pressure elicits decerebrate posture when the brain stem is contused or compressed.

misconstrued to represent anterior chest trauma caused by the original injury. This can lead to confusion about a cardiac contusion or sternal injury.

By utilizing this objective data it is possible to evaluate the critically injured patient's level of consciousness. If the level of consciousness is progressively increasing at a steady rate no further evaluating procedures may be necessary. If the level of consciousness is increasing rapidly but then suddenly the patient shows deterioration, one must immediately begin to evaluate factors causing such deterioration. Anoxia or space occupying lesions are the chief offenders in such clinical states. Airway patency must be re-evaluated. Tracheobronchial toilet done and bronchoscopy if indicated. An endotracheal tube or tracheostomy may be necessary. Obstructed breathing in patients with minor brain injuries may produce hypoxia and cerebral edema sufficient to suddenly compress the brain stem and cause loss of consciousness even though initially the patients level of consciousness was improving progressively.

Close observation and recording of size inequality and reaction of pupils to light is the next most reliable sign in the patient who has sustained cranio-cerebral trauma. Agents to dilate the pupils must always be avoided. Fundoscopie examination can be done without the benefit of pharmacologically dilated pupils. As cerebral compression increases pupillary response to light becomes slower and the size of the pupil becomes larger. When dealing with large numbers of casualities, Meirowsky[4] states that changes in the quality of pupils may set forth priority for neurosurgical intervention.

If ventilation is assessed to be adequate yet level of consciousness is decreasing, space occupying lesions must be excluded. Signs of increasing intracranial pressure are evaluated.[5] Rising blood pressure, slowing of pulse rate and respiratory rate, papilledema, unilateral pupilary dilatation, headache, localizing weakness, and decreasing state of consciousness, singularly or in combination, should arouse suspicion and lead to cerebral angiography.

When intracranial pressure is sufficient to cause a herniation of the medial part of the temporal lobe (uncus) through the tentorial notch the neurologic findings are fairly classic: decerebrate posture, a motor weakness contralateral to the herniation and oculomotor nerve paresis ipsilaterally. If the dilated pupil and hemiparesis are found on the same side of the patient, the dilated pupil is given the greatest localizing significance.

It must be remembered that signs of increasing intracranial pressure may be due to cerebral edema rather than intracerebral hemorrhage or an extracerebral space occupying lesion. The differential of the underlying pathology cannot be determined from clinical neurologic examination alone and when there is definite manifestation of increasing intracranial pressure the patient must be investigated with cerebral angiography (see Chapter 14). Cerebral angiography is the test of greatest value in the diagnosis of intracranial hematomas after head injuries.[6] Troupp[7] advocates continuous and direct recording of intraventricular pressure in patients with severe brain injury.

Evaluating the motor system is the next important assessment in patients with injuries to the nervous system. It provides invaluable information localizing the sites of brain damage. There are three general categories of motor disturbances in the acute phase: (1) paralysis or paresis, (2) convulsions, (3) decerebrate rigidity.

Paresis

Weakness or paralysis of muscles on one side of the body result from injury to the opposite side of the brain. It can therefore be a very important localizing sign and each patient with head trauma should be carefully evaluated for muscle strength. The most important appraisal is to determine whether motor power is equal between the right and left sides of the body, then between upper and lower halves of the body. Any evidence of focal weakness is important and should be recorded as baseline on a "Neurologic watch sheet" (see Chapter 13).

If the disturbance of power is present immediately after the injury, brain injury, either contusion or laceration, is invariably present. If it develops subsequently the disturbance in motor power is the result of hemorrhage, cerebral edema or hypoxemia.

As a general guideline to use in evaluating these patients paralysis resulting from laceration or contusion usually involves one entire side of the body. Paralysis or paresis due to hematoma is more apt to express itself in one part such as the arm, the leg or the face. An exception to this general rule is the weakness caused by a very well localized depressed skull fracture over the motor strip.

Any assessor of critically injured people should check motor function frequently and record their findings for the next individual who assumes responsibility for the patient. A reliable and repeatable method is simply to ask the patient to support the weight of his own extremities in the air or comparing the power of the hand grip on the two sides. If the patient is unconscious or uncooperative, motor power can be estimated by observing the patient pattern of movement during periods of restlessness, or the degree of movement of a part in response to or withdrawal from pain.

Convulsions

Intracranial hemorrhage is the leading cause of convulsions after acute head injuries. When the seizures are focal (Jacksonian Seizures) cerebral arteriography and/or surgical exploration are mandatory. If the seizures are generalized the physician is still obligated to prove an intracranial clot is not the cause. This can usually be done with cerebral arteriography. Only then is it fair to the patient to relegate him to non-operative or conservative management.

Decerebrate Rigidity

Contusion of the brain stem produces a clinical syndrome that is strikingly obvious. It occurs most frequently after closed head injuries and usually does not occur for several hours after the trauma. The patient is unconscious and many stimuli such as pain, noise, rotation of the head, or even bright light, can initiate the paroxysms of decerebrate posturing. There is external rotation and adduction of the arms with volar flexion of the wrists and fingers. The thighs are adducted and the knees extended. There is plantar flexion of the feet; the ankles are internally rotated. It resembles the righting reflex of a decerebrate cat. There are periodic variations in sweat; at times the sweating is excessive; at other times the skin may be dry and flushed. The pupils fluctuate in size but are usually equal. The head is thrown back and extension of the spine may become so pronounced that the vertex of the head nearly approximates the buttocks.

Decerebrate posturing usually occurs in paroxysms. Between such paroxysms there is relative relaxation of the extensor muscles. But if forcibly flexed they gradually return to the extended position. Defecation and spurts of urination may occur, but penile erection is not a part of this complex as it is in the spasticity syndromes after injury to the upper spinal cord. The prognosis for survival is not good. Patients who are fortunate enough to recover from decerebrate rigidity are usually left with rather severe intellectual deficits.[13]

Spastic Hemiplegia

The complete loss of voluntary control of one side of the body is designated hemiplegia. Its greatest effect is on one side of the body and can usually be demonstrated soon after injury. Infrequently it may delay its appearance for several hours. Sometimes hemiplegia is present early after injury and is followed in a few hours by decerebrate posturing. This indicates brain damage to a focal area has occurred and then with increasing cerebral edema the uncus has been pushed through the incisura of the tentorium compressing the brain stem. Contrawise hemiplegia may be transient after brain injury and in two or three days disappear as cerebral edema subsides.

Spastic hemiplegia appears more frequently after penetrating head injuries or in situations where brain tissue is instantaneously[8] destroyed as by a depressed skull. The threat to survival from injuries producing hemiplegia is not as great as it is in the trauma producing decerebrate rigidity.

The head often remains rotated toward the unaffected side of the body. There are two reasons for this: (1) homonynmus hemianopsia frequently accompanies hemiplegia and makes vision on the affected side impossible. The extraocular muscles are not affected, but the eyes may be held toward the unaffected side to improve vision. (2) The neck muscles on the hemiplegic side are weak and turning the head toward the unaffected side aids vision.

The upper arm is internally rotated at the shoulder and held close to the trunk. The elbow is flexed and the forearm pronated. The wrist is kept at slight volar flexion, and the palm and fingers are cupped. The thumb is adducted and flexed so that it lies in the palm. The index finger is usually more strongly flexed than the other fingers.

The hemiplegic leg remains slightly flexed at the hip and knee while the foot is slightly plantar flexed and internally rotated at the ankle.

OCULAR MOVEMENTS

Evaluation of ocular movements in unconscious patients can aid in localizing the function loss of the brain in a rostral-caudal direction (Table 7-II). Two reflexes are especially important: (1) oculocephalic reflex (2) oculovestibular reflex.[9]

The oculocephalic reflex (Doll's Eye Phenomenon) provides a reliable method of assessing the integrity of extraocular movements. In normal subjects with the oculocephalic reflex intact, rapid passive turning of the head causes contralateral conjugate deviation of the eyes. The Doll's Eye phenomenon is tested in unconscious patients by holding the eyelids open and rapidly turning the head to one side. If the eyes move opposite to the head movements the oculocephalic reflex is intact. When the oculocephalic reflex is absent, that is, no ocular response occurs to rapid passive head turning in either direction a severe brain stem injury is present. If concealed hemorrhage has been positively excluded and this patient shows evidence of shock. The brain stem injury can be indicted as responsible for the "neurogenic shock" but as previously discussed brain stem injuries account for shock in only 3 percent or less of injured patients. The absence of the oculocephalic reflex can be very helpful in detecting brain stem injuries in the critically injured patient.

TABLE 7-II

ROSTRAL-CAUDAL LOCALIZATION
DIENCEPHALIC DYSFUNCTION

—consciousness depressed
—Cheyne-stokes respiration
—pupils small
—pupils react briskly to light
—facile withdrawal to painful stimuli
—progressing to immobility and decorticate posturing
—roving eye movements
—full range of eye movements in response to doll's head maneuver or ice water
  irrigations

MIDBRAIN SIGNS

—central neurogenic hyperventilation
—decerebrate rigidity
—pupils fixed
—ABSENT DOLL'S HEAD MANEUVER

LOW PONS

—flaccid quadriplegia
—no ocular movements to doll's maneuver or calorics
—pupils fixed to light in midposition
—respiratory rate returns to normal (an occasional pause at full inspiration)

MEDULLARY DYSFUNCTION

—falling blood pressure
—unpatterned or "gasping" respirations
—death imminent

If the reflex is normal and the patient is in shock a brain stem injury must not be blamed for the shock and an extremely aggressive search for concealed blood loss must be done.

Brain stem injuries can also be detected by caloric stimulation tests. Before this evaluation is done the previously discussed otoscopic inspecting of the ears should have been completed and cerebrospinal fluid leaks, ruptured tympanic membranes and impaction of cerumen checked for. If any of these are present caloric stimulation tests should not be done.

The method of caloric stimulation is simple. A standard 30 or 50 ml syringe can be used or a special irrigating ear syringe if available. With the head elevated 35° above the horizon the external ear canal is irrigated with ice water for up to three minutes—unless an ocular response occurs before this time. If needed a small straight red rubber catheter can be cautiously inserted into the auditory canal for irrigation purposes.

The caloric stimulation of normal subjects causes the eyes to deviate conjugately toward the side stimulated and a coarse

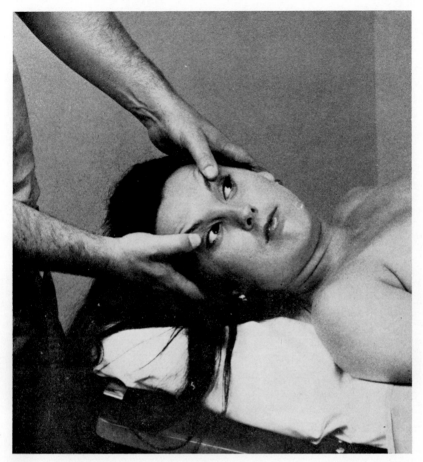

Figure 7-3. Testing the oculocephalic reflex (Doll's Eye Phenomenon) in unconscious patients.

horizonal nystagmus most pronounced when the patient looks to the side opposite the ear stimulated. The nystagmus has a fast component in the direction opposite to the ear being irrigated with ice water. In addition the normal subject pass-points to the side of stimulation. Occasionally nausea accompanies the above responses. After a five minute interval the opposite ear canal can be stimulated with ice irrigation.

An absent ocular response to irrigation with ice water on both sides is frequently associated with brain stem injury.

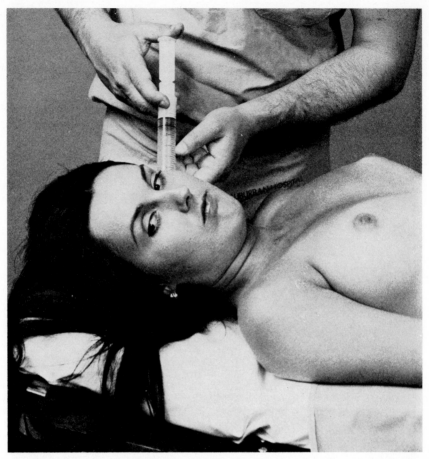

Figure 7-4.   Testing the oculo vestibular reflex by caloric stimulation.

SKULL FRACTURES

Roentgenographic evaluation of the skull should be deferred until priorities of airway obstruction, hemorrhage, repletion of blood volume, and stabilization of the vertebral column are managed. It is rare for the course of treatment of a patient with a head injury to be influenced by the presence or absence of a skull fracture. Classification of fractures based on descriptions of the line of fracture or even on the part of the skull involved is of little value.[10] Of course it is important to determine if the fragments of cranium are depressed against the brain, if the line of fracture crosses major vascular channels and if it is an open fracture.

Roentgenographic evaluation usually discloses fractures of the vault of the skull but basilar skull fractures are difficult to visualize. Fractures of the base of the skull must be detected by clinical signs. Bleeding from the auditory canal, blood behind the tympanic membrane, cerebrospinal fluid rhinorrhea are all manifestations of basilar skull fractures. Caution must be taken to exclude direct injury to the nose or ear and the drainage of blood from a face or scalp laceration into these orifices. A battle sign is a good clinical indication of fracture of the base of the skull (Fig. 7-5). This clinical sign is the result of bleeding into the tissues about the base of the skull and the mastoid process from the site of fracture in the base of the skull. Delayed periorbital ecchymosis is a sign of extravasation of blood from fracture sites that traverse the anterior fossa.

As a general rule brain injury is more severe if there has been fracture of the skull. The fracture per se is rarely responsible, it is only an indicator of the degree of the wounding force. The vault of the adult human skull is composed of dense strong laminated and resilient membranous bone. The base of the skull is formed of several inelastic cartilaginous bones. It is difficult for the base of the skull to sustain direct force. The convexity of the skull must experience tremendous force and transmit it to the base or undergo extreme deformity in order to disrupt the base of the skull.[10]

Fractures of the skull ordinarily form radiating lines outwardly from the point of impact and extending toward the opposite pole of the skull. A great force applied rapidly to a small area of the skull usually produces local depression. Most depressed skull fractures are open or compound, even though depression can occur without an open wound of the scalp. Depression of the skull along a linear fracture line may also occur but ordinarily these do not require surgical elevation because they are only 1 to 3 mm depressed. Comminuted fractures are usually depressed to a much greater degree.

The soft malleable skull of infants and young children absorb forces in a much different way than the rigid skull of adults.

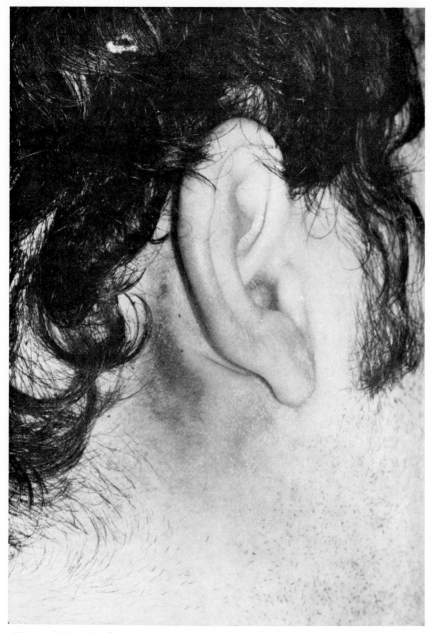

Figure 7-5.   Battle sign after head trauma indicates a basilar skull fracture.

Because of the pliability the wounding forces may be dampened and the brain protected to some extent. Many times fractures of children's skulls are overlooked and it may not be called to parents' or physicians' attention for several days or weeks when a hematoma or localized collection of spinal fluid signify a predisposing fracture. In infancy after initial forces deform the skull it may return quickly to normal contour once the force has stopped acting. As the skull bones unite, calcify and become rigid the forces delivered to the cranium are transmitted to the brain.[11]

If the head is suddenly set in motion by force or if the head is already in motion and suddenly experiences deceleration the cranial bones absorb some of the force but a great deal is transmitted to the brain. This makes the general rules about skull fractures of little value in assessing actual and potential damage to the brain. Brain injury must be appraised by clinical signs.

BRAIN INJURY

The brain may sustain either concussion or parenchymatous damage as a result of injury. Concussion is usually defined as a physiologic change produced by trauma leading to the loss of consciousness, which may occur without evidence of anatomic disruption of brain tissue In 1964 an ad hoc committee to study head injury nomenclature further defined concussion as "a clinical syndrome characterized by immediate and transient impairment of neural function, such as alteration of consciousness, disturbance of vision, equilibrium, etc. due to mechanical forces."[12] In concussion, the duration of unconsciousness after injury is usually measured in minutes. Ordinarily there is little if any evidence of neurologic or neural disabilities later. The physiologic basis of concussion is not well understood. Some studies indicate that thalamic and brain stem reticular formation have strong influence in maintaining normal waking cortical activity.[13] It is generally accepted that in concussion the electrical activity of the reticular formation is disturbed.[14]

Cerebral contusion may be focal or diffuse. When localized, contusions of the brain cause local neurologic abnormalities with or without disturbance of consciousness. But generalized contusion of the brain ordinarily is associated with immediate and long-standing coma. The morbidity and mortality are high (90%) and in those fortunate few patients who survive there are varying degrees of physical and mental disability. Local or generalized contusions of the brain can be confused with a subdural or epidural hematoma but cerebral arteriograms usually can exclude hematomas. Contusions of the summits of cortical gyri are commonly seen under the site of impact and particularly under fractures. Contrecoup injuries are contusions of parts of the brain opposite the actual site of impact. These contrecoup injuries are usually caused by deceleration forces and are typically seen at the orbitofrontal temporal or occipital poles.

Diffuse parenchymatous brain damage occurs from these decelerating injuries. Thrombosis of small vessels and small areas of hemorrhage are characteristic of these diffuse injuries. Changes in neurons similar to ischemic injury are found with pyknotic neurons exhibiting eosinophilia of their cytoplasm and shrinkage of nuclei. In addition chromatolysis and vacuolation in neurons with rapid disintegration of neurons appear to be specifically caused by trauma.[13]

In brain injury cerebral edema develops to varying degrees around areas of focal injury. As pointed out in the opening paragraphs of this chapter the degree of cerebral edema is increased by hypoxemia and shock. The edema is due primarily to swelling of the white matter of the hemispheres, but glial cells also undergo swelling.

Hemorrhage into the cerebral substance is another consequence of head trauma. It is generally regarded as the extreme index of cerebral insult as is "cerebral dissolution." A common site for these injuries is the frontotemporal region (posterior-inferior frontal and anterior temporal). Lin and associates[12] reviewed 153 intracerebral hematomas and found the majority was due to a contrecoup mechanism. They found a clinical pattern characterized by: trauma of the head, transitory unconsciousness, reorientation and residual hemiparesis. After several days drowsiness, headache and vomiting, choked disc and increasing hemiparesis ensue. There is edema of the white matter around the blood clot. Angiography usually gives the correct diagnosis.[6]

Intracerebellar hematomas result from contusion-laceration of the cerebellar cortex. The interesting clinical clue to this injury is severe opisthotonos.[13] Intracerebellar hematomas after trauma are rare compared to intracerebral hematomas. Cerebellar hematomas cause occipital headache, nausea, vomiting, ataxia and progressive obtundation with signs of brain stem compression.

Either cerebral edema or intracranial hematomas can cause herniations and secondary pontine hemorrhages. They are directly responsible for compression of the brain stem with medullary failure. Herniations of clinical significance which may be detected by cerebral angiography are: herniations of the cingulate gyrus under the free edge of the falx; herniations of the uncal gyrus through the tentorial notch with compression of the oculomotor nerve, posterior cerebral artery and midbrain; herniation of the cerebellar tonsils through the formen magnum with compression of the spinomedullary junction.[13]

In the opening paragraphs of this Chapter, I emphasized the detrimental effect of hypoxemia on cerebral edema and urged the blood gases be evaluated early in the course of the patients care and every effort made to correct the hypoxemia. A second factor that adversely influences the course of brain injuries is persistent bleeding. Brain tissue destruction cause severe defibrination. The correction of the hemostatic defects in patients with brain tissue destruction is of equal importance to correcting hypoxemia and hypovolemia. Blood should be drawn immediately for coagulation factor determination. In addition to the standard coagulation screening tests, fibrinogen concentration platelet count and protamine paracoagulation test should be done to assess the degree of defibrination. Goodnight and associates[15] found hemostatic failure due to acute defibrination in patients who had brain tissue destroyed. There were reduced levels of coagulation factors V, VIII and platelets and hypofibrinogenemia. A strongly positive protamine test was present. Defibrination was not detected in patients in whom head trauma did not destroy brain tissue. Delineating the degree of defibrination can help in differentiating actual destruction of brain tissue from other forms of head injury. Active defibrination does not persist. Therefore its correction early in the course of brain tissue destruction has the same priority as correcting hypoxemia and repletion of blood volume. In fact Goodnight and his colleagues recommend that twelve bags of cryoprecipitate (to provide fibrinogen and factor VIII) and two to four units of fresh frozen plasma should be given while waiting for the results of the evaluating tests. When the platelet count is also reduced they recommend correction with platelet concentrates.

Pontine hemorrhage is detected by quadriplegia, pin point pupils and eyes that cannot be deviated laterally even by ice water calorics. Spontaneous vertical "bobbing" movements of the eyes may occur and this indicates preservation of more rostral centers for vertical gaze.

EXTRADURAL HEMORRHAGE

The most common cause of extradural hemorrhage is laceration of a branch of the middle meningeal artery which enters the skull through the foramen spinosum and lies in a grove in the inner table of the temporal bone. Such a position makes this vessel extremely susceptible to injury. Dural sinus lacerations can also bleed into the extradural spaces. Injury of either the middle meningeal artery or the dural sinuses is usually caused by fractures of the cranium of the linear type.

The clinical pattern most often said to be associated with extradural hemorrhage is a blow to the head, usually temporal area, which may or may not produce unconsciousness. This is classically followed by a lucid interval during which the patient is symptom free. Within a short period of minutes or hours headache, vomiting, hypertension and bradycardia develop, weakness of the face, arm and leg soon follow. Sometimes there are convulsions. Then the level of consciousness begins to decrease and the pupil on the injured side dilates. When these last two changes develop the patient is near death. A tragic comment on care of critically injured patients is how frequently an undetected hematoma kills the patient (30 to 50%). Yet in its early stages if detected lends itself to a complete and permanent cure by an unusually simple and uncomplicated surgical procedure.

Many have observed and correctly so—that most patients with epidural hemorrhage do not have a "symptom free" interval, and the above picture is the exception rather than the rule. These patients are not entirely lucid but upon meticulous examination demonstrate some degree of confusion. Most have headache persisting from the time of the accident. Post-traumatic headache unrelieved by aspirin is a significant phenomenon and should not be overlooked nor minimized. If left undisturbed these patients usually sleep. Early neurologic signs are increased reflexes on the contralateral side from the trauma, with a Babinski response and a slightly enlarged pupil on the ipsilateral side. The linear fracture can be detected by X-ray but absence of a fracture does not exclude extradural hemorrhage. Cerebral angiography is usually definitive and shows displacement of vessels away from the inner table of the skull. The intermediate frontal region and posterior fossa can be misleading on arteriography especially if only anteroposterior roentgenograms are obtained (see Chapter 14). In these situations clinical signs outweigh the normal arteriography.

SUBDURAL HEMORRHAGE

In contrast to extradural bleeding subdural hemorrhage is usually from the venous side of the circulation, specifically one of the bridging veins between the cortex and the dura. Subdural bleeding can occur from very minor trauma. For purposes of classification hematomas in the subdural space are called acute, subacute, and chronic; the evolution of the different types is dependent upon the rate of bleeding and degree of associated brain injury.

Patients with acute subdural hematomas deteriorate rapidly and 90 percent or more die. The high mortality is usually due to associated brain injury more so than to amount of bleeding or volume of the hematoma. The chronic subdural hematoma can have a lucid interval of weeks or even months. The common complaint of the patient during this lucid interval is headache. Confusion is the most common sign. The paucity of signs and symptoms makes this a treacherous lesion. Any patient with head trauma who has any symptoms regardless how insignificant should at least be evaluated with brain scan and echoencephalography. Patients with additional findings that cause suspicion should then have cerebral angiography. An avascular space between the cortical vessels and the calvarium on the anteroposterior view indicate space occupying lesions.

APPRAISAL OF CRANIAL NERVES

Six percent of patients with neurologic injuries had trauma to the cranial nerves.[13] Such injuries were most often associated with fractures of the base of the skull. The most common cranial nerves injured are: olfactory, statoacoustic, fourth and sixth, facial, optic and trigeminal. The frequency of injury was in the order given.

It is imperative that the status of the cranial nerves be recorded at the time of the initial examination. Cranial nerve deficits that are present immediately after impact indicate laceration of the nerve and as noted above this usually accompanies a fracture of the base of the skull. Contrawise disturbances that appear later in head injury patients indicate the presence of an intracranial clot or severe cerebral edema. For example if the pupil is dilated and fixed immediately after a head injury it would usually be due to a laceration of the third cranial nerve but dilation of the pupil developing later, usually indicates an intracranial hematoma.

First Cranial Nerve

A fracture through the anterior fossa of the skull can injure the olfactory nerve. It can also be injured by direct contusion or laceration without fracture. Anosmia may be an unpleasant and sometimes permanent residual of head trauma but other than this small inconvenience it has little significance in assessing acute head injury.

Second Cranial Nerve

If blindness occurs immediately after an injury it is usually due to laceration of the optic nerve and frequently related to injuries in which the fracture line crosses the optic foramen. A recent patient on our trauma service had bilateral blindness from a severe skull fracture but this is rare. Decelerative forces can produce retinal hemorrhages and slow forming subdural clots may cause papilledema; they must be differentiated from optic nerve lacerations by fundoscopic examination.

Third Cranial Nerve

After head trauma the oculomotor nerve is frequently paralyzed by herniation of the temporal lobe through the incisura. This temporal lobe herniation is usually due to a space-occupying clot. The detectable result of this phenomenon is a progressive dilation of the pupil. The size of the pupil is not proportional to the size of the clot but to the degree of herination of the temporal lobe through the incisura. The size of the pupils and the reaction of the pupil to a strong light stimulus should be observed frequently and recorded on the neurologic watch sheet. In many patients the size of the pupils will vary spontaneously but they remain equal. These changes are not reliable diagnostically. It has been observed however that patients whose pupils vary in size but remain equal on the two sides seldom require surgical intervention.[10] Progressive dilatations of a pupil can as a rule be considered to indicate a space-consuming intracranial lesion.

Fourth Cranial Nerve

The trochlear nerve innervates the superior-oblique muscle and moves the eyeball downward and outward. Involvement of this nerve by intracranial hematomas, cerebral edema or herniation is rare.

Fifth Cranial Nerve

Fractures of the base of the skull rarely damage the trigeminal nerve. If injured it can be detected by loss of sensation over the skin of the face including forehead scalp cornea, orbit, nose, lips, teeth and mouth as well as the anterior two thirds of the tongue. The sensory deficits are accompanied by paralysis or weakness of the masseters and pterygoid muscles. The patients will therefore be unable to chew or move their jaw effectively. Injury of the trigeminal nerve is rarely of any specific diagnostic value in assessing the patient with a head injury.

Sixth Cranial Nerve

The abducens nerve innervates the external rectus muscle. Paralysis of the nerve results in the patient's inability to rotate the eyeball outward. Intracranial hematomas or cerebral swelling rarely cause injury to this nerve. When injured it is usually due to a severe skull fracture involving the petrous bone or cavernous sinus.

Seventh Cranial Nerve

Fractures of the base of the skull can also involve the facial nerve. It may be instantaneous after injury and involve all the muscles of facial expression. The patient is unable to close his eye, move the muscles of his cheek, or elevate the corner of his

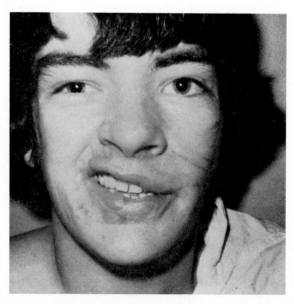

Figure 7-6.   Facial nerve paralysis after a head injury in a seventeen-year-old boy. Note inability to elevate the corner of his mouth on the left.

mouth (Fig. 7-6). Depending upon the site of fracture, taste over the anterior part of the tongue may also be affected. This peripheral type injury of the facial nerve can develop hours or a few days after the initial injury. It is more apt to occur in patients who have had bleeding from an ear or other evidence of a basilar skull fracture. The peripheral type facial nerve deficit does not reflect the presence of an intracranial clot.

Brain injury over the face area of the cerebral hemisphere produces a different kind of paralysis than basilar skull fractures. In this central type facial nerve injury only the lower half of the face is affected because there is dual innervation to the muscles about the eye and forehead. This lower facial weakness is very early evidence of a small focal hematoma over the cerebral hemisphere. It must be remembered that the cerebral hemisphere involved is opposite to the facial weakness.

Eighth Cranial Nerve

Skull fractures through the petrous portion of the temporal bone may sometimes injure the acoustic nerve. This nerve has two parts: (1) chochlear (2) vestibular. In trauma the two segments are usually equally involved. The chochlear segment innervates hearing and this can readily be evaluated by testing the patient's ability to hear. The vestibular segment innervates the equilibrium apparatus and the patient experiences vertigo and ataxia. The kinds of fractures of the base of the skull which involve this nerve also cause bleeding from the ear and cerebrospinal fluid leakage. When this combination is detected never irrigate the external auditory canal and never insert plugs of cotton or other foreign bodies.

Ninth Cranial Nerve

The glosspharyngeal nerve is part motor and part sensory. Motor fibers innervate the stylopharyngeus muscle which elevates and widens the pharynx during swallowing. It supplies sensation to the mucous membranes of the throat, tonsils, soft palate and posterior part of the tongue. It also supplies taste fibers to the posterior part of the tongue. It is rarely involved alone. Most of the patient noticed and physician detectable deficits are loss of sensation. The stylopharyngeus plays such a minor role in swallowing that very little impairment is present and usually not noticed by the patient nor detectable by the physician.

Tenth Cranial Nerve

The vagus is a long nerve. Its intracranial segment can be involved in some severe fractures of the base of the skull. In the neck it is subject to injury by gunshot wounds, lacerations, or stab wounds. On examination of the throat the palate droops on the injured side. The patient is asked to say "Ah" and the palate moves to the injured side. The palatal and pharyngeal reflex is absent. The vocal cord on the side of the injury is abducted. This can be seen with a laryngeal mirror or directly with a laryngoscope. Sensation is absent in the external auditory meatus and the pinna of the ear.

Eleventh Cranial Nerve

Traumatic injury of the spinal accessory nerve is rare. It innervates the sternocleidomastoid and trapezuis muscles. The neck loses its normal contour if this nerve is injured. The scapula is rotated downward and outward. There is inability to raise the shoulder because of weakness of the trapezuis and the arm cannot be raised above the horizontal plane. The loss of sternocleidomastoid function produces flatness of the neck on the affected side, and failure of the muscle to stand out on rotation of the neck.

Twelfth Cranial Nerve

The hypoglossal nerve is entirely a motor nerve and supplies the muscles of the tongue. The tip of the tongue tends to curl to the uninjured side; on protrusion it deviates to the uninjured side and cannot be pushed firmly against the cheek.

The 9, 10, 11, 12 cranial nerve injuries rarely have diagnostic significance in evaluating craniocerebral injuries but their function should still be evaluated in regard to extracranial lacerations, gunshot and stab wounds.

SPINAL CORD INJURIES

It has been estimated that 5,000 patients sustain spinal cord injuries each year in the United States. At least 50 percent of these patients have neurologic complications.[13] Stabilization of the spinal column is one of the highest priorities in managing critically injured patients. Once again, the physician's responsibility extends to pre-hospital care and transportation of these individuals to special centers. It is in this Phase I area that trained emergency medical technicians can make the difference between permanent cord damage and a reversible injury.

The patient must be transported without bending or extending the spine; maintaining neutral position with spine boards applied at the scene of the accident. If the patient has no sensation or movement from the shoulders down, a cervical cord injury must be suspected and the head sustained in a neutral face forward position with sandbags or other immobilizing supports on either side. When the head and neck are rigidly immobilized, great responsibility falls upon the attendants to give extreme care to clearing secretions, blood, vomit, etc., from the airway.

In assessing patients with spinal cord injuries establishing the mode of injury and careful neurological examination are mandatory. An alert patient can give his own history, but frequently information must be garnered from relatives, highway patrolmen, or EMT.

A patient who dives into unknown waters and surfaces paralyzed must be suspected of cervical cord injury. A construction worker or mine worker buried in a cave-in and is removed from the shaft paralyzed from the waist down must be suspected of thoracic cord injury. In both these situations, information regarding whether sensory or motor symptoms were present immediately or developed enroute to the hospital is critical. EMTs and rescue workers must be taught to make such initial and critical observations.

A cervical spine lesion may paralyze the intercostal muscles and accessory muscles of respiration but spare the diaphragm. Inspection of respiratory patterns shows no intercostal movement and diaphragmatic breathing is present. High spinal cord injuries may also produce autonomic paralysis with subsequent hypotension. Hypotension *per se* does not mean shock. If there is evidence of decreased peripheral perfusion tachycardia, cold, clammy skin and pallor, attention should be directed to repletion of blood volume and detecting sites of concealed blood loss.

The spine should be palpated carefully one vertebrae at a time without turning the patient. Hematomas and seat belt marks should be noted. Motor power is assessed by asking the conscious cooperative patient to move his limbs, the unconscious or uncooperative patient must be given a painful stimulus and movement of the extremity carefully observed. Are these movements purposeful? Motor power at the shoulder, elbows and wrist should be recorded in specific descriptive terms or a grading system that is simple and universally understood.

Levels of hypoalgesia must be established by response to pinwheels or needle sticks. A hypoalgesic level just above the nipple indicates an injury betwen C-4 and T-5. There is some overlapping of the supraclavicular nerves in this area. Later a more specific localization can be determined by axillary and arm examination.

A saddle hypoalgesia from a cauda equina injury will be missed unless the sensory evaluation includes the perineum and back of the legs. Perineal sensation is also important in paraplegic injuries as sacral sensation is sometimes spared. Posterior column sensation should be assessed by position and vibration sense from the toes upward. These modalities are preserved in the anterior cord syndromes.

Deep tendon reflexes are helpful in evaluating cord injuries. Such reflexes persisting below a sensory and motor level several hours after injury may indicate an incomplete lesion and suggest early neurosurgical consultation regarding decompressive laminotomies. In the first few hours after an injury deep tendon reflexes below the level of a complete cord transection are usually absent. The plantar response is usually flexor in the acute phase of spinal cord injury.

There are numerous ascending and descending tracts in the

spinal cord. In evaluating injuries of the spinal cord there are three that all clinicians should remember:

1) Spinothalamic Tract—at any given level this tract conducts sensory impulses of temperature, pain and crude touch from the OPPOSITE side of the body.

2) Posterior Columns—conduct impulses of light touch vibration and position sense from the SAME side of the body.

3) Corticospinal Tracts—conduct impulses for voluntary motor control of the SAME side of the body.

Since the spinal cord is a segmented organ with lower motor neurons arranged in a rostro-caudal manner, the clinician should remember the relationship in Table 7-III. Vertebral injuries below Lumbar 1 are usually associated with injuries of the roots of cauda equina because the spinal cord terminates at the lumbar 1 or 2 level in most people.

Two kinds of injuries usually occur in the spinal cord itself: complete and incomplete.[16] The complete type means either an anatomical or functional transection of the cord producing a total loss of motor and sensory dysfunction caudal to the injury. Associated with the total sensory and motor loss is autonomic dysfunction producing priapism, absence of sweating, loss of bowel and bladder control. Vasomotor tone is absent below the level of transection and causes significant reduction in blood pressure. If there is evidence of any function below an injury, the spinal cord lesion must be considered incomplete.

Incomplete injuries of the spinal cord can produce several different patterns. For the purposes of this book only two will be described. The first is the anterior cord syndrome.[17] The anterior two-thirds of the cord function is absent. This would include the spinothalamic tracts and corticospinal pathways

TABLE 7-III

TOPOGRAPHY	SKELETON	SPINAL CORD
Neck	C1—C4	C2—C4
Arms	C5—T1	C5—T1
Thorax, Abdomen	T2—T10	T2—L1
Legs	T10—L1	L2—S2
Sphincters	L1	S2—S4

bilaterally; voluntary motor activity, deep pain and temperature sensation are lost below the injury. Light touch, vibratory and position sense are retained bilaterally because the posterior columns are spared. A deceleration injury, ventral mass or ischemia due to interruption of the anterior spinal arteries produces the anterior cord syndrome.

A classic incomplete cord injury is known as the Brown-Seguard syndrome due to spinal cord hemisection. There is ipsilateral loss of motor power, light touch, position and vibration sense below the level of injury and contralateral loss of pain and temperature sensation.

The central cord syndrome results from hyperextension in the cervical area.[17] Peripheral tracts in the cord are spared. The corticispinal, spinothalamic and posterior columns to the lower extremities are frequently intact. When the patient is evaluated, there is profound weakness of the arms, with more strength in the lower extremities including intact position sense. Anterior-posterior compression of the spinal cord by infolding of the ligamentum flavum occurs with extreme extension of the neck.

The shorter the time between injury and neurologic deficit, the graver the outcome. In like manner, a prolonged interval after injury before onset of the neurologic deficit indicates in most instances a better prognosis for recovery. Hence, it is important in evaluating these patients to approximate the time interval between injury and symptoms. The completeness of the neurologic deficit on initial evaluation is also prognostic. Incomplete motor weakness and spotty sensory loss are encouraging whereas total sensorimotor deficiencies portends minimal recovery. On the other hand, early return within twenty-four to forty-eight hours after injury suggests the patient may even improve to the point of full recovery.

Age of the patient is a major factor in assessing spinal cord injuries. Beyond the seventh decade the mortality is 50 percent regardless of the level of injury, and 100 percent in the eighth decade. The level of spinal cord injury is highly prognostic. Total transection above the fourth cervical level produces 50 percent mortality within thirty days whereas an injury at the fifth cervical level had a thirty day mortality of only 19 percent. Gol[19] has divided cervical spinal cord lesions into two main categories based on whether there is X-ray evidence of fracture or dislocation (Table 7-IV).

SPINAL TAP AND MANOMETRICS

There are actually very few indications for spinal taps and manometrics in evaluating neurologic injuries. Sometimes in children with an obvious spinal cord deficit. If a history of trauma cannot be elicited or is denied an appraisal of cerebrospinal fluid and pressure changes can be helpful. A non-traumatic spine tap with blood in the CSF is strong evidence in favor of trauma. When there is an open fracture of the vertebral column and meningitis is suspected a spinal tap can be helpful in evaluating the patient.

Extradural compression of the cord by large intervertebral disc fragments, bone fragments or extradural hematomas may be detected by a spinal tap with manometrics and myelography. Rarely edema alone may be the cause of a complete manometric subarachnoid block. Drake[18] advocates myelography to detect blocks, feeling that manometrics are unreliable.

The greatest problem is in the patient with at least some function and evidence of a cerebrospinal fluid block. If there is no definite evidence that a bone fragment or disc material is compressing the spinal cord, and reasonably good function is present the patient is immobilized with traction and observed. Any functional deterioration indicates surgical exploration. Discography has been helpful in some instances.[18] If the discs are intact the major problem is most likely edema. If discography shows nucleus pulposus material is extruded operative intervention is indicated.

PERIPHERAL NERVE INJURIES

Nerve injury is suggested by pain, paresthesias, or intense burning in the sensory distribution of the injured nerve. Symptoms are increased by palpation of the suspected nerve.

TABLE 7-IV
CLASSIFICATION OF CERVICAL SPINAL CORD INJURY
A. No neurological deficit

	Category I Without X-ray Evidence of Dislocation or Fracture	Category II With X-ray Evidence of Dislocation or Fracture
Acute and Subacute	Traction—physiotherapy.	a. *Dislocation*: Traction with tongs to fifty-five pounds, reduce to three to six hours. Sometimes fusion. b. *Fracture*: Tongs to twenty-five pounds, possibly myelography and laminectomy later.
Chronic	as above.	Traction as above—usually little change. Myelography and surgical reduction or laminectomy if indicated.

B. Neurological deficit improving

Acute Subacute and Chronic	Traction—physiotherapy; myelogography if recovery incomplete; surgery if significant compressing lesion demonstrated.	As in *a* above, but myelography if recovery incomplete and surgery if significant compression lesion shown.

C. Neurological deficit increasing

Acute and Subacute	Traction, hourly checks. If no improvement in three hours in acute or twelve hours in subacute, or deterioration continues, emergency myelography and surgery if indicated.	Tong traction as in *a* until reduced. If still deteriorating over a period of hours, myelography and surgery if indicated.
Chronic	As for acute, but prior of observation up to twenty-four hours.	Tong traction. If no improvement in twenty-four hours, myelography and surgery if indicated.

D. Neurological deficit stable

Acute	Traction. If no improvement in twelve to twenty-four hours, myelography and surgery if indicated.	Tong traction as in *a*. If no improvement or a plateau reached, myelography and surgery if indicated.
Subacute and Chronic	As for acute, but period of observation of up to two days.	Tong traction. If no improvement in two to three days, myelography and surgery if indicated.

E. Apparent cord transection

Acute	Emergency myelogram or with open manometric test may observe two to three hours, with traction. If no change, myelography and surgery if indicated.	Tong traction as in *a*. If no change three hours after reduction, myelogram and surgery if indicated.
Subacute	Myelogram, and surgery rarely indicated.	Tong traction as in *a*. If no improvement in twelve hours, myelography, and surgery rarely indicated.
Chronic	Make comfortable.	Make comfortable.

Reproduced by permission Gol, A.: *J Trauma*, vol. 5, 1965, p. 379.

Careful scrutiny of the traumatized limb for nerve injury is an important part of evaluating critically injured patients. Significant neurologic deficits are easily overlooked unless one examines the extremity with the idea of nerve deficits in his mind. Examination for motor deficits in the acutely injured patient is frequently unrewarding because of the pain associated with the original trauma.

Obvious injuries leading to wrist drop or foot drop are quickly observed and recorded. Examination with a pinwheel or pin prick looking for sensory deficits is a reliable means of evaluating injuries to peripheral nerves. Another objective observation is the absence of sweating over the distribution of the involved nerve.

Where nerve injury is complete, evaluation is fairly easy, but assessment of crushed, contrused, stretched or partially transected nerves, presents difficult problems and requires astute observations because the signs of deficits in these injuries are not always clear-cut.

Peripheral nerve injuries are generally categorized by three descriptive terms.[20]

Neurontomesis indicates both neural and connective tissue elements of the nerve are completely divided. This represents complete anatomic transection of the nerve.

Axontomesis implies injury to only the axon with the supporting structures intact. Even the Schwann cell tube is intact in this kind of peripheral nerve injury.

Neuroproxia occurs when no anatomic interruption of nerve function has occurred, but conduction of neural impulses is blocked.

Neurontomesis results in immediate flaccid paralysis of the muscles supplied by the nerve and progressive atrophy of denervated muscles.

BRACHIAL PLEXUS

This complex structure of nerve roots has been the nemesis of several generations of medical students dissecting out and memorizing its various components (Fig. 7-7). Injuries to the

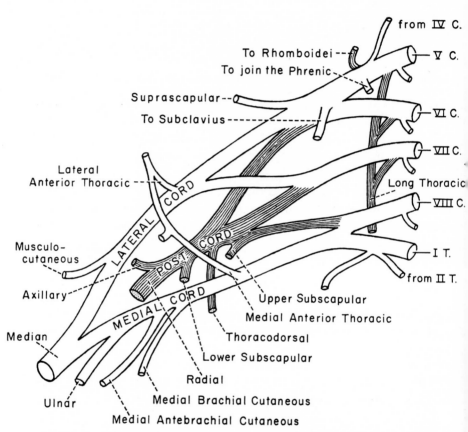

Figure 7-7. Comprehension of the plan of the brachial plexus is essential in evaluating injuries to this complex structure of nerves. (Reproduced with permission from *Gray's Anatomy of the Human Body,* 29th Ed. Philadelphia, Lea and Febiger, 1974.)

brachial plexus are important and serious injuries. Profound and significant neurologic deficits follow disruption and trauma of this plexus of nerves. Some can produce very perplexing neurologic pictures. Plexus injuries are important for another reason. It has an intimate relationship with the subclavian artery and vein and the dome of the pleura otherwise known as Gibson's fascia.

Penetrating wounds in this region need operative exploration after clinical evaluation (see Chapter 12). Closed injuries of the brachial plexus have been divided into three types: 1) total, 2) upper (Erb-Duchenne type), and 3) lower type (Klumpke).

The upper type (Erb) results from injury to C5 and C6, usually by extreme lateral bending of the head away from the side of injury and depression of the ipsilated shoulder. There is inability to abduct the arm (deltoid), to flex the arm (biceps, brachialis, supinator longus), to rotate the arm outward (supra and infraspinati) and to supinate the forearm. Sensation is lost in a shield-like area over the deltoid and across the arm and forearm.

The lower type brachial plexus injury is detected by examining the patient for function of the flexor digitorum (flexion of the fingers) weakness of flexion at the wrist (flexor carpi ulnaris), paralysis of abduction and adduction of the fingers (interossei) and for abduction, adduction and flexion of the thumb. It is obvious from this examination of the patient that the Klumpke or lower type injury of the brachial plexus results in denervation of the median and ulnar nerves.

The complete injury to the brachial plexus implies a total loss of function throughout the area supplied by the plexus or a combination of the upper (Erb) and lower type (Klumpke). A treacherous injury and one that must be carefully watched for because the patient may be accused of being hypochondrical or hysterical is an incomplete injury combining both the upper and lower type and the patient has dissociated loss so that sensation may be present and motor function absent. These patients should not be labeled "crocks" and disregarded. The reason for such dissociated losses in peripheral nerves is the greater susceptibility of large motor fibers to stretch injury. The classic findings of dissociated loss of motor power from sensation should establish the diagnosis of an incomplete injury to the brachial plexus.

UPPER EXTREMITY

Five major nerves should be evaluated in injuries of the upper extremities (Table 7-V). The axillary nerve (circumflex n.) supplies the deltoid muscle and a small oval area of sensation over the deltoid. Abduction of the arm and shoulder is the test to determine motor function of this nerve. One must remember, however, that the first 15° of abduction is initiated by the supraspinatus, and it is only when attempting to abduct the arm beyond 15° that deltoid innervation can be assessed. The patient with injury to the axillary nerve when attempting to abduct the arm and shoulder will tilt his trunk away from the affected side in an effort to abduct the denervated shoulder.

Flexion of the arm at the elbow is the crucial test in evaluating injury to the musculocutaneous nerve. The sensory loss is over the radial side of the forearm. The musculocutaneous nerve is derived from the lateral cord of the brachial plexus. It accompanies the median nerve through the axilla and passses to the radial side of the arm traversing the coracobrachialis muscle and from thence, descends between the biceps and brachialis supplying all three muscles. At the elbow the musculocutaneous becomes the lateral cutaneous nerve of the forearm. Some amount of flexion of the forearm may still be present because the brachioradialis is innervated by the radial nerve. The coracobrachialis draws the humerus forward and inward.

The median nerve innervates most of the flexor muscles of

TABLE 7-V

FIVE MAJOR NERVES TO EVALUATE IN
UPPER EXTREMITY INJURIES

1. Axillary (Circumflex N.)
2. Musculocutaneous
3. Median
4. Ulnar
5. Radial

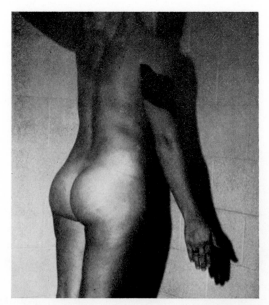

Figure 7-8. Inability to abduct the arm more than 15' degrees indicates axillary nerve injury. Sensory loss is confined to area shown in solid black.

the forearm and the thenar eminence. Wrist and finger flexion is impaired when this nerve is injured and ability to touch the thumb to the little finger is lost. There is also weakness in pronation of the forearm (pronator teres). When the patient is asked to make a fist, only the ring and little fingers flex. When the patient is asked to flex the wrist, ulnar deviation of the wrist occurs.

The ulnar nerve accompanies the brachial artery in the arm, then passes posteriorly to reach the groove in the medial epicondyle of the humerus at the elbow; here it is very susceptible to injury. It supplies motor function to the flexor muscles of the ulnar side of the arm and the intrinsic muscles of the hand. The interossei and lumbricals of the third and fourth fingers. Trauma to the ulnar nerve renders the patient unable to abduct and adduct the fingers. The patient should also be asked to flex the wrist and if ulnar nerve function is absent the wrist deviates radially due to paralysis of the flexor carpi ulnaris. The sensory loss results in numbness over the dorsal and palmar surface of the little finger (Fig. 7-10a and 7-10b).

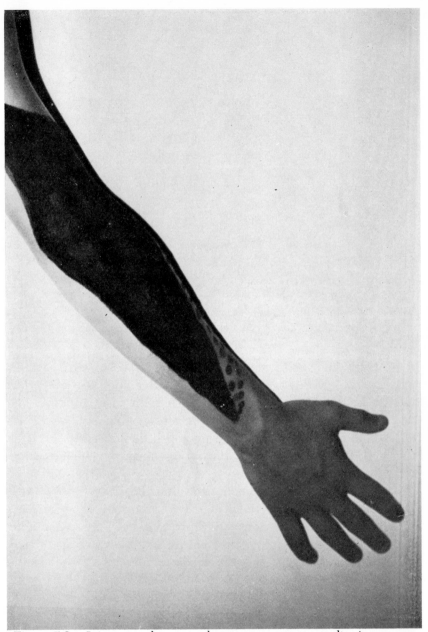

Figure 7-9. Injury to the musculocutaneous nerve results in sensory deficit supplied by the lateral antebrachial cutaneous nerve (stippled area). Radial nerve injury causes loss of sensation to the dorsum of the arm as illustrated in black (posterior antebrachial cutaneous nerve) wrist drop and sensory loss to the hand as depicted in Figure 7-10.

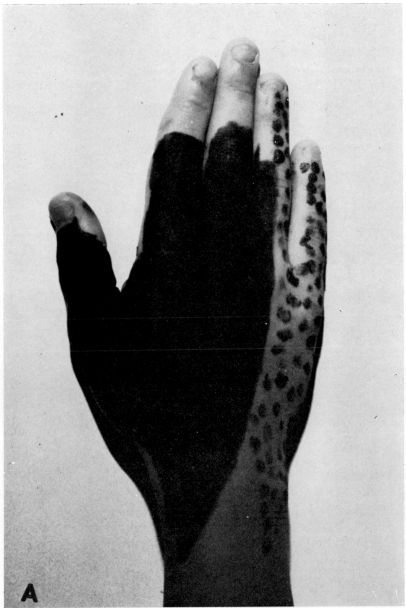

Figure 7-10. Radial nerve injury results in loss of sensation over dorsum of hand as illustrated in solid black. The stippled area shows sensory loss in ulnar nerve injuries and the unshaded tips of the finger have loss of sensation after median nerve injury (a). The palmar surface of the hand shows sensory loss from ulnar nerve injury (solid black) and median nerve injury (stippled area) (b).

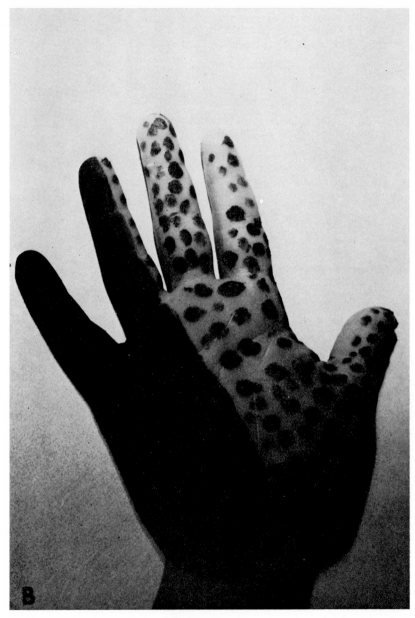

Figure 7-10b.

The radial nerve is the main branch of the posterior cord of the brachial plexus and is very susceptible to injury as it passes in front of the lateral epicondyle of the humerus between the brachialis and brachioradialis muscles. It is chiefly a motor nerve and clinical evaluation is mainly assessment of motor function. The radial nerve is the main extensor innervator of the arm, wrist and fingers. It supplies the triceps, anconeus, supinators extensor carpi radialis longus, extensor carpi radialis brevis, extensor communis digitorum and the extensor pollicis longus and brevis muscles.

Injury to the nerve above the branch supplying the triceps muscle results in loss of extension of the forearm, loss of extension of the wrist with subsequent wrist drop, inability to extend the fingers, loss of extension of the thumb, and weakness of flexion of the elbow. The triceps reflex is absent and there is loss of sensation over the dorsum of the hand (Fig. 7-11).

Injury to the radial nerve below its bifurcation into a deep motor branch which passes under the origin of the extensor carpi radialis and a superficial sensory branch which passes over this muscle results in almost a pure motor syndrome. The dorsal interosseous nerve alone is damaged at this point and results in finger drop because of weakness of extension of all fingers. When the patient is asked to extend the wrist, the wrist deviates to the radial side because of weakness of the extensor carpi ulnaris.

The most frequent site of trauma to the radial nerve is in the arm resulting from a fracture of the humerus. All patients with fractures of the humerus should be suspect and should be evaluated for wrist drop, loss of extension of fingers and thumb, weakness of flexion of the forearm at the elbow and weakness of supination.

Trauma to the radial nerve below the branch to the supinator longus gives the same picture except flexion of the forearm and supination are uninvolved.

LOWER EXTREMITY

There are three major nerves in the leg that should be evaluated clinically (Table 7-VI).

The femoral nerve (L2, 3, 4) is susceptible to injuries by

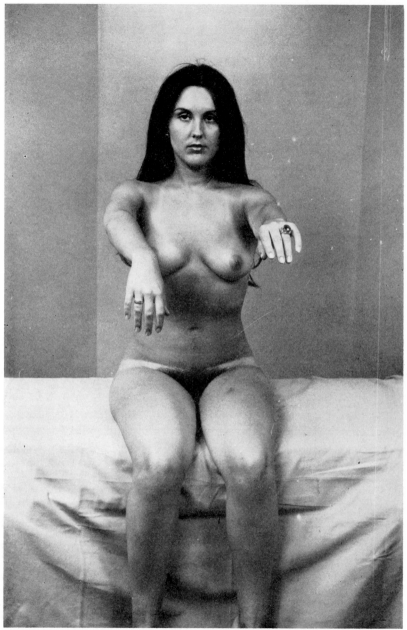

Figure 7-11.   Trauma to the radial nerve causes an obvious wrist drop on the injured side.

TABLE 7-VI

THREE MAJOR NERVES TO LOWER EXTREMITY
REQUIRING ASSESSMENT

1. Femoral
2. Obturator
3. Sciatic
      Posterior tibial
      Peroneal

gunshot and stab wounds of the groin. It supplies motor function chiefly to the quadriceps, femoris, startorius, and pectineus muscles. The patient with this injury is unable to extend his knee and has bouts of sudden falling when attempting to walk or stand. Anesthesia is present along the medial aspect of the thigh, leg and foot. The knee jerk is abolished (Figs. 7-12a and 7-12b).

The sciatic nerve may be damaged by penetrating injuries or in association with fractures about the hip, pelvis or thigh. The sciatic nerve (L, 5 and S1, 2, 3) is the largest nerve in the body and supplies motor functions to most of the muscles of the thigh and leg. It provides innervation to the main flexors of the leg on the thigh (hamstrings).

It divides into common peroneal and tibial at varying points between the sciatic notch and the popliteal space. The common peroneal eventually dividing into the superficial and deep peroneal nerves. The common peroneal is most vulnerable at the knee where it winds around the head of the fibula.

The deep *peroneal nerve* innervates the dorsiflexors of the foot and toes (tibialis anterior, extensor digiroum longus, extensor hallucis longus, and peroneus tertius). Injury to this nerve or the common peroneal leads to foot drop and a high stepped gait. Should the injury miss the common peroneal and spare the superficial peroneal, the patient would tend to evert his foot when attempting to walk. Sensory loss is illustrated in Figure 7-13 and is limited.

The superficial peroneal nerve supplies the evertors of the foot. When isolated injury to this nerve occurs the patient is asked to dorsiflex the foot and the foot has a tendency to invert. Eversion of the foot is weak. The sensory deficit is over the

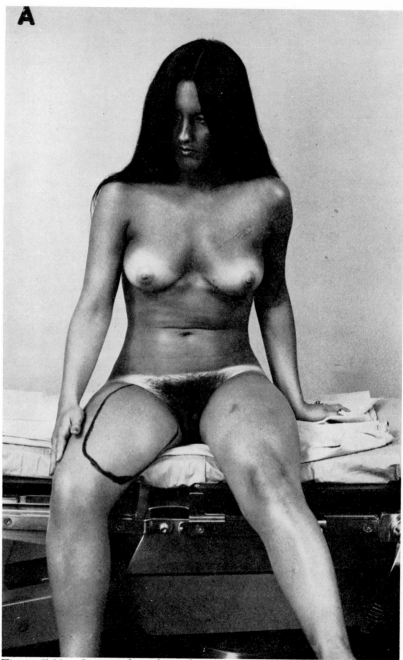

Figure 7-12.   Sensory loss from femoral nerve injury is to the medial thigh and the patient is unable to extend her knee (a).   Saphenous nerve sensory deficit is over lateral foreleg and the patient is unable to dorsiflex the foot (b).

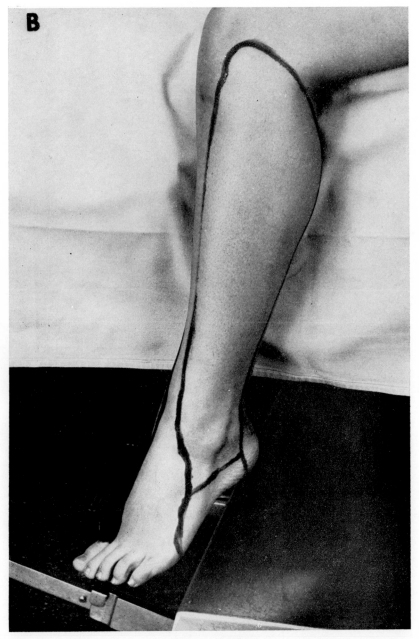

Figure 7-12b.

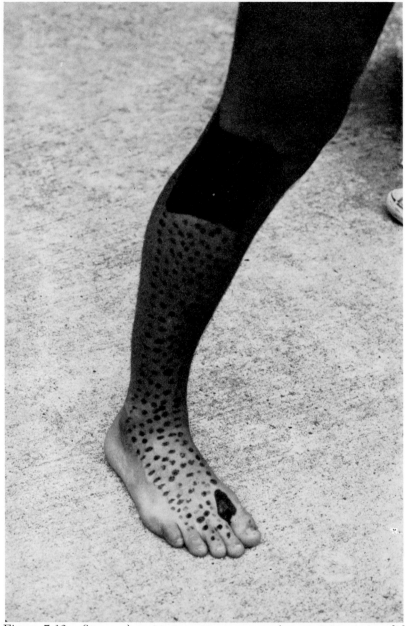

Figure 7-13.   Sensory loss due to common peroneal nerve injury is in solid black and the deficit due to superficial peroneal is shown by the stippled area.   (Note: common peroneal injury produces a loss of sensation of a triangle between the first and second toes.

lateral aspect of the lower half of the leg and the dorsum of the foot sparing the region between the first and second toes as previously described for the common peroneal (see Fig. 7-13).

Injury to the common peroneal produces the sum of the defects described above for the isolated deep peroneal and superficial peroneal.

The tibial nerve is fairly well protected from injuries since it lies deep in the popliteal fossa. The most common type of injury to this nerve is a penetrating wound of the popliteal space and it will often occur in combination with injury to the popliteal artery. The tibial nerve is the main flexor nerve of the leg and foot. In the popliteal fossa it supplies the gastrocnemius plantaris, soleus, and popliteus and usually the tibialis posterior.

At the level of the fibrous arch of the soleus muscle the tibial nerve becomes the posterior tibial nerve and its branches supply the soleus and tibialis posterior as well as the flexor digitorum longus. The posterior tibial nerve terminates by dividing into the medial and lateral plantar nerves.

A patient with a tibial nerve injury has weakness when attempting to flex the toes. This results in a characteristic deformity best described as claw foot. There is also weakness of abduction of the first and second toes. Cupping of the foot is ineffective. The sensory loss is limited to the heel (Fig. 7-14). An anastomotic branch of the tibial nerve joins with an anastomotic branch of the peroneal nerve contributing to the sural nerve which is purely sensory function over the lateral aspect of the leg and foot (see Fig. 7-14). When injury of the tibial nerve occurs above the origin of the nerves to the gastrocnemius, plantaris, soleus and popliteus, there is weakness of plantar flexion of the foot.

If the major trunk of the sciatic nerve is injured, the patient has no motion of the foot or toes and has an anesthetic foot.

The obturator nerve supplies the abductor muscles of the thigh. This nerve is usually injured when there is serious trauma to the medial aspect of the thigh. Penetrating injuries are the most frquent mode of trauma to this nerve. There is sensory loss along the upper medial aspect of the thigh. The obturator nerve arises by three roots from the ventral portions of the second, third and fourth lumbar nerves. It emerges from the medial

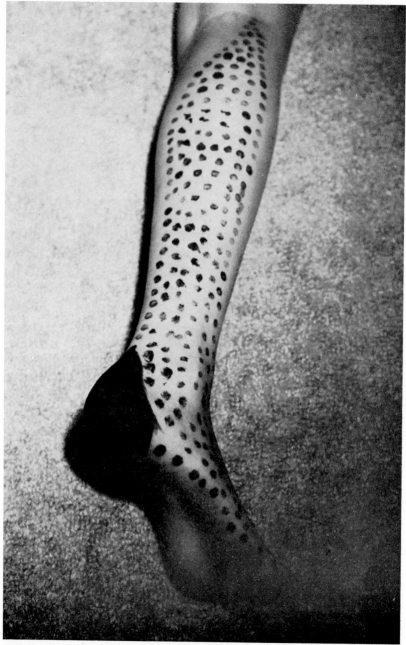

Figure 7-14. Sensory loss from tibial nerve injury shown in solid black. Injury to sural nerve produces sensation loss in stippled area.

border of the psoas major near the brim of the pelvis, under cover of the common iliac vessels, passes lateral to the ureter and runs along the wall of the lesser pelvis to enter the obturator foramen with the obturator vessels. It may be injured in penetrating wounds of the perineum. Injury to the obturator nerve results mainly in motor loss as the sensory loss is usually difficult to detect if the femoral nerve is intact because of combined innervation to the medial thigh through the femoral nerve by its anterior cutaneous and saphenous branches. The motor loss in obturator nerve injury is inability to adduct the thigh.

The general plan of the lumbar and sacral plexuses are illustrated in Figures 7-15a and 7-15b.

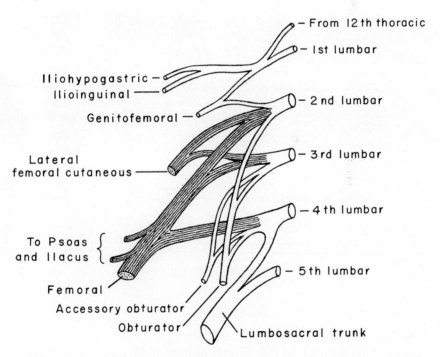

Figure 7-15. Comprehensive of the lumbar and sacral plexuses is essential to understanding specific peripheral nerve injuries of the legs. (a) lumbar plexus, (b) sacral plexus. (Reproduced with permission from *Gray's Anatomy of the Human Body*, 29th Ed., Philadelphia, Lea and Febiger, 1974.)

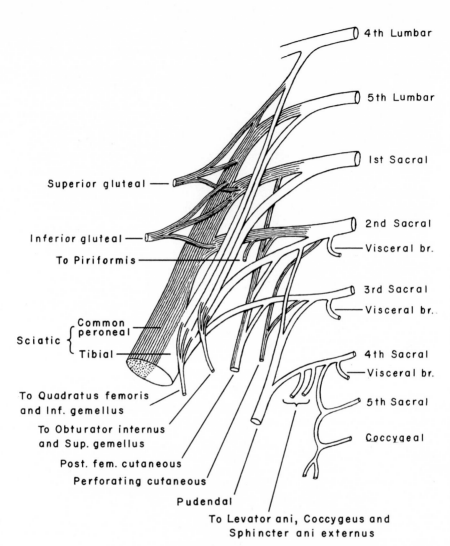

4th Lumbar

5th Lumbar

1st Sacral

2nd Sacral
Visceral br.

3rd Sacral
Visceral br.

4th Sacral
Visceral br.

5th Sacral

Coccygeal

Superior gluteal

Inferior gluteal
To Piriformis

Sciatic { Common peroneal / Tibial

To Quadratus femoris and Inf. gemellus
To Obturator internus and Sup. gemellus
Post. fem. cutaneous
Perforating cutaneous
Pudendal
To Levator ani, Coccygeus and Sphincter ani externus

Figure 7-15b.

REFERENCES

1. Sinha, R. P.; Ducker, T. B., and Perot, P. L.: Arterial oxygenation. Findings and its significance in central nervous system trauma patients. *JAMA, 224*:1258-1260, 1973.
2. Campbell, E., and Whitfield, R.: Emergency management of injuries of the head and spine. *Surg Clin N Ann, 36*:1295, 1956.
3. Youmans, J. R.: Causes of shock with head injury. *J Trauma, 4*:204, 1964.
4. Meirowsky, A. M.: *Neurologic Surgery of Trauma*. Washington, D.C.

Office of the Surgeon General, Department of the Army, 1965.

5. Cushing, H.: Some experimental and clinical observations concerning states of increased intracranial tension. *Am J Med Sci, 124*:375, 1902.

6. Carton. C. A.: Cerebral angiography in the management of head trauma. *American Lecture Series No. 336.* Springfield, Thomas, 1959.

7. Troupp, H.: Intraventricular pressure in patients with severe brain injury. *J Trauma, 5*:373-378, 1965.

8. Heimburger, R. F.: Spasticity arising from lesions in the brain. In: *Neurologic Surgery of Trauma.* Washington, D.C. Office of the Surgeon General, Department of the Army, 1965.
   Nathanson, M., and Bergman, P. S.: Newer methods of evaluation of patients with altered states of consciousness. *Med Clin N Am,* 701-709, May, 1958.

9. Nathanson, M.; Bergman, P. S., and Anderson, P. J.: Significance of oculocephalic and caloric responses in the unconscious patient. *Neurology, 7*:829-832, 1957.

10. Mayfield, F. H., and McBride, B. H.: Craniocerebral trauma. In: *Neurologic Surgery of Trauma.* Washington, D.C., Office of the Surgeon General, Department of the Army, 1965.

11. Campbell, J. B., and Cohen, J.: Epidural hemorrhage and the skull of children. *Surg Gynecol Obstet, 2*:3, 1951.

12. Report of Ad Hoc Committee to Study Head Injury Nomenclature. Clinical Neurology. Proceedings of the Congress of Neurologic Surgeons. Baltimore, Maryland, Williams and Wilkins, 1966.

13. Clark, K., and Grossman, R. G.: Trauma to the nervous system. *Care of the Trauma Patient.* McGraw-Hill, New York, 1966, p. 270.

14. Magoun, H. W.: Cardal and cephalic influences of the brain stem reticular formation. *Physiol Rev, 30*:459, 1950.

15. Goodnight, S. H.; Kenoyer, G.; Rapaport, S. L.; Patch, M. J.; Lee, J. A., and Kurze, T.: Defibrination after brain-tissue destruction. *N Eng J Med, 290*:1043-1047, 1974.

16. Schneider, R. C.: The syndrome of acute anterior spinal cord injury. *J Neurosurg, 12*:95-122, 1955.

17. Schneider, R. C.; Cheery, G., and Pantek, H.: The syndrome of acute central cervical spinal cord injury: with special reference to the mechanisms involved in hyperextension injuries to the cervical spine. *J Neurosurg, 11*:546-577, 1954.

18. Drake, C. G.: Cervical spinal cord injury. *J Neurosurg, 19*:487-494, 1962.

19. Gol, A.: Severe cervical spine injuries. *J Trauma, 5*:379-385, 1965.

20. Seddon, H. J. (Ed.): Peripheral nerve injuries. Medical Research Council, Special Report Series No. 282, London, Her Majesty's Stationery Office, 1954.

CHAPTER 8

EVALUATION OF UROLOGIC INJURIES

"It cannot be contradicted that accurate urological diagnosis is a prerequisite to scientific management."

SIR GORDON TAYLOR

1. Insert Urethral Catheter
2. Exam Urine Early After Trauma
3. Always Investigate Hematuria
4. Urethrogram
5. Cystograms
6. Infusion Pyelography
7. Arteriography
8. Retrograde Pyelography

THE APPRAISAL OF the urinary tract has been separated from the evaluation of the abdomen to help establish a very important axiom in the mind of the examining physician. Roentgenograms are of minimal aid in evaluating abdominal injuries, but assessment of urinary tract trauma is totally dependent on roentgen examinations.

The physical examination of the external genito-urinary organs is still fundamentally important even though most investigation is done with radiography. Inspection of the perineum often reveals whether a urethra is ruptured anteriorly or posteriorly to the triangular ligament simply by the difference in diffusion of the hematoma. Skin discoloration and diffusion of hematoma in the perineum indicates an anterior rupture of the urethra. Note the normal perianal area (Fig. 8-1). Exactly the opposite happens in posterior disruptions of the urethra. The ecchymosis is limited to the area around the anus while the perineal area

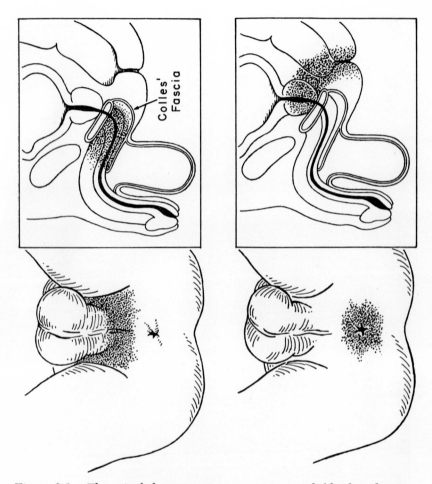

Figure 8-1. The stippled area represents extravasated blood and urine in relation to anterior rupture of the urethra (upper drawing) and posterior rupture of the urethra (lower diagram).

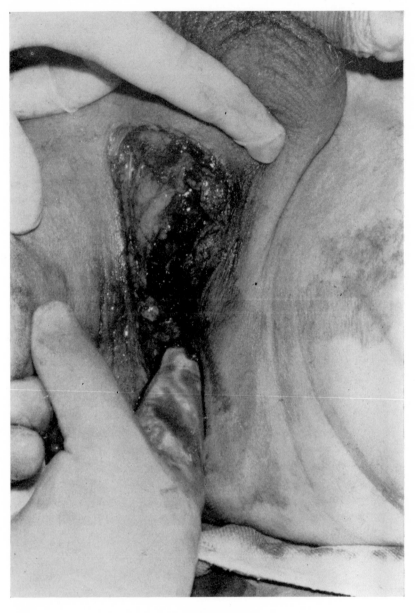

Figure 8-2. Rectal examination in the male can detect a "floating prostate" a reliable indication of urethal avulsion.

remains normal. This peculiar partioning of blood and urine is due to the insertion of Colles fascia on the posterior border of the triangular ligament (urogenital diaphragm), thus containing anterior hemorrhage inside its limits.

Rectal examination is important in the male. Should the prostate gland be palpated in a much higher position than normal, avulsion of the urethra at the urogenital diaphragm is probably present. Vermooten[1] considers such a "floating prostate" as a reliable indication of urethral avulsion (Fig. 8-2).

Continuing the physical examination one must look for contusions and avulsions over the flanks and costoverebral angle as indications of blunt trauma or wounds as indications of penetrating trauma. Just as low posterior rib fractures on the left point to splenic trauma so posterior low rib fractures on the right and vertebral body or transverse process fractures point to renal trauma. An enlarging flank mass is highly significant and should lead one to suspect renal injury.[2]

Fundamental problems in evaluating injury to the urinary tract are: (1) determination of degree of disruption of the parenchyma of the kidney, bladder and their allied conducting systems, (2) degree of hemorrhage, (3) detection of extravasated urine, (4) presence of pre-existing disease.[3]

In the early chapter on general preparation the importance of inserting a Foley catheter into the urinary bladder was emphasized. At that stage catheterization of the urinary bladder was chiefly to monitor urinary output. But the passage of a urethral catheter also gives much information regarding the urethra and bladder. If the Foley catheter does not pass easily into the urinary bladder it is not forced. Upon withdrawal of the catheter if there is bright red blood one must suspect urethal or bladder disruption.

If, however, the catheter passes freely into the urinary bladder and there is excessive but bloody urine, an injury higher up the urinary tract must be searched for. If the catheter passes rapidly into the urinary bladder and there is little or scant bloody urine a bladder or renal injury or both must be investigated.

It is important never to forcibly insert a catheter into the urinary bladder because one loses the ability to assess the original trauma that brought the patient to the hospital. In some older male patients it becomes difficult to decide whether the catheter won't pass because of urethral disruption or prostatic hypertrophy. A skilled maneuver in this situation is to fill a 10 ml syringe with lubricant jelly and inject this under minimal pressure in the urethra prior to attempting to pass the urethral catheter.

The external genitalia should be inspected carefully for contusions, avulsions, tears that might suggest further evaluation of the urinary system.

The urinary bladder and urethra are best evaluated as a unit. After insertion of the Foley catheter 250 ml of Renograffin® 30 percent is instilled into the bladder. If extravasation of contrast material is not visualized on a standard anteroposterior roentgenogram an additional 150 ml of Renograffin is instilled by gravity and a second anteroposterior roentgenogram is taken. If there is no extravasation the catheter is removed and the patient is asked to void while an oblique roentgenogram is made. This voiding cystourethrogram allows a thorough evaluation of the lower urinary tract. After voiding a final roentgenogram is taken and extravasation or retention of contrast material is assessed.

If the bladder has been established to be intact but concern about a male urethral injury remains, a retrograde urethrogram should be done. A lubricated "Christmas tree' adaptor is attached to a 20 ml syringe filled with Renograffin 30 percent and the adaptor inserted into the urethral meatus. The contrast material is injected under pressure in a retrograde fashion. Roentgenograms are taken during the injection and after voiding. These films are evaluated for urethral extravasation.

When the urethral catheter passes easily into the urinary bladder and clear profuse urine flows readily, microscopic evaluation of the urine is helpful. Microscopic hematuria is frequently the only indication of injuries to the urinary tract. The amount of blood is a poor indicator of the extent of injury. The presence of either gross or microscopic hematuria after trauma mandates searching and studying the urological system until the precipitating cause is delineated.

After completing the assessment of the lower genito-urinary system, the upper tract is evaluated. This is begun with an infusion pyelogram.[4] Renograffin (30%) 60 ml is inserted into a liter of 5 percent Dextrose in water and rapidly infused into a peripheral vein while anterior posterior roentgenograms are taken at five, ten, fifteen minutes after state of infusion.

The infusion pyelograms are evaluated for kidney function, extravasation of contrast material from ureters, pelvis or calyces, displacement and/or disruption of ureters. The chief contribution of intravenous pyelography in suspected renal trauma is to determine function and presence of kidneys. Occasionally, however, the pyelogram will portray a ruptured kidney (Fig. 8-3).

Too great emphasis must not be placed on the intravenous pyelograms. There is a 30 to 34 percent incidence of normal excretory urograms in patients with serious renal injury (Guerriero, Scott, Carlton).[5] The usefulness of excretory pyelography in suspected renovascular trauma is to document the functional status of the uninjured kidney.

Because there is a significant false negative intravenous pyelography in about a third of urological injuries, added dimensions of diagnosing renal injuries are necessary particularly in renovascular injuries.

Selective renal angiography is an extremely reliable method of evaluating renal trauma. The femoral artery is catheterized percutaneously and a vascular catheter passed under fluroscopic control into the renal artery. Renograffin is injected at the rate of 8 to 12 ml/sec and rapid sequence filming done. Blunt trauma frequently causes internal disruption and thrombosis of the renal artery (see Chapter 14). Aside from complete occlusions of the major renal artery the films are inspected for intrarenal distribution of contrast and extravasation of contrast, either inside or outside the capsule. A venous phase can be obtained and is also valuable.

The left renal vein was the most commonly injured structure in nineteen patients (Carlton).[6] This is logical since it transverses the rigid spinal column in a relatively exposed position.

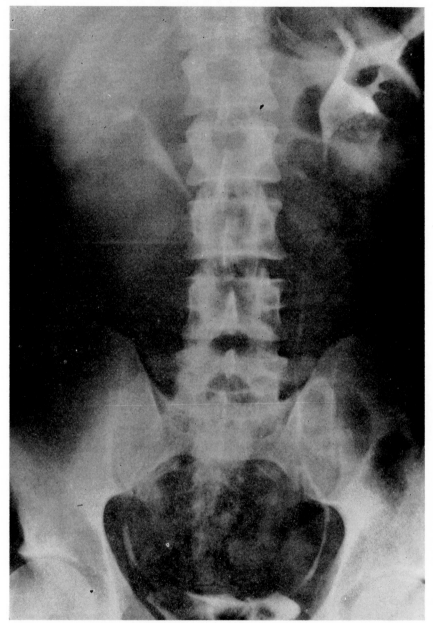

Figure 8-3.   Infusion pyelogram of a twenty-three-year-old physician injured in an automobile collison shows rupture of the inferior pole of the
right kidney.

Selective arteriography is the most reliable evaluating method for delineating precisely the extent and nature of renal injuries. The indications for selective renal arteriography in trauma patients are: (1) intravenous pyelography fails to show excretion of contrast medium, (2) extravasation of contrast medium, (3) retroperitoneal bleeding.

Renal scanning has been advocated by some for assessing renal injury (Kazim,[8] Samuels[9]). Although renal scanning provides no additional information not obtainable on angiography its chief proponents point out it is accomplished without preparation and is rapid and easily repeatable with very low radiation exposure.

BLADDER TRAUMA WITH PELVIC FRACTURES

Fracture of the pelvic girdle and rupture of the urinary bladder form such a specific clinical entity that they must be discussed separately and in greater detail. The mortality rate is so high (44.2%) [Cass[10]] that increased emphasis must be placed on early recognition of ruptured bladder in patients with pelvic fractures. Bladder and urethral injuries occur in association with approximately 8 to 17 percent of fractures of the pelvis.[11, 12] Symphyseal or sacroiliac separation, displacement comminution or bilateral pubic arch fractures are associated with more severe bladder and urethral injuries. Pubic arch fractures usually indicate underlying trauma to the urinary bladder.

Excretory cystography is unreliable. Every patient with a fracture should have a cystogram as described in the early paragraphs of this chapter. There is one addition. If the initial insert of 250 ml of contrast doesn't demonstrate extravasation, then bladder distention with 400 ml should be done and a post-washout roentgenogram obtained. Cystograms done in this fashion are so simply carried out and so reliable that they should always be done in patients with pelvic fractures (Fig. 8-4a and 8-4b).

Two kinds of bladder rupture occur: (1) intraperitoneal, (2) extraperitoneal. Where there is intraperitoneal rupture the contrast material inserted into the bladder enters the free peritoneal

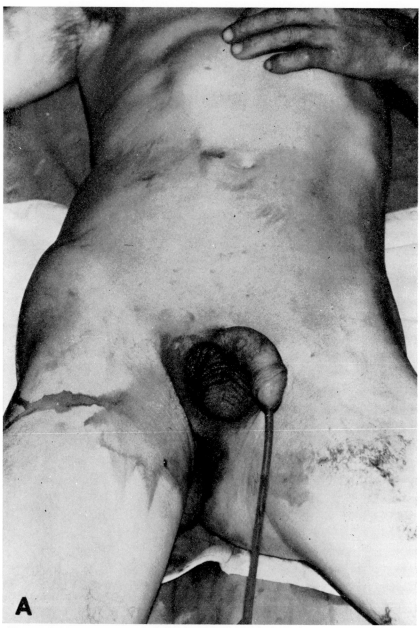

Figure 8-4. Asymmetry of pelvic girdle associated with hematuria and soft tissue contusion suggests a pelvic fracture in this workman (A). Cystogram showed extraperitoneal extravasation and confirmed rupture of the urinary bladder (B).

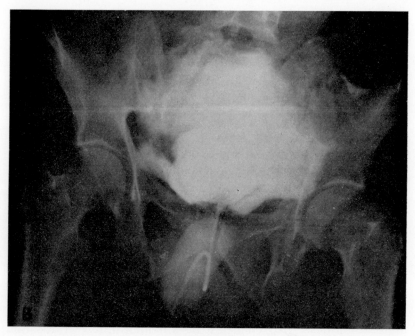

Figure 8-4b.

cavity and outlines the loops of intestine. Approximately 20 percent of bladder ruptures occur intraperitoneally.

The more common extraperitoneal ruptures occur in 80 percent and often causes a "tear drop" shaped bladder.[13] This tear drop shape is due to bilateral compression of the bladder by hematoma. Lateral displacement of the bladder "half moon" results from a unilateral hematoma.[14]

URETERAL INJURIES

These are perhaps the most uncommon injuries in the urological system but by far the most difficult to recognize. Most result from penetrating trauma. They are rare after closed trauma. Salvatieria and associates reported that only 27 percent of ureteral injuries were recognized and treated at the initial operation This means that complications of ureteral injury are the chief source of raising suspicion of ureteral injury. The complications of unrecognized ureteral injury are: (1) urinary fistula, (2) urinary ascites, (3) perinephric or iliac abscesses, (4) extraperitoneal cysts, (5) hydronephrosis.

This is most unfortunate and modern physicians should be unwilling to accept first manifestations of an injury to be complications of that injury. Our goal must be to detect ureteral injuries early prior to the onset of such complications.

Intravenous pyelography is entirely unreliable in detecting ureteral injuries. If by chance it does demonstrate extravasation or defects in the ureter one should feel fortunate. On the other hand, a normal infusion pyelogram does not exclude ureteral defects.

The above factors leave one and only one conclusion. Penetrating injuries should be explored with the intent of demonstrating an intact ureter. During the course of exploration injection of a dye marker may be helpful, but surgeons must develop skills in identifying the ureters quickly, and tracing their course without stripping them of their blood supply. Exploration for ureteral injuries will be further discussed under the chapter "Laparotomy as an Evaluating Method."

REFERENCES

1. Vermooten, V.: Rupture of the urethra: A new diagnostic sign. *J Urol, 56*:228, 1946.
2. Reiser, C.: Diagnostic evaluation of suspected genito-urinary tract injury. *JAMA, 199*:124, 1967.
3. Del Villar, R. G.; Ireland, G. W., and Cass, A. S.: Management of renal injury in conjunction with the immediate surgical treatment of the acute severe trauma patient. *J Urol, 107*:208-211, 1972.
4. Morse, T. S.: Infusion pyelography in the evaluation of renal injuries in children. *J Trauma, 6*:693, 1966.
5. Guerriero, W. G.; Carlton, C. E.; Scott, R., and Beall, A. C.: Renal pedicle injuries. *J Trauma, 11*:53-62, 1971.
6. Carlton, C. E.; Scott, R., and Goldman, M.: The management of penetrating injuries of the kidney. *J Trauma, 8*:1071-181, 1968.
7. Scott, R.; Carlton, C. E., and Goldman, M.: Penetrating injuries of the kidney: An analysis of 181 patients. *J Urol, 101*:247, 1969.
8. Kazmin, M. H.; Brosman, S. A., and Cockett, A. T. K.: Diagnosis and early management of renal trauma: A study of 120 patients. *J Urol, 101*:783, 1969.
9. Samuels, L. D., and Smith, J. P.: Kidney scanning in pediatric renal trauma. *J Trauma, 8*:583-592, 1968.
10. Cass, A. S., and Ireland, G. W.: Bladder trauma associated with pelvic fractures in severely injured patients. *J Trauma, 13*:205-212, 1973.
11. Kaiser, T. F., and Farrow, F. C.: Injury of the bladder and prostato-membranous urethra associated with fracture of the bony pelvis. *Surg Gynecol Obstet, 120*:99-112, 1965.
12. Rieser, C., and Nicholas, E.: Rupture of the bladder: Universal features. *J Urol, 90*:53-57, 1963.
13. Prather, G. C., and Kaiser, T. F.: The bladder in fracture of the bony pelvis; the significance of a "tear drop bladder" as shown by cystogram. *J Urol, 63*:1019-1030, 1950.
14. Morehouse, D. D., and Mackinnan, K. J.: Urological injuries associated with pelvic fractures. *J Trauma, 9*:479, 1969.

CHAPTER 9

EVALUATION OF
MUSCULOSKELETAL INJURIES

ALTHOUGH ONE OF the simplest to accurately evaluate, the musculoskeletal system leads to the greatest confusion in priority and judgement decisions. Most injuries to this system are obvious and striking. A bare bone sticking through the skin is perhaps the most frightening injury the physician encounters. Yet if he is not able to perceive a difference between an isolated open femoral shaft fracture and a femoral shaft fracture in a patient with a ruptured spleen, flail chest and closed head injury, there are dangers ahead and the quality of his patients lives, if they survive, are dependent upon his ability to establish priorities.

The assignment of low priority to the skeletal system is not a comment on the importance of physicians who limit themselves to the practice of orthopaedics. The American Academy of Orthopaedics is a leader in upgrading the care of injured patients. They publish an excellent text on the subject.[1]

Physicians are again dependent upon the quality of pre-hospital care (Phase 1) in the ultimate outcome of injuries to this system. A closed spiral fracture of the femoral shaft may be converted to an open contaminated femoral fracture enroute from the scene of injury to the hospital simply by deficiencies in transporting the patient properly splinted in an adequate vehicle. How many fractures that were initially closed are converted to open contaminated fractures by jostling an injured patient with an unprotected fracture side to side or against the wall of a speeding, recklessly driven vehicle, will probably never be known!

For this reason the physician is forced to involve himself and extend his abilities to the scene of injury by helping to train and educate emergency medical technicians to properly splint and protect fracture sites before transporting patients to definitive care centers. If adequate provisions for transporting, these patients are not available, the physician must involve himself in governmental and societal organizations to obtain such for the public.

Priorities outlined in the preceding chapters must be adhered to. Because concealed blood loss in and around fracture sites can seriously compromise the circulation, estimation of blood in each fracture site should be a first priority. That volume must be restored before sending the patient with compromised circulation off to have multiple x-rays of his broken bones.

An estimated 1,000 ml of volume may be lost from the circulation in a severe pelvic fracture. Some that involve iliac and pelvic vessels may represent 2,000 to 3,000 ml deficits by the time they come under the care of a physician.

In femoral shaft and severe fractures above the knee, 500 to 800 ml of volume may be lost to the circulation. Lesser volumes of 250 ml may occur in serious humeral and elbow fracture sites.

One of the most frequent mistakes in evaluating patients with multiple severe fractures is to neglect the volume losses. Because the blood is not visible at the scene of injury or on the stretcher or hospital bed it is very easy to simply forget that fracture sites conceal significant blood loss (Fig. 9-1).

The next order of priority in evaluating musculoskeletal injuries is vascular deficiencies. There are certain fractures in which the incidence of compromised circulation is greater than in others. These will be pinpointed later. The importance of a judgement decision in evaluating the circulation distal to fracture sites cannot be over emphasized. Assessing the patency of blood vessels must take precedence over x-ray evaluation of fractures.

Sites where capillary filling can be evaluated must be examined thoroughly, pulses should be carefully checked and recorded, then rechecked in sequential order. Where more sophisticated equipment is available and personnel are familiar

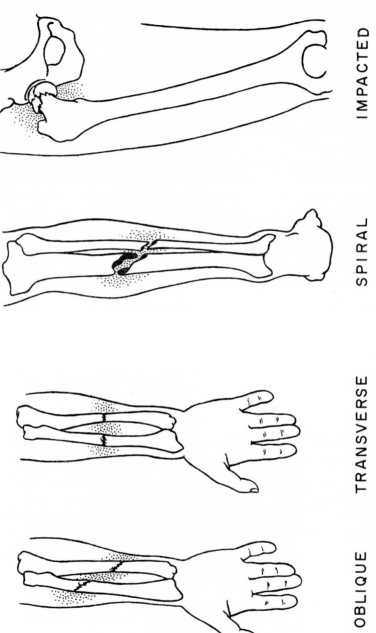

IMPACTED

SPIRAL

TRANSVERSE

OBLIQUE

Figure 9-1. Kinds of fracture lines commonly encountered.

to interpret results, ultrasonic arteriography and plethysmography may be helpful.

Absence of pulses distal to a fracture site in a cool pale extremity which is numb, with voluntary loss of motion indicates the possibility of major arterial injury. Arteriography then becomes a first priority evaluating tool and should be done quickly. In certain suspicious fractures especially those classically known to involve arteries arteriography should be done as part of clinical assessment of that fracture even though pulses may be palpable. Drapanas and colleagues reported 27 percent of 128 patients with injuries to major extremity arteries had palpable pulses distal to the injury.[2] The use of arteriography as an important clinical tool in assessing arterial injuries will be discussed in greater detail in later chapters.

Although this text is not primarily involved with treatment we would be remiss if we did not mention that many times gentle manipulation and immobilization of a fracture site at the scene of injury or upon arrival at the hospital often restores an absent pulse, and saves an extremity that otherwise may have been loss. Sometimes the physician can correlate the appearance and disappearance of a pulse with the gentle manipulation of a fracture. In these situations the fracture should be meticulously immobilized before any additional x-ray studies or arteriograms.

Once the examiner is certain that the circulating blood volume is adequate and peripheral perfusion of tissues is taking place, the third priority is to prevent additional contamination of open fracture sites. Again this is a priority that hopefully was begun at the scene of the accident and followed through until the patient is on the operating table and prepared for definitive debridement.

If this precaution has not been accomplished in Phase 1, the physician should institute it as soon as blood volume is restored and arterial obstructions are corrected. The skin surrounding the fracture skin is quickly washed with surgical soap and irrigated with saline, then covered with a sterile occlusive dressing. This is not definitive care. This must not be misconstrued as representing definitive care it is only a precaution to reduce additional contamination as the patient moves from stretcher to stretcher, to the X-ray department, in waiting and holding areas until he finally arrives in the operating room for definitive care of his open fracture.

Just as in evaluating the genito-urinary system, roengtenography was the basic primary tool, so in evaluating skeletal injuries, the ultimate, definitive appraisal has to be radiological. But we will not deal with the technical or interpretive aspects of X-ray diagnosis of fractures. This must be left to the discretions of the physician who provides the definitive care. Rather we will deal with initial appraisal by the physician. This is necessary in the care of seriously injured patients because it pinpoints the areas that require further delineation with roengtenograms. There are several cogent reasons why such an appraisal of the musculo-skeletal system must precede definitive roentgenographic delineation of fractures. Total body irradiation is hazardous. Multiple X-ray studies consume valuable time that can be better utilized. A careful examination by an alert physician can prevent many unnecessary X-ray studies and save valuable time. He detects the injury and simply uses roentgenograms to delineate the more detailed aspects of the problem. In the non-osseous injuries roentgenograms will mislead the physician who has not done a careful inspection and palpation of his patient.

The following paragraphs are written with these preliminary thoughts in mind. It is understood that when the following examinations have been completed, the task is only half done. Suspicious areas detected by physical examination are then subjected to scrutiny by roentgenologic technics. After physical examination X-rays are necessary to delineate kind of fracture and locate or exclude foreign bodies.

DEFINITIONS

Definitions often seem so elemental that some prefer to omit them, but a basic language organizes the mind of the examiner in a systematic fashion. Understanding definitions creates awareness of what the examiner is expected to search out and discover (Figs. 9-2a and 9-2b).

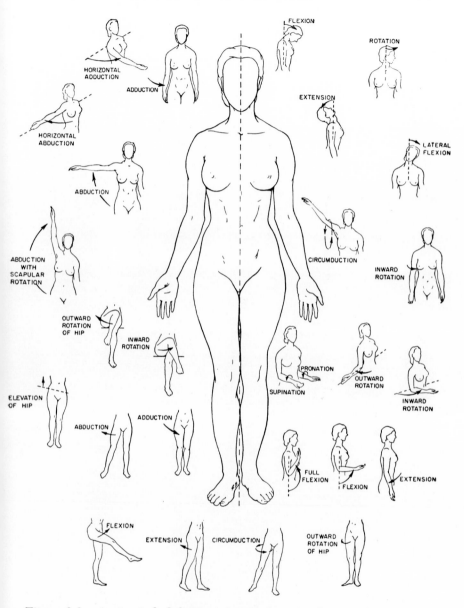

Figure 9-2. Anatomical definitions important in evaluating the musculo skeletal system. (Reproduced with permission from *Trauma*. Copyright 1959 by Matthew Bender and Co., Inc.)

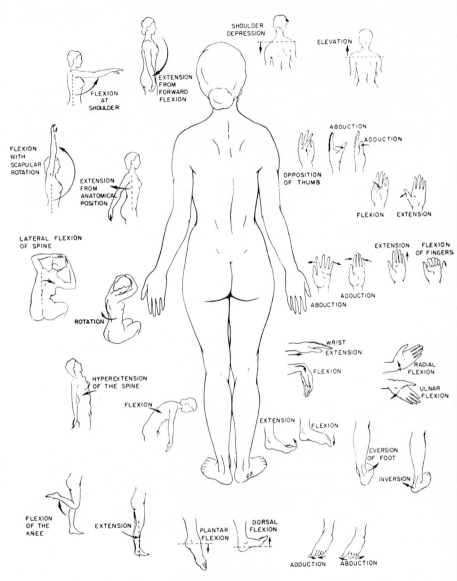

Figure 9-2b.

A fracture is any break in the continuity of bone or cartilage, but in evaluating fractures there are modifying terms that must be constantly in the physician's mind. Modifying terms can be briefly outlined:

1. Complete or incomplete.
   Fractures do not always involve both cortices.
2. Closed or open.
   Open fractures communicate externally through broken skin.
3. Kind of fracture line.
   a) TRANSVERSE:
      line of fracture is roughly transverse in relation to longitudional axis of the bone.
   b) SPIRAL:
      the fracture line describes a spiral in relationship to the longitudinal axis of the bone.
   c) OBLIQUE:
      line of fracture is obliquely oriented in relation to the longitudinal axis of the bone.
   d) IMPACTED:
      One fragment is telescoped upon a second fragment. Hip and vertebral fractures are particularly prone to this mechanical phenomenon and produces some degree of stability (Fig. 9-3).
4. Location within the bone.
   a) fracture of proximal or distal portion of a long bone
   b) fracture of the shaft of long bone
   c) fractures involving epiphysis of actively growing bone
   d) fracture involving articular surfaces
   e) fracture of a process of a bone.

A clinical description or observation of deformities caused by fractures can call attention to areas that need further study by X-ray and is useful in planning treatment. Such categorization of fractures helps the physician remember what to evaluate in particular areas:

1. DISPLACEMENT:
   Fracture fragments may sometimes show complete loss of

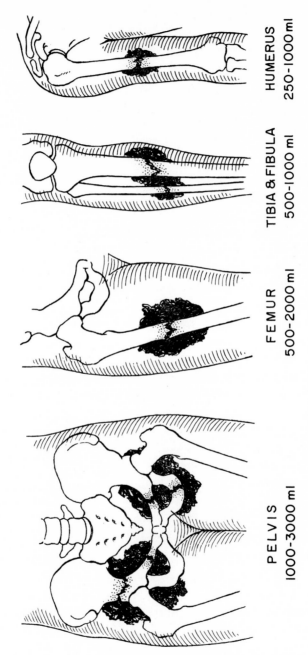

HUMERUS
250-1000 ml

TIBIA & FIBULA
500-1000 ml

FEMUR
500-2000 ml

PELVIS
1000-3000 ml

Figure 9-3.   Range of blood volume loss in several common fractures.

apposition or varying degrees of partial displacement between this extreme and the non-displaced fracture.

2. ANGULATION:

This is generally present to some degree in fractures of the long bones. The best way to remember this deformity is to describe the distal fragments longitudinal relationship to the proximal fragment.

3. ROTATION:

This deformity is frequently overlooked or missed. It depends upon the relationship of the distal fragments in its rotatory orientation to the proximal fragment.

4. SHORTENIING:

Impacted fractures often show some degree of shortening. When displacement is complete shortening is usually present. In spiral oblique and severely comminuted fractures shortening may develop in the absence of complete displacement.

Inquiry into the history and mechanics of injuries can often raise suspicion and help in the diagnosis of certain fractures. The clinical assessment is usually as important as the radiographic diagnosis in determining degree of deformity. There is always a temptation to depart from a methodical examination of the total patient and focus on a more striking and obvious fracture. This should be resisted in favor of a systematic complete examination of the entire musculoskeletal system. He should adapt a sequence proceding from the proximal to distal portion of each extremity, inspecting for swelling, ecchymosis, deformities and palpating for tenderness, crepitance and instability; then testing for range of motion.

Inspection of the nude patient should include a search for open wounds and small puncture sites. In some injuries a sharp fragment of bone may penetrate the skin some distance from the fracture site. Injuries always occur in a dynamic state and when the patient comes to rest on the examining table, the sharp fragment of bone retracts inside the skin and comes to lie some distance from the site of the small puncture wound. This may be missed. The examiner should compress any hematoma around the fracture site. If dark blood is expressed from the skin wound the two most likely communicate and represents an open fracture just as much as if the bone were still protruding.

There are two areas of evaluation often neglected in examining the patient with multiple fractures. One of these, vascular obstruction, has already been discussed at length. The other is motor and sensory function of the nervous system. Because certain fractures are known to be frequently associated with specific nerve injuries, the physician should always give a little extra attention to these trouble spots during his examination:

1. HUMERAL HEAD DISLOCATIONS:
   The axillary nerve is injured about 15 percent of the time. The examiner should look for sensory impairment over the lateral surface of the shoulder and inability to abduct the arm beyond 15 degrees.
2. HUMERAL SHAFT FRACTURES:
   The radial nerve is often entrapped or severely contused as it spirals the shaft. The patient has wrisp drop and when tested is unable to extend his wrist.
3. SUPRACONDOLYLAR FRACTURES AT ELBOW:
   The median nerve is frequently compressed. The flexors of the wrist and fingers are impaired, but not complete if the ulnar nerve is intact. Sensory loss over the hand and fingers is present except one half of the ring finger and all of the little finger. The abductor brevis and opponens are paralyzed. Pronation of the forearm is paralyzed.
4. DISLOCATIONS OF THE LUNATE:
   The median nerve is often injured when the lunate is forcefully impinged on the nerve at the wrist, again there is sensory loss over the thumb, index, middle and the distal half the ring finger.
5. DISLOCATIONS OF THE ELBOW:
   Forces that displace the forearm forward or into valgus position frequently injures the ulnar nerve as it passes behind the medial condyle of the humerus. The ulnar nerve is not injured as frequently as the median in supra-

condylar fractures. The flexor carpi ulnaris is paralyzed as are the terminal phalanges of the ring and little finger, the muscles of the hypothevar eminence, all the interossei, the ulnar two lumbricals, the abductors of the thumb and the short head of the flexor pollicis brevis. There is sensory loss over the ulnar side of the hand and little finger.

6. DISLOCATION OF THE HEAD OF FEMUR:
   The sciatic nerve is often injured and there is paralysis of muscles below the knee.

7. FRACTURES OF PROXIMAL TIBIA AND FIBULA:
   Varus injuries about the knee with rupture of the lateral soft tissues often injuries the peroneal nerve. Sensory loss is present over the dorsum of the foot. The peroneal muscles and the muscles of the anterior compartment are paralyzed, consequently there is inability to lift the foot. (Foot drop.) Sensory loss is also present over the lateral aspect of the foreleg, the instep and the dorsal surface of the four medial toes at their most extreme tip.

GENERAL SURVEY

Before obtaining roentgenograms of obvious fractures there should be a quick but systematic and careful evaluation of the entire musculoskeletal system. All moving joints should be tested for spontaneous motion and active motion against resistance applied appropriately by the examiner. Remember tendons and soft tissues do not visualize on radiographs and the inability to move against resistance may be the only indication of tendon injuries.

Shoulder

The shoulder joint is stabilized by muscles and their various tendinous attachments. There are two groups. The intrinsic muscles give support anteriorly and superiorly. They are: subscapularis, supraspinatus, infraspinatus and the teres minor. The extrinsic muscles stabilizing the shoulder joint posteriorly and inferiorly are: pectoralis major, deltoid, long head of triceps, long head of biceps, latissimus dorsi and the teres major.

There are important surface landmarks which the examiner should learn from a normal subject before proceeding to evaluate the injured. These landmarks are: acromion process, the tuberosities and head of the humerus, the coracoid process, the acromial and sternal articulations of the clavicle.

A posteriorly displaced humeral head can be discovered by palpating the bone in the soft tissue after noting asymmetry between the two shoulders and a concavity beneath the acromion process. The glenoid fossa appears empty to visual inspection.

More commonly the humeral head is displaced anteriorly and comes to rest beneath the coracoid process. The possible involvement of the axillary nerve by the displaced humeral head has already been discussed. As the humeral head is displaced the greater tuberosity may be torn off. This can be detected later by X-rays.

Injuries to the acromioclavicular joint and sternoclavicular joint can seldom be detected on radiographs, but are very accurately determined by physical examination.

In sternoclavicular separations the proximal clavicle is displaced forward and can be easily palpated beneath the skin in front of the sternum. Remember that complete dislocation means complete rupture of the costo clavicular ligament and may point to more serious involvement of the subclavian vessels and brachial plexus.

Trauma to the acromioclavicular joint will usually evolve in three distinct patterns: simple strain, subluxations and complete dislocations. Simple strains are detected by slight swelling and well localized tenderness over the joint. There is a mild tearing of the acromic clavicular ligament.

In subluxation of the acromioclavicular joint the articular extremity of the clavicle can be palpated as it rises above its normal position. This creates a distinct step, which is visible to careful inspection, between the clavicle and the acromion process. There is local edema with tenderness well localized to the acromioclavicular joint. There is complete or at least nearly complete rupture of the acromioclavicular capsule.

Often the examiner can grasp the clavicle between his fingers and attempt to move it above the acromian and anterioposteriorly.

This motion is not possible in subluxation as it is in complete dislocation.

In complete dislocations the lateral clavicle is torn free of all its attachments including the coracoclavicular ligaments. The clavicle then rides free and can be grasped by the physician's fingers and moved in all planes.

Fractures of the clavicle are common. They usually occur in the middle third and the deformity and swelling are obvious to inspection and palpation. Incomplete fractures can be detected by careful palpation along the entire length of the bone. Fractures of the medial and lateral third are less common but can be detected by careful palpation and inspection. More important than the disruption of the bone itself is the possible injury of contiguous structures such as the subclavian vessels and brachial plexus. The pulse in the axillary and brachial vessels should be checked when this injury is present. If the pulses are absent a percutaneous transfemoral arteriogram should be done (see Chapter 14).

The scapula is seldom fractured. It requires severe crushing injuries or high energy impacts to disrupt this well protected bone. Soft tissue swelling and discoloration over the scapula and splinting of the shoulder and arm should lead to further investigation with roentgenograms. When fracture of the scapula is proven it is almost certain that there are associated rib fractures and contusion of the lungs. It is these associated injuries that make detection of scapular fractures pertinent.

Fractures of the glenoid fossa range from simple linear fractures to explosive disruption with associated humeral head displacements. These fractures usually result from direct injury to the side of the shoulder. The shoulder is gently rotated passively by the examiner and pain of motion and resistance to motion assessed.

Humerus

Dislocations of the humeral head have already been discussed under the section on shoulder. Fractures of the humerus usually involve either the tuberosities, the neck, the shaft or the condyles.

Local swelling and tenderness over the greater tuberosity

after a direct blow on the side of the shoulder indicates either a contusion fracture or avulsion fracture of the greater tuberosity. Attempts at active abduction causes pain to the local area.

The humeral neck is divided into the surgical neck and the anatomic neck. Each may be injured separately or both may be comminuted. They are detected by the marked swelling over the entire proximal portion of the arm, tenderness is diffuse. There is pain when any active motion is attempted. The examiner can further evaluate this injury by gentle passive rotation of the shoulder joint and observing for grating, crepitance, or pain.

Fractures of the shaft of the humerus are usually apparent if looked for. Inspection shows deformity and swelling. Angulation is often striking, shortening may be present. Both humeri should be looked at together and each compared to the other. In the absence of swelling and angulation the shaft should be palpated with the arm of the patient in the hands of the physician and the thumbs of each hand applying firm pressure on each side of the suspected site of fracture. Crepitance is often present in complete fractures. When the fracture is incomplete exquisite pain when thumb and finger pressure are applied will uncover the fracture site. As previously mentioned the innervation of the radial nerve should also be evaluated.

The elbow is a complex joint. It is composed of the extremities of three separate bones forming three articular joints: ulnohumeral, radiohumeral, and proximal radioulnar. When evaluating this joint there are bony landmarks formed by the prominences of the humerus, radius and ulna that must be seen and must be felt in every suspected elbow injury. These landmarks form a triangle with which every physician should acquaint himself. These structures can almost always be palpated even in the presence of considerable swelling.

The examiner must also remember that the distal humerus flattens into a broad articular surface that angulates forward from the shaft of the humerus at an angle of 30 degrees. A strong circular band of ligamentous fibers encircles the head of the radius and maintains the circumferential surface of the radial head in the radial notch of the humerus. This annular ligament is attached to the ulna at the anterior and posterior margins of the radial notch. The upper border of the annular ligament blends with the joint capsule.

In full extension the forearm forms a obtuse angle with the arm. This angle is approximately 15 degrees and directed laterally from the midline. It is more commonly known as the carrying angle. In flexion the forearm is directly opposed to the arm in the true anteroposterior plane. The examiner should check each of these angles in normal subjects and become so familiar with them that abnormalities in injured patients will be immediately obvious.

Supracondylar fractures are the most common elbow fractures. These frequently happen in children. Vascular impairment, leading to Volkmann's contracture is a major tragedy in these injuries. Thus evaluation of circulation is a first priority in suspected elbow fractures. The earlier the diagnosis is made the quicker the deficiencies can be corrected. Inspection of the elbow shows swelling and deformity, the carrying angle and the angle of the condyles with the shaft is either abnormally exaggerated or absent. On palpation of the joint, tenderness is well localized over the fracture site. If there is displacement the forearm is shortened and the elbow projects posteriorly. The triangle made by the olecranon, the medial and lateral condyles is normal. This differentiates a fracture from a dislocation of the elbow.

After the initial evaluation the pulses and capillary filling in the nailbeds should again be observed and recorded.

Fractures of either the medial or lateral humeral condyles is usually apparent from inspection. The exact type must be later determined by roentgenography. A common type is when the fracture line extends into the joint and forms either a Y or T. The olecranon is driven into the humerus splitting off the condyles to either side. Three fragments result. Sometimes comminution may be so severe that the fragments and Y and T are not distinguishable. Again vascular and nerve patency are the first priority and require repeated assessment.

Dislocations of the elbow present such a striking picture on physical examination that they are not usually missed. Soft tissue associated injuries are important and since these do not show on X-ray the physician who confines his evaluation to radiographs alone does his patient a great disservice. The disruption of the triangle formed by the medial epicondyle, lateral epicondyle and olecranon is very reliable as a diagnostic criteria. Whereas in supracondylar fractures this triangular relationship is preserved.

In a dislocation the olecranon projects on a plane behind the two epicondyles. This exaggerated position of the olecranon is quite evident on inspection and palpation. The tendon of the triceps is stretched tight like a guitar string over its bridge and is more apparent than in the normal elbow. The articular process of the humerus is palpable in the antecubital fossa. Again vascular patency is first priority. The brachial artery is often entrapped or avulsed. Careful evaluation of distal pulses and arteriography, if indicated, must be done before attention is focused on the dislocated bones.

In very young children the forearm is often jerked suddenly by an adult or older child. This usually forces the elbow into extension and the forearm into pronation. The radial head, which is very small in children is pulled down under the annular ligament. Inspection shows the child is holding the forearm in some flexion and pronation. Upon palpation the radial head is tender and very prominent. In children the radial head is not ossified and roentgenograms show no abnormality. The history is very important in detecting this injury.

Forearm

The relationship of the ulna and radius are such that when one bone is fractured or severely displaced there is nearly always displacement, fracture or some disturbance in the normal relationship of the two bones at either their proximal or distal articulation.

The fracture described by Monteggia is an example of this relationship and the reader will encounter many others if he is suspicious enough to look for them. In the Monteggia fracture the ulna is fractured and bowed forward. The radial head is anteriorly displaced from its normal position just distal to the capitellum into the antecubital fossa. The displacement of the radius may stretch the motor branch of the radial nerve and the patient should be checked for evidence of wrist drop, inability to extend the fingers, loss of extension of the thumb and weakness of flexion of the elbow.

The radius and ulna are often fractured in combination. The ulna is subcutaneous and the entire length of this bone can be palpated by the examiner making it very easy to detect fractures of this bone. In examining the forearm the physician should remember certain important points of reference. These are: The olecranon process and radial head proximally and the styloid processes of the ulna and radius distally. In its distal third the radius is palpable beneath the tendon of the brachio radialis, the abductor pollicis longus and the extensor pollicis brevis.

The radius and ulna may fracture at the same level, but the examiner must remember that it is not uncommon to find one bone broken at one level and a second fracture of the opposite bone at a higher or lower level. In children the fracture line is often incomplete giving this particular fracture the "greenstick" terminology. Inspection alone usually picks up fractures of both bones of the forearm. Again careful examination for nerve and vascular injuries must be carried out. The ulna and radius are then palpated gently with the thumbs and index fingers while supporting the forearm with the hands. Careful evaluation of rotation, angulation, shortening is noted and recorded.

Fractures of a single bone also occurs as noted previously the ulna is subcutaneous and can be easily inspected and palpated throughout its length. Since the radius is the heavier of the two it is broken less frequently than the ulna. These are roughly transverse fractures. Swelling and tenderness with hematoma formation are evident at the fracture site upon inspection. The patient experiences pain when trying to actively rotate the arm.

A good technic of assessment is for the examiner to take the patient's hand in a handshake position. He then supports the patient's forearm with his free hand and carefully rotates the hand and wrist passively, the fractured proximal fragment does not follow and the patient experiences pain.

The distal radioulnar joint is often disrupted in fractures of distal third of the radius, just as the proximal radioulnar joint is disrupted in the Monteggia fracture.

Wrist

Perhaps the best known fracture to the medical profession is that described by Colles. In most instances it is the result of a fall on the outstretched palm. These fractures may sometimes be incomplete and do not always give the classic "silver fork" deformity that most physicians are fully acquainted with.

The distal fragment of the radius is usually displaced and rotated dorsally. Sometimes there is lateral displacement and varying degrees of impaction producing some shortening of the bone. Fracture of the ulnar styloid and navicular bone are frequent coexisting injuries.

In children the distal radial epiphysis may be displaced dorsally and backward. The line of fracture runs through the zone of provisional calcification.

When there is no displacement of the radial fragment, there is no "silver fork" appearance upon inspection. In these situations the fracture can be detected by palpation of the distal radius and ulnar and the styloid processes of these bones. Well localized tenderness over the distal radius should cause suspicion of a fracture. If compared to the uninjured side there will often be some degree of swelling. Injuries of the distal radial epiphysis may show nothing on roentgenograms and the diagnosis is dependent on clinical evaluation.

A fall on the dorsum of the hand with the wrist in flexion produces a fracture almost the reverse of Colles. A Smith's fracture line extends from the volar surface of the radius approximately an inch above the articulation extending distally and dorsally in an oblique manner. If this fracture is displaced the deformity swelling and angulation is evident upon inspection of the wrist and the diagnosis is obvious. In the absence of displacement, tenderness, as detected by gentle palpation and manipulation of the wrist is suggestive of a fracture and roentgenograms will delineate the direction of the fracture line.

Barton's fracture can be a co-existing injury of the Colles fracture or it may occur as an isolated injury. This is a fracture of the posterior margin of the distal radius and tends to permit the wrist to sublux dorsally. This tendency toward dorsal subluxation plus swelling and tenderness leads to the suspicion of this particular fracture. A roentgenogram will either confirm or exclude this diagnosis.

Fractures of the navicular bone are common. They must be thought of and searched for otherwise they will be overlooked in the critically injured patient. The fracture occurs most frequently in young adult males. It is usually the result of a fall on the outstretched arm. This same fall in an elderly individual produces a Colles fracture. This is another fracture which is always diagnosed clinically. Initial roentgenograms seldom show the fracture site. If the physician's clinical evaluation suggests this fracture the roentgenogram should be repeated in six weeks and at this time the diagnosis can usually be confirmed. The fracture line is most commonly across the waist of the bone. Less frequently the distal tubercle or the proximal pole may be broken.

To evaluate a patient for a navicular fracture the physician looks for swelling distal to the radius. Then with his thumb he exerts firm pressure over the radial styloid, tenderness at this point indicates the swelling is due to a fracture of the radial styloid. If tenderness is absent over the radial styloid the examiner slids his thumb into the patient's anatomical snuffbox and again exerts firm pressure. If tenderness is present a tentative diagnosis of navicular fracture is made and the wrist immobilized in plaster. At six weeks a roentgenogram is obtained and the fracture line may be apparent or the proximal navicular may appear dense due to the interruption of its vascular supply by the fracture.

Other carpal bones are much less commonly injured than the navicular, but any combination or single injury can occur. Clinical findings of well localized swelling and tenderness indicate injury and are treated as such.

The most commonly dislocated carpal bone is the semilunar (lunate). It is protected by the radius and capitate but when a patient falls on the dorsiflexed hand or tries to break the force of impact by placing both hands against the dashboard, the semilunar bone is forcefully impinged between the capitate and radius and "popped" into the carpal canal. This volar dislocation of the semilunate produces swelling over the volar wrist. The physician can detect this swelling by careful inspection of the wrist and comparing it with the uninjured wrist. If the injury occurs bilaterally the value of comparison and degree of swelling is lost and then the examiner must look for the fingers to assume a flexed position and check for median nerve compression. The dislocated semilunar bone compresses these latter structures when it is forced into the carpal canal.

In a few injuries the semilunar retains its anatomical position and the remaining carpal bones along with the hand are displaced dorsally and to the radial side of the forearm. This is usually referred to as perilunar dislocation of the carpus. The deformity is more obvious. The solitary dislocation of the lunate requires careful examination of roentgenograms to be detected but the perilunar dislocation of the carpus can be detected by inspection. The marked dorsal and radial deformity with swelling leads the physician to suspect this injury.

Hand

Fractures of the metatarsals are best evaluated as to whether the neck, shaft, or base is involved. The most common fracture of the metacarpal bones is the fifth and it is most commonly broken through the neck. This is referred to as a Boxer's fracture because it usually results from a blow to the head of the bone while the fist is clenched. The head of the metacarpal is displaced volarly and this angulation is maintained by the interosseous and lumbrical muscles. This injury is detected by the local swelling and tenderness present over the head and neck of the bone. Firm pressure can be applied by placing one thumb of the examiner over the volar head of the metacarpal and pressure in an opposite direction by the other thumb over the shaft of the metacarpal. This test illicits pain and tenderness if a fracture is present.

The next most common injury of the metarcarpals is fracture of the base of the first metacarpal. This usually results from direct trauma to the metacarpal forcing it toward the ulnar side of the hand. Localized swelling and tenderness to pressure over the base of the metacarpal are indications of fracture.

If the direction of the force is longitudinal an oblique fracture line of the base of the metacarpal occurs. This usually enters the carpometacarpal joint. The triangular fragment of the base of the metarcarpal resulting from this oblique fracture remains in normal anatomical position at the joint and the distal fragment including a small portion of the articular surface is displaced radially and proximally. This is commonly called Bennett's fracture dislocation. Inspection shows deformity angulation and swelling. Palpation and passive motion disclose tenderness and severe pain.

Fractures of the phalanges commonly involve the proximal and middle phalanges in their proximal third. The fracture line is usually transverse and the insertion and pull of the tendons produces dorsal angulation of the distal fragment. These fractures are detected by applying firm pressure over the phalanx and assessing for pain. The fingers are inspected for swelling and hematoma formation.

The distal phalanges are also commonly fractured. Very frequently these are comminuted resulting from crushing forces. Industrial plants and automobile doors are the common distributors of such forces. When the extensor mechanism to the distal phalanx is pulled away a small triangular fragment of bone is often avulsed from the base of the joint. The resulting deformity is early recognized because the patient is unable to extend his distal joint. Lacerations of the extensor mechanism without bony fracture also produces this deformity which has been labelled Baseball finger.

The carpometacarpal, metacarpophalangeal and interphalangeal joints should also be carefully inspected for dislocations. The diagnosis is usually apparent upon careful inspection of the individual joints and passive motion assessing the range of motion and degree of discomfort.

After assessment of bone injuries the hand must also be evaluated for nerve and tendon injuries. Inspection of the patient's hand should lead to the diagnosis of flexor tendon injuries. The arm and hand are placed in a relaxed position on a table or armboard with the palm up. In this position the fingers spontaneously assume a partially flexed position. Any finger which doesn't assume this normal position of partial flexion is then further assessed for ability to flex against resistance. The absence of this ability confirms disruption of the flexor mechanism.

The extensor tendons are evaluated in a similar manner. Here the ability to extend the wrist and fingers against resistance is tested. Failure to complete extension indicates extensor tendon disruption.

The innervation of the hand is checked with pin pricks and light cotton contacts for sensory deficits. In the unconscious patient these tests are low in priority and should be omitted, until a later appropriate time.

Pelvis

The human pelvis constitutes a firm heavy ring which is normally non-compressible. It protects pelvic organs from much trauma, and when the pelvic girdle is disrupted injuries to these organs is usually more significant than fracture or dislocation of the bony girdle.

The intactness of the incompressible pelvic ring can be quickly evaluated by placing one heel of the palm of the hand against each iliac crest and pushing firmly toward the midline (Figs 9-4a and 9-4b). This allows the examiner to view the patients facies for evidence of pain and determine whether there is some abnormal compressibility of what is normal a firm non

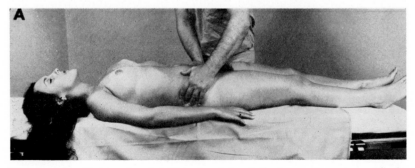

Figure 9-4.   Testing for stability of pelvic girdle by compression with the heel of the hands. Pressure exerted toward the midline (a) then pressure exerted away from mid-line (b).

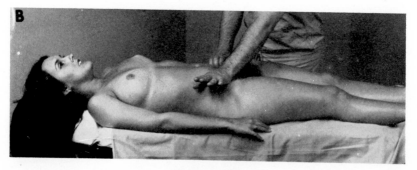

Figure 9-4b.

compressible ring. This maneuver evaluates the intactness of the pelvis in its lateral to medial plane.

Next the compressibility of the pelvis in its antero-posterior structure is evaluated by placing the heel of the hand over the symphysis pubis and pushing firmly toward the table in an antero-posterior direction (Fig. 9-5). While exerting pressure in this direction the physician evaluates the degree of compressibility and the amount of discomfort.

Since the pelvic girdle represents an architecturally incompressible ring any abnormal motion or crepitance indicates fracture. Simple non-displaced fractures of one or both pubic

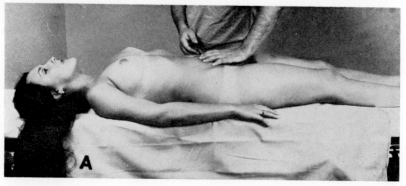

Figure 9-5. Testing for anterior-posterior compressibility of pelvic girdle by pressing firmly on the symphysis pubis with the heel of the hand. (A) Any abnormal motion or pain indicates fracture.

rami may occur as an isolated injury but in most patients when there is severe fracture with wide separation of the pelvic ring anterior to the acetabulum there is frequent separation or fracture of the posterior ring or sacroiliac joints. An example of this is the Malgaigne fracture of the pelvis. In this particular injury there is an anterior fracture line through the symphysis or both pubic rami and the posterior or second line of injury is represented by disruption of the sacroiliac joint or a fracture through the ilium. Various combinations of these fractures occur and must be carefully searched for in the injured patient.

Although I have already discussed the peril of concealed hemorrhage in earlier chapters and the problem of hemorrhage associated with fractures in the opening paragraphs of this Chapter I am repeating portions of these discussions here. The association of concealed life threatening hemorrhage in pelvic fractures is so common that it must be re-emphasized.

Braunstein and his associates[4] reviewed ninety patients who were admitted with pelvic fractures and found twenty-one of them to have blood loss severe enough to cause death or contribute substantially to a fatal outcome. This concealed hemorrhage should always be assumed to be present. Careful inspection of the perineum, scrotum, buttocks and inquinal region may also reveal ecchymoses or hematomas suggesting more extensive hemorrhage into the retroperitoneal space. In several of Braunstein cases the blood loss was as great as 3,000 ml.

This blood loss takes priority over the injury to the skeletal system and must be replaced before any minute diagnosis of fracture lines are undertaken.

I also discussed injury to the urinary bladder in earlier chapters, but again it must be emphasized that all patients with fracture or separation of the pelvic girdle should have a cystogram and urethrogram as part of their evaluation.

Rupture of the posterior urethra is almost exclusively related to fractures of the pubic rami.[5] When the posterior urethra is completely ruptured, rectal palpation of the membranous urethra and prostate, discloses that the prostate is easily displaced or at least difficult to feel. If hematoma has had sufficient time to

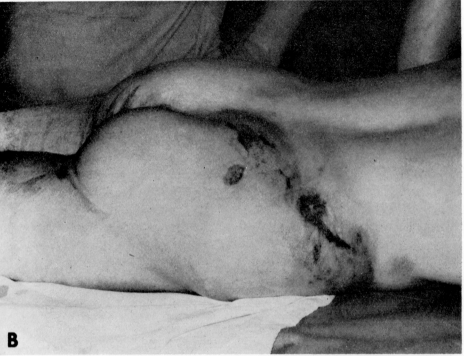

B

Figure 9-5b. Contusion asymmetry (B) and lateral compressibility suggested pelvic girdle fracture later confirmed by x-ray (C).

accumulate the prostate is not palpable and the perineum should
be inspected for ecchymoses and hematomas (see Chapter 8).
The urine must be examined for blood and both a cystogram
and urethrogram obtained.

In addition to hemorrhagic and urologic complications, fractures of the pelvis often have neurologic complications. Patterson
and Morton[7] reviewed 633 patients with pelvic fractures and
dislocations. They found twenty-two patients (3.5%) with neurologic injuries and recommend repeated neurologic assessment
and when indicated electrodiagnostic tests to confirm the clinical
observations and evaluating the prognosis. Motor and sensory
deficits must be evaluated as described in Chapter 7. Weakness
or paralysis of the hip adductors is especially significant as is
weakness or sensory deficits in the thigh, leg and ankle. Nerves
injured frequently are: pudenal, sciatic and femoral.

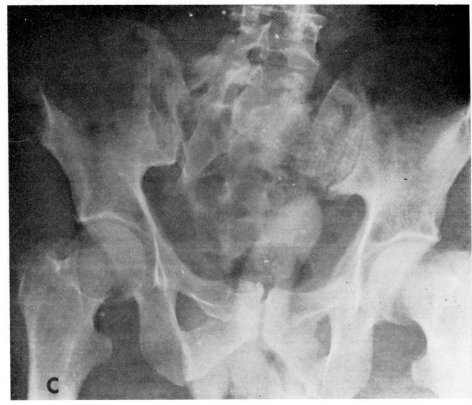

Figure 9-5c.

Hip

Proper assessment of the hip joint in the injured patient requires astute inspection of the nude patient, recording carefully the position the patient spontaneously assumes and looking for evidence of shortening, adduction and flexion.

Posterior dislocation of the hip frequently occurs when an occupant in a motor car is thrown forward violently striking one of both his knees against the dashboard. The femoral head is driven through the posterior capsule and comes to rest posterior and cephalad to the acetabulum (Fig. 9-6).

In patients presenting with this kind of history the physician should inspect the lower extremities. If the leg is in a position of flexion, adduction and internal rotation with some degree of shortening the physician should palpate the region posterior and cephalad to the acetabulum and if the head of the femur is present in this abnormal location the diagnosis of posterior dislocation of the hip is made.

Anterior dislocations of the hip are less frequent but do occur. The extremity is maintained in external rotation and slight abduction.

A small fragment of the acetabulum frequently accompanies the head of the femur. Soft tissue damage in these dislocations is severe. In posterior dislocations the sciatic nerve is often compressed or stretched. Paralysis or weakness in the distribution of the sciatic innervation denotes this complication.

Central dislocations of the femoral head are difficult to detect. There is no shortening, adduction, internal rotation as seen in posterior dislocations. Suspicion is aroused by passive motion of the hip joint. The physician holds the patient's foot with his right or left hand, depending on which hip he is examining and supports the posterior knee with his other hand, while gently flexing, rotating, adducting and abducting the hip. A central dislocation is suspected if there is significant pain produced by this motion. A rectal examination discloses edema and tenderness opposite the floor of the acetabulum (Fig. 9-7).

Before leaving the examination of the hip three questions must be answered: 1) Is the leg shortened? 2) Is the greater trochanter of the femur elevated? 3) Is the trochanter abnormally close to the mid-line of the pelvis?

Shortening can often be detected by simple inspection of the patient. When greater accuracy is indicated the length should be measured. An accurate method is to place one end of a tape measure on the anterior superior iliac spine and stretching the tape over the medial malleolus at the ankle. The position where the tip of the malleolus strikes the tape measure is recorded and the opposite side measured in a similar fashion. Normally the two extremities have no greater difference than a quarter of an inch. Very rarely a difference of half an inch may be normal (Fig. 9-8).

Elevation of the trochanter is determined by palpating the ischial tuberosity and the anterior superior iliac spine. A line is drawn between these two points (Roser-Nelaton line) (Fig.

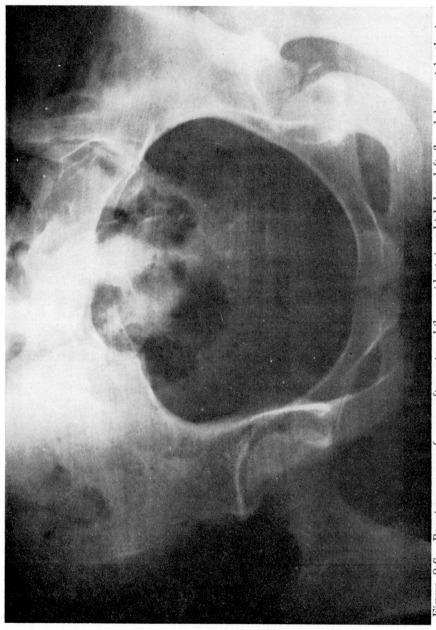

Figure 9-6.   Roentgenogram of nurse after automobile accident in which her left flexed knee violently impacted against the dashboard. Note femoral head cephalad and posterior to the fractured acetabulum.

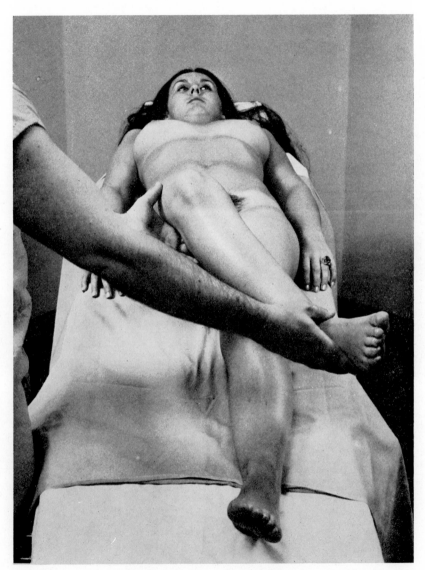

Figure 9-7. Testing for central dislocations of the femoral head.

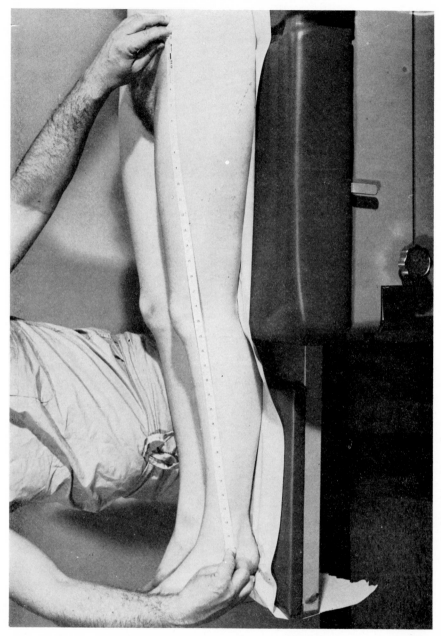

Figure 9-8.   Testing for shortening of the leg.

9-9). A convenient and accurate way of determining this line is to have the patient lie on the opposite side with the hip next to the table slightly flexed. An umbilical tape or tape measure is stretched from the anterior superior iliac spine to the tip of the tuberosity of the ischuim. The tip of the greater trochanter is determined and marked for identification. In normal non-injured subjects the tip of the greater trochanter of the femur lies just distal to (below) the Roser-Nelaton line. When the trochanter is elevated its tip can be palpated on the line or proximal to (above) it.

The distance of the greater trochanter to the midline of the pelvis is determined by palpating the posterior border of the trochanter and measuring the distance from this point to the symphysis pubis. The two extremities must be in the same position and the patient must be flat, supine and relaxed. Large calipers or a tape measure are useful in this evaluation. If they are not available an umbilical tape can be used and marked appropriately with an ink marker. To increase the accuracy of this measurement the mid-line of the pelvis can be determined by dropping a perpendicular line from a line between the anterior superior iliac spines. The trochanter on the side of the dislocated femoral epiphysis or neck fracture will be found to be closer to the median plane. This evaluation is often referred to as Morris' measurements.

Head of Femur

The head of the femur is very firm dense cancellous bone and is protected in its bed in the acetabulum. Consequently it is rarely fractured but displacement of the head of the femur on the proximal end of the neck of the femur does occur. It is limited to the adolescent age period and sometimes called adolescent coxa vara. The clinical picture resembles a fracture through the neck of the femur. To evaluate a patient for this injury the physician looks for shortening of the leg and external rotation with slight adduction. Active movement of the hip is impossible. The physician inspects Scrapa's triangle for swelling. Passive motion of the hip produces severe pain and cartilaginous crepitus and must always be applied gently.

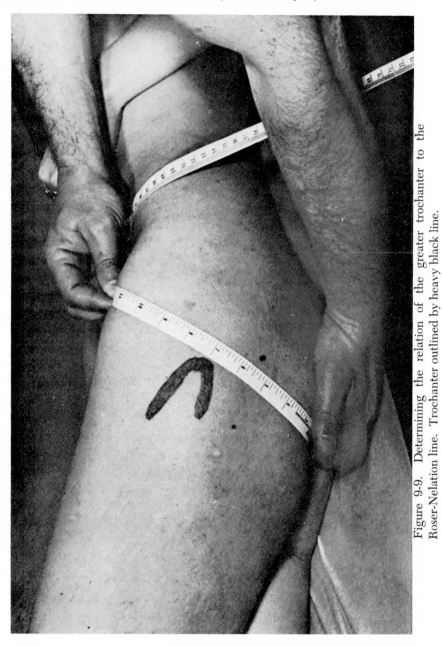

Figure 9-9. Determining the relation of the greater trochanter to the Roser-Nelation line. Trochanter outlined by heavy black line.

Neck of Femur

Fractures through the neck of the femur present such a typical picture that the physician can detect them by simple inspection of the patient. The injured side assumes a position of external rotation and slight abduction. The extremity looks like it suffers a flaccid paralysis. There is often some degree of shortening. Localized swelling may be present directly over the hip joint. Movement of the hip is very painful and there is usually no need to demonstrate it as the diagnosis is usually evident without this. The trochanter is elevated above the Roser-Nelaton line. Tenderness to palpation is also a very useful diagnostic sign. It is most easily detected over the front of the joint in Scarpa's triangle. This injury produces an abnormal looseness of the fascia lata between the iliac crest and the trochanter. depending on the amount of shortening. This relaxation of the fascia allows the physician to press his fingers in more deeply over the trochanter on the fractured side than on the normal side. This is known as Allis' sign. It is not reliable unless there is considerable shortening of the distance of the greater trochanter to the iliac crest.

Assessment of false motion at the hip is done by placing the thumb on the anterior superior spine and the tips of the fingers of the same hand on the trochanter. The other hand alternately makes slow traction and upward pressure on the thigh. If the fragments of the neck fracture are not impacted the trochanter moves up and down on the pelvis without producing much pain.

Greater Trochanter

This is generally a rare injury and may take the form of either a fracture in the adult or epiphyseal separation in the child. The mechanism is usually a direct blow or kick on the greater trochanter. The history of injury is important in the diagnosis. The physician searches for well localized tenderness to palpation and swelling on inspection. Occasionally the examiner may be able to palpate the separated loose fragment of the bone.

Lesser Trochanter

The tenderness and swelling are on the upper inner aspects of the thigh in fractures of the lesser trochanter. These injuries are usually the result of hyperextension and abduction injuries of the hip or sudden unusual strain on the iliopsoas muscle which is attached to this prominence. The insertion of this particular muscle makes possible a good evaluation test. The patient in the sitting position is asked to flex the hip. Inability to perform this motion should lead the physician to suspect a fracture of the greater trochanter. This is frequently referred to as Ludloff's sign of fracture of the lesser trochanter.

The differential between a fracture of the neck of the femur and fractures of the greater or lesser trochanter often requires roentgenographic assessment. There is frequently the same amount of pain disability and deformity. The location of the swelling and tenderness are usually helpful. In fractures through the neck of the femur the swelling and tenderness are most often limited to the region over the front of the joint usually referred to as Scarpa's triangle. In trochanteric fractures the swelling and tenderness are more marked in the region around the trochanter. This differentiation added to Ludloff's sign, palpation of the greater trochanter, relationship of trochanter to Nelaton's line and Morris' measurement, external rotation, abduction, and shortening will usually provide a reasonably accurate clinical differentiation between neck and trochanteric fractures.

Shaft of Femur

The shaft of the femur is broken in any part of its length but the majority occur in the middle third of the bone because this is the apex of a normal anterolateral bowing of the shaft. In the average case the diagnosis is self evident. There is shortening which may vary from a fraction of an inch to four or five inches. The femoral shaft fracture can be differentiated from the neck fractures by the physician if he will simply note the tip of the greater trochanter and observe that in shaft fractures the tip of the trochanter is in its normal position below the Roser-Nelaton line.

The circumference of the thigh is increased in shaft fractures and the amount of increase is directly related to amount of volume lost from the circulation and must be replaced.

The fractured femur has lost its normal anterolateral bowing and presents an exaggerated angular deformity. The level of the fracture can usually be determined by evaluating maximum tenderness after gently palpating the length of the thigh and noting the level at which false motion occurs. False motion can be evaluated by gently raising the foot and leg and moving it from side to side all the while maintaining traction on the extremity with the other hand placed on the thigh.

Another method is to grasp the greater trochanter in one hand then with the other hand rotate the leg and knee. If the greater trochanter does not rotate with the leg, this is false motion and indicates disruption of the shaft of the femur.

Distal Femur

Injury to the lower end of the femur usually occurs after a fall from a height or automobile accident. The resulting supracondylar fractures vary over a wide range, from a simple undisplaced transverse fracture to a severely comminuted fracture with a vertical line running into the intercondylar notch displacing the condyles.

The distal fragment of femur is often displaced posteriorly because of the pull of the gastrocnemius muscle. The detection of this injury is usually obvious by inspection alone. Angular deformity is frequently obvious and edema is well localized to the knee joint. Blood and fluid are usually present in the joint. Measurement discloses some shortening. The tips of the broken bones can occasionally be palpated in the popliteal space or beneath the quadriceps tendon.

The intercondylar fracture is usually referred to as a T fracture. The proximal fragment is driven into the distal fragment and splits the condyles apart. This produces increased broadening of the lower end of the femur which is visible and palpable. Unless the proximal fragment comes to rest between the two condyles, they can be squeezed back together by lateral pressure. This movement of the condyles indicates a T fracture of the distal femur.

As described previously the examination must evaluate distal circulation and innervation. Associated injury to the popliteal artery or vein must be excluded. Sensory and motor function of the foreleg and ankle must be checked.

Although the diagnosis of a fracture of the distal femur is usually detected by physical assessment, whether or not there is a fracture between the condyles (T fracture) must be determined by roentgenographic study.

A single condyle of the distal femur may be fractured. There is no shortening and no false motion. Localized tenderness can be palpated over the involved condyle. If a intra-articular fragment is present there is some limitation or blocking of motion at the knee joint.

Patella

Fractures of the patella may occur with no displacement of fragments. The knee appears markedly swollen and the joint is distended with fluid. The swelling of the knee is characteristic in that it is symmetrical and dome-like with maximum edema over the region of the patella. On palpation the patella is tender, but false motion and deformity are absent. Active motion by the patient causes pain.

Other fractures lines may cross the patella medially and laterally and extend into the quadriceps retinaculum causing wide separation of the fragments. On palpation the sulcus between the separated fragments can be detected. False motion is present and can be demonstrated by moving the two fragments independently from side to side. There is loss of ability to actively and forcefully extend the knee.

Disruption of the patellar ligament is detected when the patient is unable to extend the leg on the thigh and there is localized swelling and tenderness over the front of the knee. The knee may be distended with fluid. More importantly there is subcutaneous swelling at the site of rupture in the ligament. By palpation this is demonstrated to be below the patella while the intact and nontender patella can be palpated in an abnormally cephalad position. There is a definite depression in the tissues below the patella.

The quadriceps tendon may be ruptured without skeletal fracture. There is localized pain tenderness and swelling over the torn tendon and the patient is unable to extend the leg on the thigh. The patella is intact, nontender and in its normal position. The knee joint is distended with fluid. By palpating carefully the sulcus between the torn tendon and the patella can be demonstrated.

The patella may be displaced intact without a fracture line. It usually comes to rest on the lateral condyle and can be palpated in this abnormal position. In more rare situations it may be dislocated medially or rotated on its long axis in such a manner that one of its lateral borders is engaged between the condyles of the femur. The anterior surface of the knee appears flat and the smooth edges of the femoral condyles can be felt beneath the skin and subcutaneous tissues while the patella can be palpated in its abnormal position.

Knee

Complete dislocations of the knee produces such a striking deformity that the diagnosis is usually made by inspection alone. The large size and subcutaneous location of the bones makes palpation of identifying landmarks an excellent means of confirming the dislocation. When the dislocation is incomplete, swelling obscures the deformity and the diagnosis is more difficult. Palpation of the condyles of the femur and tibia disclose the abnormal relationship of the tibia and fibula to the femur.

In both complete and incomplete dislocations the cruciate and lateral ligaments are ruptured and very gentle manipulation delineates abnormal mobility of the knee. The circulation and nerve supply to the leg must be given careful attention.

The term "internal derangement of the knee joint" was used by Hay in 1784 to include an alteration of the joint preventing the condyles of the femur from moving in the hollow of the semilunar cartilages and depressions of the tibia. The principle causes of internal derangement of the knee are shown in Table 9-1.

Injuries of semilunar cartilages are the most common cause of internal derangement of the knee. The mechanism is usually sudden forceful internal rotation of the femur on the flexed and fixed tibia. This movement is usually combined with abduction of the knee opening the inner side of the joint. The anterior horn of the cartilage is torn loose and displaced. It usually comes to rest in the center of the joint and is caught between the condyles and the tibia when the knee is extended. The posterior horn is rarely involved. It is thought due to external rotation of the femur on the tibia followed by flexion. A longitudinal or bucket handle type tear is produced when the cartilage is broken near its middle and this portion of the cartilage is torn loose from the lateral ligament then caught between the condyles and the tibia.

On examination there is acute tenderness over the anterior portion of the semilunar cartilage and active motion of the knee is painful. The physician must test for passive extension by supporting the thigh with one hand and using the other hand to gently extend the knee. Extension is limited by ten to thirty degrees. In the early hours after injury there is little if any edema or effusion. If the patient is examined several hours after injury the normal contour of the joint is obscured by bleeding and effusion into the joint. The limited extension of the knee is the most characteristic sign and is almost pathognomic of a dislocation of the semilunar cartilage. When locking in extension is not present and tenderness to palpation and swelling with joint effusion causes the physician to be suspicious of semilunar cartilage injury, he then must inject air into the knee joint

TABLE 9-I

CAUSES OF INTERNAL DERANGEMENT
OF THE KNEE

1. Injuries of semilunar cartilages.
2. Sprain or rupture of the lateral ligaments.
3. Ruptures of cruciate ligaments.
4. Tibial spine fracture.
5. Loose bodies.

and obtain a roentgenogram. Without air injection the radiograph will be negative because the cartilage does not show in roentgenograms.

The lateral ligaments of the knee are simply condensed and thickened portions of the joint capsule. Disruption of the lateral ligaments is accompanied by effusion into the joint. In some situations the ligament is torn from its attachment to either the femur or tibia and a small segment of bone is frequently avulsed with the ligament. In a sprain fracture tenderness to palpation is most acute over the involved osseous attachment of the ligament and sometimes the careful examiner can palpate the segment of avulsed bone beneath the skin and subcutaneous tissue. There is a variable degree of edema locally over the torn lateral ligament and the knee is distended with fluid. The normal contour of the joint is obliterated by the edema. The patella floats. Flexion of the knee joint is painful and limited by the degree of effusion. If the semilunar cartilages are intact extension of the knee is free and unlimited. The tenderness is well localized and limited to the area of the disrupted ligament which is well posterior on the side of the knee. Lateral mobility of the knee joint is increased particularly if complete disruption of the ligament is present. The lateral mobility of the knee joint is away from the side of the injury. For example, when the internal lateral ligament of the knee is disrupted the leg can be abducted (moved outward) on the thigh to an abnormal degree. The joint is stable in the anteroposterior plane. To detect this increased lateral mobility of the knee joint, the physician stands to the side of the examining table and fixes the thigh with one hand while supporting and trying to move the leg outwardly with the elbow and his other hand (Figs. 9-10a and 9-10b). Lateral ligament injuries are commonly called sprains. Semilunar cartilage injuries are also frequent associated problems because they are so intimately bound to the lateral ligaments.

The cruciate ligaments are protected from injury by their location in the center of the knee. They are rarely injured. But when injured, extreme instability of the knee is present. The anterior cruciate ligament is injured more frequently than the posterior. When the knee is fully extended the anterior cruciate

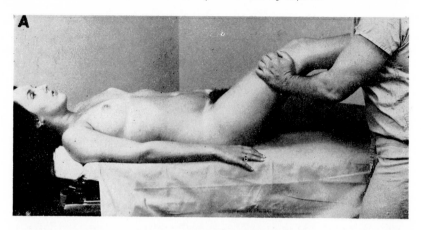

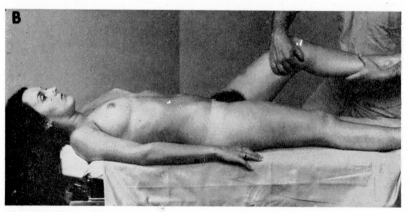

Figure 9-10a & 10b.   Testing for lateral and medial instability of knee joint.

ligament is taut and prevents hyperextension of the knee. The anterior cruciate also prevents forward slipping of the tibia on the femur when the knee is fully extended. If the internal lateral ligament has been torn the intact cruciate ligament prevents abduction and external rotation of the tibia on the femur. The posterior cruciate ligament is taut when the knee is flexed. The posterior cruciate prevents the flexed tibia from slipping upward on the femur.

The physician detects torn or disrupted cruciate ligaments of the knee by loss of stability in the anteroposterior plane.

To test for the presence of instability the physician stands in front or to one side of the injured patient. He grasps the leg just below the knee joint. With the knee extended he tries to move the tibia backward and forward on the femur. Next, he tries to gently hyperextend the knee. When these tests are positive the anterior cruciate ligament is stretched torn or actually avulsed. The examiner then flexes the knee and tries with passive pressure and motion to move the tibia up and down on the femur (Fig. 9-11). If abnormal motion is present the posterior cruciate ligament is disrupted. If false motion is present on both the above examinations both cruciates are injured. This method of evaluating cruciate ligament function is extremely reliable and in the absence of complete fractures about the knee this lack of stability in the anteroposterior plane is pathognomonic of cruciate ligament disruption.

After examining the knee thoroughly if the cruciate and lateral ligaments are proven intact yet there is pain, effusion and edema in the knee joint, injury of the tibial spine must be suspected. The most important diagnostic sign is a firm bony block greatly limiting extension of the knee. The limitation of extension must be differentiated from semilunar cartilage injuries. This is possible because there is a very slight but perceptible difference in the elastic block resulting from semilunar cartilage disruption and the firm concrete bony limitation of extension due to tibial spine fracture. A second differentiating point is that the localized tenderness is not over the cartilage region of the knee but is palpable beneath the patellar tendon.

The presence of blood or effusion within the knee joint carries such critical diagnostic implications that the knee must be specifically assessed for hydroarthoris and hemarthrosis. This is done by balloting the knee. Pressure is exerted with one hand on the quadriceps pouch. The tips of the fingers of the opposite hand press and release the patella. If fluid or blood is present in the joint space the patella is floated upward on the condyles and ballottment is detected by pressing it downward and releasing (Fig. 9-12).

When ballottment indicates fluid within the knee joint the excess blood or effusion should be aspirated with a syringe and

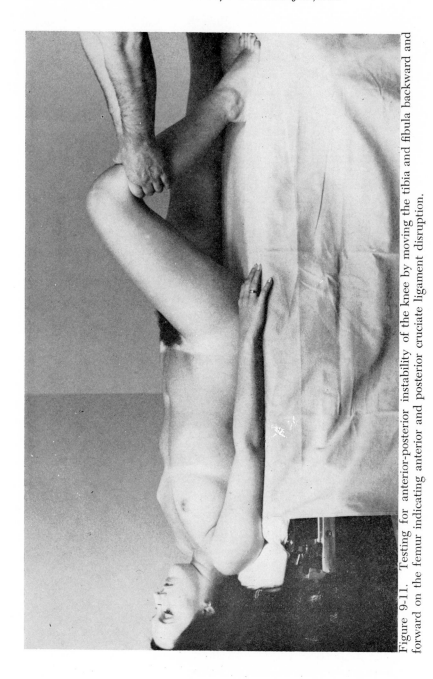

Figure 9-11.   Testing for anterior-posterior instability of the knee by moving the tibia and fibula backward and forward on the femur indicating anterior and posterior cruciate ligament disruption.

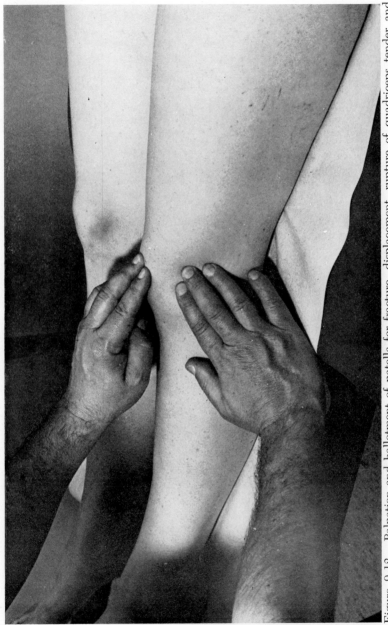

Figure 9-12. Palpation and ballotment of patella for fracture, displacement, rupture of quadriceps tender and joint fluid,

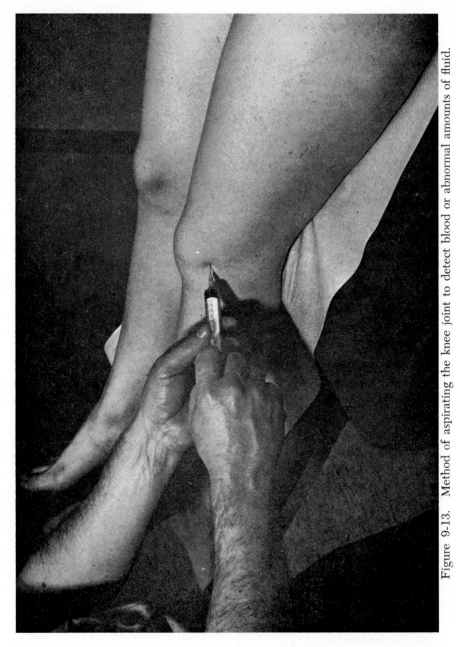

Figure 9-13.   Method of aspirating the knee joint to detect blood or abnormal amounts of fluid.

needle. This tells the assessor whether the trauma has been severe enough to disrupt blood vessels or whether the fluid is clear indicating an effusion. The knee joint can be entered laterally or mesially to the patella. The skin is prepared with a standard surgical scrub and painted with a bactericidal solution. The needle is inserted as illustrated in Figure 9-13, just deep to the patella and quadriceps tendon and the joint penetrated. The syringe is aspirated until the excess fluid is removed. Sometimes pressure against the opposite side of the joint with the other hand helps localize the fluid and makes aspiration easier.

Although Koenig's etiological term, "osteochrondritis dessicans" is the most widely known and popular explanation of loose bodies within the knee most authorities agree that direct trauma is the most common cause. In fact Key and Conwell[8] state that in some instances the injury is followed almost immediately by symptoms and signs of a loose body in the joint. In this Chapter I am concerned only with those loose bodies which are the direct result of trauma. Such loose bodies can be multiple or single. They are usually composed of cartilage and some smaller segment of underlying bone which has been detached from the articular surface of the several bones composing the knee joint. The most characteristic sign which the physician should look for is momentary locking of the joint with sudden severe pain. If the physician palpates the knee carefully he can often feel a protrusion at the joint line. In other patients a large loose body may be palpable beneath the skin and subcutaneous tissue. Such large loose bodies tend to localize in the quadricips bursa.

Tibia and Fibula

Because the proximal tibia and fibula are close to the joint, fractures of these bones are difficult to diagnose. Many of these fractures are incomplete and this makes clinical evaluation even more difficult. The patient is unable to bear weight or move the joint actively. Passive movement of the joint by the examiner is free but painful. Edema and deformity are present in variable amounts. If there has been a compression fracture of the external condyle the leg is usually in a varus or knock knee position. An avulsion fracture of the external condyle of the tibia may cause the leg to assume a valgus or bowleg position. If the examiner finds shortening of the tibia he must assume there is a fracture of the shaft of the tibia with upward displacement because this shortening is absent in fractures of a single condyle.

The examiner must palpate the tibial condyles and spine and if there is tenderness extending entirely around the bone a diagnosis of fracture is considered. If the external condyle has a compression fracture there is abnormal mobiilty of the leg outward (valgus) and tenderness is fairly well localized over the external condyle. In an avulsion fracture of the internal condyle, there is abnormal mobility of the leg inward (varus) and tenderness is again localized over the condyle. Such avulsion and compression fractures of the tibial condyles show a clinical pattern very similar to that described previously under internal derangements of the knee. A major differentiating point is that tenderness is localized over the proximal tibia in the compression and avulsion fractures of the tibial condyles.

Because of edema it is difficult to assess displacement of the fragments in proximal tibial fractures. In a T fracture, if there is definite separation of the fragments, it is possible to delineate a broadening of the condyles of the tibia. It is sometimes possible to demonstrate independent motion of the condyles of the tibia by squeezing them together or holding one condyle firmly and attempting to move the other condyle gently backward and forward with the other hand. Transverse fractures of the proximal tibia permit the examiner to demonstrate false motion in all directions. This should be done gently and with great care.

In severe fractures of the proximal tibia both condyles may be split off and driven downward creating an inverted V or Y fracture. In these severe fractures the upper third of the fibula is usually broken. The fibula is so accessible to evaluation in its proximal third that such injuries are easily detectable. There is localized pain and tenderness over the proximal fibula. A good test is to squeeze the tibia and fibula together with the hands. If pain is produced over the upper fibula it is probably broken. The examiner must remember that the peroneal nerve is often injured in proximal fibular fractures and the popliteal vessels in proximal tibial fractures.

Fractures of both bones of the leg are a very common traumatic injury. They usually involve the shafts of the tibia and fibula are nearly always complete. In most patients there is both shortening and angulation of the leg and some degree of rotation of the foot. By palpation and passive motion the examiner can nearly always find abnormal mobility. One should not fear testing for abnormal mobility in these injuries. If the examiner is careful there is relatively little pain or additional trauma to soft tissue. He should support the upper leg and knee with one hand and with the other hand gently lift the foot from the table and carefully move it from side to side. If there is a fracture the leg will bend abnormally at the fracture site. In greenstick fractures in children where the periosteum remains intact, this test does not bend the leg. The diagnosis in this age group depends upon point tenderness to palpation over the shaft of the tibia and fibula.

The amount of shortening in these injuries can be determined by measuring the distance from the external condyle to the tip of the external malleolus and (Fig. 9-14) comparing it to the opposite leg. Circulation and neural innervation of the leg distal to the fracture site must be evaluated.

Ankle

Sprain of the ankle is probably the most frequent injury of extremities. On examining the ankle there is edema anterior to and below the external malleolus. In severe sprains the swelling involves the entire foot, ankle and lower leg. A helpful test to differentiate sprain from fracture is to press the foot directly upward against the articular surface of the tibia. If severe pain is elicited there is usually a fracture because in a sprain this manipulation can be done without eliciting pain. Fractures of the external malleolus in which there is little or no displacement are difficult to diagnosis without the aid of roentgenograms. In severe fractures of the ankle with displacement of the foot on the leg inspection alone makes the diagnosis obvious.

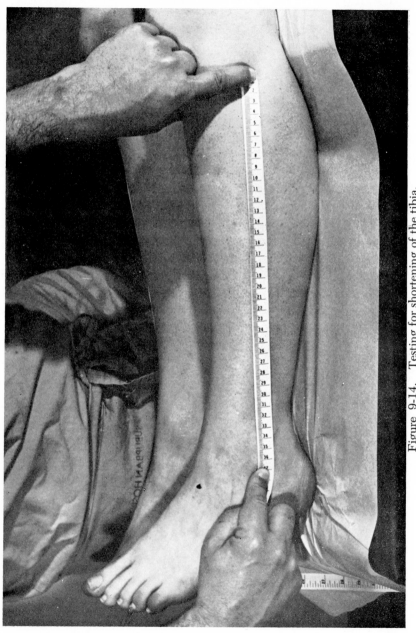

Figure 9-14.   Testing for shortening of the tibia.

Most surgeons refer to all fractures in the region of the ankle as Pott's or Dupuytren's fractures. A better classification is given by Ashhurst and Bromer[9] (Table 9-II). The examiner should inspect the foot carefully comparing it to the other foot. If the foot occupies its normal position on the leg the injury is either a sprain or a fracture with no displacement. The degree of edema is not a reliable evaluating tool. The examiner should especially check to see if there is a rotation deformity or lateral or posterior displacement of the foot. When lateral displacement is detected there must be either an abduction or an external rotation fracture. When inward displacement is detected there is an adduction fracture. Posterior displacement can be present with severe abduction or external rotation fractures. Forces which compress the ankle in the long axis of the leg can also cause posterior displacement of the ankle.

The foot and ankle should be gently palpated to assess points of tenderness. Acute tenderness around either malleolus usually means a fracture of that malleolus. Tenderness in the shafts of the tibia and fibula above the malleolus means a fracture of those bones. During this meticulous and gentle palpation the physician should take note of the position of the tips of the malleoli and confirm his suspicion of deformity that he saw upon inspection.

The examiner then manipulates the foot to assess the present or absence of false motion and whether normal motion is limited. As described before, a good way to start is by making direct pressure upward on the foot while the leg is fixed. As mentioned before this does not elicit pain in sprains of the ankle, but a fracture of even one malleolus causes pain (Fig. 9-15).

Next the leg is fixed and lateral mobility is determined. This is best done by grasping the heel and ankle firmly with one hand supporting the leg with the other hand and attempting to move the ankle outward and inward on the tibia. If lateral mobility is present there is obviously a fracture either in the lower third of the leg or one or both malleoli. Inversion and exersion of the foot are evaluated next. These motions are painful but they are useful in detecting the presence of a supramalleolar fracture.

TABLE 9-II

CLASSIFICATION OF FRACTURES, SPRAINS, AND
DISLOCATIONS ABOUT THE ANKLE

	No.	Percent
A. Fractures by External Rotation		
1. First Degree: Lower end of fibula only ("mixed oblique")	79	(26%)
2. Second Degree: Same plus rupture of internal lateral ligament of fracture of internal malleolus ("low Dupuytren")	100	(33%)
Viz.,		
(a) Internal lateral ligament, uncomplicated 13		
Internal lateral ligament complicated by posterior marginal fragment of tibia 13		
(b) Internal malleolus, uncomplicated 32		
Internal mallecolus complicated by posterior marginal fragment of tibia 42		
3. Third Degree: Same plus fracture of whole lower end of tibia, representing the internal malleolus.	5	(1.7%)
Total Fractures by External Rotation......	184	(61%)
B. Fractures by Abduction (Fibular Flexion)		
1. First Degree: Internal malleolus only	41	(13.7%)
2. Second Degree: Same plus fracture of fibula (transverse, above or below tibiofibular joint)		
(a) Below inferior tibiofibular joint (no diastasis) ("bimalleolar fracture") 13	20	(6.6%)
(b) Above inferior tibiofibular joint (with diastasis) (Pott's fracture, "Dupuytren type") 28		
3. Third Degree: Internal malleolus represented by whole lower end of tibia	2	(0.66%)
Total Fractures by Abduction	63	(21%)
C. Fractures by Adduction (Tibial Flexion)		
1. First Degree: External malleolus only, transverse, at or below level of tibial plafond	27	(9%)
2. Second Degree: Same plus		
(a) Internal malleolus below level of tibial plafond ("bimalleolar facture") 3		
(b) Median surface of tibia up and in from joint surface 8	11	(3.6%)
3. Third Degree: Same, plus whole lower end of tibia (supramalleolar fracture by adduction")	2	(0.66%)
Total Fractures by Adduction	40	(13.3%)
D. Fractures by Compression in Long Axis of Leg		
1. Isolated Marginal Fractures 1		
2. Comminution of tibial platform 3		
3. T or Y-fractures ("V-fractures of Gosselin")......4		
Total Fractures by Compression in Long Axis of Leg	8	(2.7%)
E. Fractures by Direct Violence (Supramalleolar types)	5	(1.7%)

* Taken from Ashhurst and Bromer, *Arch Surg*, vol. 4, 1922, pp. 51-129.
(Used by permission.)

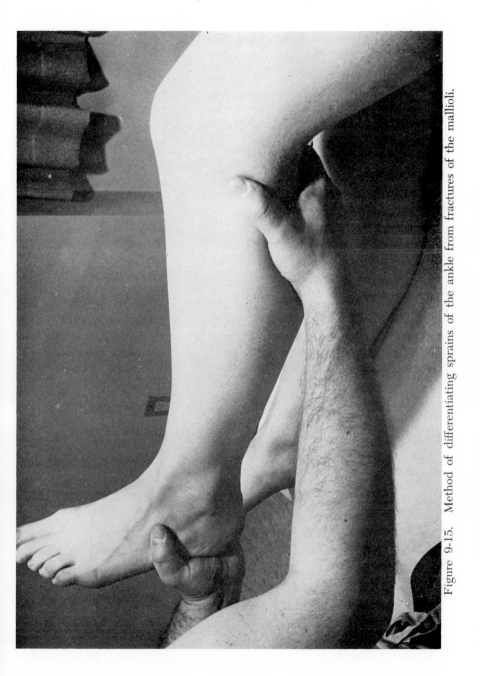

Figure 9-15. Method of differentiating sprains of the ankle from fractures of the mallioli.

Finally the range of motion at the ankle is evaluated. If there is no posterior displacement of the foot dorsiflexion is normal. It may be slightly limited by extreme swelling. If the foot is displaced posteriorly dorsiflexion is limited. Limitation of dorsiflexion suggests a posterior marginal fracture with backward displacement of the foot.

Dislocations of the ankle without fractures are rare. However, they do occur. The most frequent dislocation is posterior, the next is the anterior dislocation and the most rare is dislocation upward. A dislocation of the ankle in the lateral plane without fracture is practically impossible.

In a complete posterior dislocation the abnormal relation of the foot to the bones of the leg is usually obvious upon inspection of the ankle. The lower ends of the tibia and fibula can be palpated beneath the skin over the front of the ankle. If swelling is minimal they are also visible. The distance between the anterior border of the tibia and the heel is greatly increased. In minor posterior displacements there is loss of dorsiflexion and the lower end of the tibia is prominent. The forefoot appears definitely shortened. Lengthening of the heel can be assessed by direct measurement.

In anterior dislocations the abnormal relation of the foot to the leg is once again obvious. The heel is shortened. The tips of the fibula and tibia are prominent posteriorly. The foot is maintained in a position of dorsiflexion. The smooth articular surface of the astragalus is in front of the lower end of the tibia and the examiner can recognize this smooth articular surface by palpation.

Foot

The os calcis is not only the largest bone in the foot but is more frequently injured than any other tarsal bone. About 90 percent of the fracture lines involve the body of the os calcis. The fractures may vary from a simple crack in the bone without displacement to severely comminuted fractures. Swelling occurs soon after injury and involves the entire heel and mid portion of the foot and ankle. The heel is broadened by the bony deformity and swelling. The tissues on each side of the heel are infiltrated with blood which gives them a bluish discoloration. The long arch of the foot is flattened and the malleoli are lowered. The infiltration of blood into the surrounding soft tissues imparts a peculiar semifluctuant consistency that can be palpated on either side of the heel. Motion at the ankle joint is free, but lateral motion is limited and painful. By careful palpation the examiner can often detect the presence of excess bone behind and below the external malleolus.

Dislocation of the astragalus is rare, but can occur after severe compression and leverage injuries. There is great swelling and complete disability. The displaced astragalus is often visible beneath the skin. It can almost always be plapated in its abnormal position beneath the skin. The os calcis and malleoli are usually intact but not always. The malleoli are lowered on the os calcis.

In subastragaloid dislocations the foot is fixed in an abnormal position on the leg. The circulation of the foot is embarrassed. The malleoli are intact and motion at the ankle joint is possible, but very painful. Determining the position of the os calcis is the key to deciding the direction and degree of dislocation. Posterior dislocations of the foot shortens the forefoot and the head of the astragalus is palpable in front of the ankle. Anterior displacement of the foot shortens the heel and there is a prominence palpable beneath the Achilles tendon.

Dislocation through the midtarsal joint produces marked edema of the entire foot and ankle. The malleoli and ankle joint are intact. The forefoot is grossly displaced and the foot is shortened. The examiner should be able to palpate the head of the astragalus and the proximal borders of the displaced anterior tarsal bones in their abnormal position. Motion is possible at the ankle, but the forefoot is fixed in its abnormal position.

Fractures of the scaphoid cause the foot to be held in a position of eversion and attempts on the part of the physician to invert or dorsiflex the foot cause pain at the site of fracture. The patient is unable to bear weight on the foot. The physician should palpate the area of pain and swelling searching for the fragments of bone which are usually present in the subcutaneous tissue.

Dislocations at the tarsometarsal joints may be accompanied by such extensive edema that the deformity of the dislocation is overlooked. Palpation is important in these situations. Many times the deformity is visible especially in dorsal dislocations where the heavy base of the metatarsals causes a marked prominince on the dorsum of the foot. The extensor tendons of the foot are drawn tightly over this prominence.

To detect fractures of the metatarsal bones the examiner attempts to demonstrate false motion. The physician immobolizes the proximal end of the metatarsal with one hand then grasps the distal fragment between the thumb and fingers of the other hand. The distal metatarsal is moved in flexion and extension searching for crepitus and false motion.

Achilles Tendon

The most impressive statistic regarding rupture of the Achilles tendon is the delay in diagnosis There is little to explain this delay in diagnosis other than lack of proper evaluation of patients. The lesion is often misdiagnosed as ankle sprain, peritendinitis, "tennis leg," plantaris rupture or periostitis.

Disability of the patient is increased by both the delay in diagnosis and the misdiagnosis.

Sudden unexpected dorsiflexion of the ankle and violent dorsiflexion of a plantar-flexed foot rupture the tendon either at its insertion, or the museulotendinous junction. In some there is an avulsion of a fragment of the os calcis accompanying the tendon.

The detection of this injury is fairly simple and the statistics regarding delay in diagnosis and misdiagnosis in the face of an accurate means of detection must mean that physicians forget to evaluate patients for this injury. The course of the tendon can easily be palpated in its subcutaneous location. The examiner palpates carefully for a defect or a difference in tension between the two sides. Then he applies a very reliable test. Grasping the gastrosoleus mechanism with his hand he squeezes. Failure of the foot to respond with plantar flexion invariably means rupture of the Achilles tendon. Thompson described this test,[10] and others have found it reliable in differentiating complete from incomplete ruptures.[11] The physician must not misinterpret an ankle jerk nor active plantar flexion of the foot by the patient. In the presence of complete rupture of the Achilles tendon these can be accounted for by the long toe flexors, peroneals and tibialis posterior. However, the strength of plantar flexion will be significantly less than the intact side. Another diagnostic sign is the excessive dorsiflexion at the ankle that can be produced by passive motion on the side of the rupture.

ROENTGENOGRAPHIC APPRAISAL

It is only after the preceding meticulous evaluation of the musculoskeletal system has been concluded that roentgenographic aid is sought. These are only to aid the physician and confirm what he has discovered by his assessment. To do otherwise is to abdicate a primary responsibility that the patient entrusts to his physician. Too many seriously injured patients spend excessively long hours under a cathode tube receiving total body irradiation because their physicians have relegated their role as diagnostician to a machine.

The irrational and complete trust in total roentgenographic evaluation of critically injured patients precipitates in actuality what the doctor is futilely hoping to prevent: the overlooked injury, the missed diagnosis. Yet the common practice is to obtain total body radiographs first and then come back when there is time and look at the patient. This process must be reversed. The assessments described in this chapter must be done first, then and only then are roentgenograms obtained. They are to confirm and further delineate the injuries, displacements, dislocations and fractures that have been disclosed by his evaluation. Of major importance are those injuries that roentgenograms are unable to divulge. I have tried to emphasize them and I have probably omitted some in doing so. Once the physician eradicates his blind faith in roentgenographic diagnosis such injuries will be easily remembered.

These statements must not be misconstrued to reduce the

importance of roentgenographic evaluation of the musculoskeletal system. But in a time when the customary method is to survey injured patients with total body irradiation there must be some effort to restore the physician to his primary position. His judgement based on his findings will then allow him to order not only the radiographs needed by his patient but also direct the timing and order in which this roentgenographic assessment is done. If in his judgement there is no need on the day of admission to X-ray a nondisplaced humeral shaft fracture in a seriously injured patient with hypovolemia, ruptured liver, flail chest, and arterial hypoxemia, then as team captain he must establish priorities. After correcting hypovolemia repairing the ruptured liver, stabilizing the flail chest and increasing the arterial pO_2, thorough roentgenographic assessment of the humeral fracture can be done twenty-four to seventy-two hours later in a stable patient.

IMMOBILIZATION

An integral part of appraising injuries of the musculoskeletal system is proper splinting before and after evaluation has been done. In the ideal emergency medical system this will be initially instituted at the site of injury. Within the hospital the physician removes the splinting device and evaluates the fracture, status of peripheral circulation and nervous innervation. After evaluation appropriate splinting devices are re-applied before the patient is sent to the X-ray department or jostled about the hospital from stretcher to table to stretcher.

If no attempts have been made to immobilize fracture sites before the patient's arrival at the hospital it then becomes the physician's responsibility to see that such fractures are adequately immobilized even though the splinting may be very temporary. Any open skin or puncture wounds should be quickly scrubbed with surgical soap. A sterile occlusive dressing is applied over the wound before the splinting device is applied.

Immobilization of fractures before and after clinical evaluation is important because it prevents closed fractures from becoming open fractures while the patient is turned, examined and transported. It prevents unstable displaced fractures from incar-

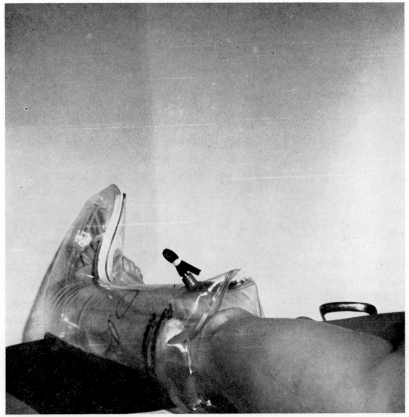

Figure 9-16. Temporary immobilization of fractures by various kinds of splinting devices is essential. The pneumatic splint is helpful in some leg fractures.

cerating arteries and nerves. It reduces the patient's pain, discomfort and suffering. Immobilization plus sterile occlusive dressings prevent additional contamination of open fractures by environment and hospital microorganisms (Fig. 9-16).

REFERENCES

1. American Academy of Orthopedic Surgeons: *Emergency Care and Transportation of the Sick and Injured.* George Banta Co., Menasha, Wisconsin, 1971.
2. Drapanas, T.; Hewitt, R. L.; Weichert, R. F., and Smith, A. D.:

Civilian vascular injuries: A critical appraisal of three decades of management. *Ann Surg, 172*:351, 1970.

3. Mayer, J. H.: Colles' fracture. *Br J Surg, 27*:629-642, 1940.

4. Braunstein, P. W.; Skudder, P. A.; McCarroll, J. R.; Musolino, A., and Wade, P.: Concealed hemorrhage due to pelvic fracture. *J Trauma, 4*:832-838, 1964.

5. Levine, J. I., and Crampton, R. S.: Major abdominal injuries associated with pelvic fractures. *Surg Gynecol Obstet, 116*:223-226, 1963.

6. Wiggishoff, C. C., and Klefer, J. H.: Urethral injury associated with pelvic fracture. *J Trauma, 8*:1042-1047, 1968.

7. Patterson, F. P., and Morton, K. S.: Neurological complications of fractures and dislocations of the pelvis. *J Trauma, 12*:1013-1023, 1972.

8. Key, J. A., and Conwell, H. E.: The management of fracture dislocations and sprains. St. Louis, C. V. Mosby Co., 1934.

9. Ashhurst, A. P. C., and Bromer, R. S.: Classification and mechanism of fractures of the leg bones involving the ankle. *Arch Surg, 4*:51-129, 1922.

10. Thompson, T. C., and Doherty, J. H.: Spontaneous rupture of tendon of Achilles: A new clinical diagnostic test. *J Trauma, 2*:126-129, 1962.

11. Ljungquist, R.: Spontaneous partial rupture of the Achilles tendon. *Acta Orth Scand Suppl, 113*:1-86, 1968.

FACIAL INJURIES

———————————————————————————————————————

$\mathbf{F}$ ACIAL INJURIES ARE almost never fatal and ordinarily are very low in priority of treatment. Reduction and fixation of facial fractures usually do not need to be considered an emergency.[1] Facial bones are membranous and healing begins with fibrous union. Although healing begins immediately, facial bone fractures can be readily reduced within a two week period following injury! Soft tissue injuries of the face can be put off twenty-four hours without jeopardizing the functional and esthetic result, providing bleeding has been controlled and wounds properly cleaned and dressed.

Although these are principles proposed by authorities, they are often neglected or overlooked. I reported several patients who had cardiac arrest from hypvolemia while scalp wounds were being cleaned and sutured.[2] Facial wounds are so obvious that it is difficult for physicians and nurses not to be impressed with their severity. The neglected facial injury is indeed a real tragedy but an even worse tragedy is death or brain necrosis resulting from hypovolemia and hypoxemia from subtle hidden, but more serious injuries. After first priorities have been managed facial injuries should be given the skilled and careful treatment they rightly deserve. In order for patients to receive appropriate management facial injuries must be detected and appraised by careful thorough examination of the face.

The automobile provides modern society with a weapon capable of mutilating the face in a manner previously unimagined. Although many other accidents injure the face, none are as

Clinical Evaluation of the Critically Injured

TABLE 10-I

CAUSES OF FACIAL INJURY

Cause	*No. of Patients*	*Percent*
Automobile Accidents	565	54
Home Accidents	171	17
Athletic injuries	118	11
Animal bites	60	6
Other	55	5
Intended injury	46	4
Work injury	27	3
TOTAL	1042	100

From *Facial Fractures* by Schults, R. C., Copyright 1970 by Year Book Medical Publishers, Inc., Chicago. Used by permission.

frequent nor so severe as those resulting from high velocity vehicular acceleration and deceleration injuries (Table 10-I). The type of injury appears related to the position of the victim within the automobile. The front seat non-driver passenger seems the most vulnerable. Proper application of seat belts could quickly reduce the degree and frequency of these injuries.

Varying degrees of respiratory embarrassment accompanies nearly all facial injuries. Airway obstruction is a frequent complication. As we have discussed in previous chapters establishing a patent, functioning airway is the first priority. In the ideal emergency medical system this is done at the scene of the accident. If physicians discover this is not being done, they have a responsibility to society and critically injured patients to begin whatever steps are necessary to see that adequate airways are established in Phase 1 management of patients. The most excellent technique of a skilled plastic surgeon in careful and meticulous coaptation of facial wounds in a beautiful young female patient may be cancelled completely if anoxic brain damage for lack of proper airway thrusts the young lady into a bleak, dark nursing home where her lovely face along with imperceptible scars can never grace the company of friends and admirers ever again.

The mouth, nasopharynx, and pharynx should be suctioned at the scene of injury and the airway palpated for foreign bodies, broken dentures, etc., with the index finger. When finally under the care of a physician in Phase II management the initial airway established by the emergency medical technician should be re-evaluated; suctioning of the mouth and pharynx repeated. A more complete and thorough inspection is now done with illumination and direct visualization. Smaller foreign bodies that could not be detected by gross unilluminated inspection in a muddy, snow covered field or rocky ledge, must be searched for: bits of bone, teeth, dental prosthetics, aspirated meat and vegetable fibers must be removed.

The tongue receives major support from the mandible. A disrupted mandible allows the tongue to occlude the airway. Swelling and bleeding reduce the amount of posterior displacement of the tongue needed to obstruct the airway. The alert physician must not underestimate this.

A more efficient or durable airway may need to be substituted for the initial airway established at the scene of injury. This is especially important before the physician sends his patient riding around the hospital to X-ray departments and elsewhere with a temporary airway that may be easily dislodged.

The need for doing tracheostomies in poorly illuminated and inadequately equipped areas outside the operating suite is disappearing. The easy availability of disposable endotracheal tubes of varying size and laryngoscopes whose batteries and bulbs are maintained and replaced on a regular basis should continue to reduce the hurried, scarry, blind type tracheotomies. The insertion of tracheal tubes either by nose or mouth is not an exclusive technique of those trained in anesthesiology. It is a sad commentary on medical education and training today that this procedure has been uniquely considered a highly specialized area. Every physician regardless of his area of interest should master and be prepared to instruct nurses and emergency medical technicians in the technic.

The next major complication of facial injuries that takes priority over all other aspects maxillofacial trauma is hemorrhage. The vascularity of the face is almost extravagant. Large volumes of blood can be lost instantaneously. Continued slow oozing at what appears to be a rather insignificant rate can rapidly accumulate into volumes that influence circulation. A frequent pitfall in evaluating this hemorrhage is attempting to control with hemostats each and every solitary pumping arteriole. The neophyte physician will find that he can unconsciously spend many minutes or in some instances hours futilely clamping away at a myriad of briskly bleeding arterioles. The accumulative blood loss becomes significant endangering circulatory efficiency.

Such areas of hemorrhage should be quickly assessed with an index finger for foreign bodies, fractures, crepitus and then occluded with a sterile pressure dressing while he proceeds to further evaluate the patient. If the anatomy of the area precludes achieving hemostatic levels of pressure, he should enlist the aid of an assistant and instruct them to apply firm pressure with their hands to the dressing. Most hemorrhage from facial injuries can be quickly and effectively controlled in this manner.

While arranging priorities it is important to remember that soft tissue injuries of the face can be put off twenty-four hours if necessary without compromising the final result. If this delayed management is decided upon, the wounds should be scrubbed with surgical soap, occluded with sterile dressings and the patient given antibiotics.

The appraisal of facial injuries after the priorities of airway obstruction, hemostasis and blood volume replacement are met, depends upon the detection of dislocations and fractures of the facial bones (Table 10-II). The chief method of evaluating these fractures is inspection and palpation. Roentgenograms are an aid in delineating more completely what the physician has already determined by palpation. Nearly all fractures of facial bones can be accurately diagnosed by palpation.

Bimanual palpation of the facial bones with one examining finger in the facial cavity where possible is one of the most reliable means of evaluating facial injuries. Each physician should organize and work out his own system of palpating the bony structure of the face, but it should always include the following structures: (1) teeth and alveolar ridges, (2) mandible, (3) malar eminences, (4) maxilla, (5) nasal bones, (6) zygoma, (7) zygomatic arches, (8) orbital boundaries; supraorbital, infraorbital lateral and medial orbital rims inclusive.

TABLE 10-II

FREQUENCY OF BONES FRACTURED

Type	No.	Percent
Nasal Bones	382	37
Zygoma and Arch	159	15
Mandible	112	11
Orbital Floor	112	11
Maxilla	84	8
Teeth	71	7
Sinuses	50	5
Supraorbital	36	4
Alveolus	25	2
TOTAL	1,031	100

From *Facial Fractures* by Schults, R. C., Copyright 1970 by Year Book Medical Publishers, Inc., Chicago. Used by permission.

Teeth and Alveolar Ridge

The teeth and aveolar ridge are palpated with the fingers and thumb. Completely avulsed teeth should be removed to avoid aspiration and occlusion of the airway. These teeth should be handled gently and placed in saline containing an appropriate antibiotic to await the appraisal of consultants regarding replantation. Partially avulsed teeth are replanted with care to await immobilization on a more permanent basis by a dental consultant.

Grossly displaced fractures of the alveolar ridge may occur as a solitary lesion or in association with mandibular fractures. If the segment of alveolar ridge is large and the surrounding soft tissue is not so severely avulsed as to devitalize the segment, it should be returned to its anatomical position and await future appraisal by dental consultants. When the aveolar process is avulsed and obviously devoid of its blood supply and nervous innervation it should be removed. The area can later be debrided, cleaned and prepared for definitive alveoloplasty.

Mandible

Anterior dislocation of the mandible occurs without fracture after certain kinds of blows to the face. The condylar head advances forward beyond the articular eminence. The mouth is locked in this wide open position and the patient is unable to close it. The muscles which close the jaw experience severe spasm and this produces acute pain for the conscious patient. This continuing muscle spasm of the masseter, internal pterygoid and temporalis muscles keep the jaw dislocated.

The index finger of the examiner can be placed into the patient's external auditory canal and while the patient or an assistant moves the mandible the physician cannot feel the condyle moving at the tip of his index finger. In normal subjects this movement of the condyle can be palpated in the external auditory canal.

In unilateral dislocations of the mandible, the chin deviates to the opposite side. In bilateral dislocations the jaw is held forward by the displaced condyles and there is malocclusion.

Rowe and Killey[3] report the mandibular fractures are the most common of all facial bone fractures (45%). If a fracture is detected at any point along the mandible the examiner must search carefully for a second or third fracture site, because multiple fractures of the mandible occur more than 50 percent of the time. Physicians should be aware of the common combinations of mandibular fractures (Table 10-III).

Inspection begins inside the mouth. Particular attention is paid to the floor of the mouth. Ecchymosis in the floor of the mouth is pathognomic of fracture of the body of the mandible. Hemorrhage around one or more teeth and malocclusion are also highly significant. The examiner should next inspect the external surface. Asymmetry, displacement and localized swelling are noted with care. Gross displacement and asymmetry are easy to detect by the alert examiner.

The body of the mandible can be easily palpated with one finger inside the mouth on the lingual side and the other hand

TABLE 10-III

COMMON COMBINATIONS OF MANDIBULUAR FRACTURES

Anatomic Site of Applied Force	Contrecoup Stress Injury
Symphysis	Either Angle
Body	Contralateral Angle
Symphysis	Either or Both Condyles
Body	Contralateral Condyle
Ramus	Contralateral Ramus

on the external surface of the jaw (Fig. 10-1). The two hands working in unison can apply leverage and pressure alternately. Pain crepitus and false motion indicate fracture.

Next the angles of the mandible are palpated with the fingers grasping the inner surface and the thumbs applying gentle pressure on the external surface (Fig. 10-2). Finally the condyles are palpated by placing the index fingers in the external auditory canal and asking the patient to open and close his mouth (Fig. 10-3). The amount of pain and the difference in feel between the two sides will determine the side of the injury. In the

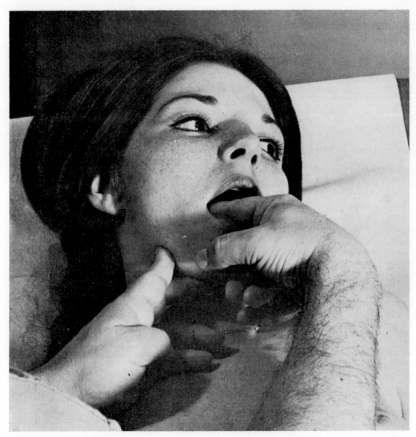

Figure 10-1. Method of bimanual palpation of the body of the mandible.

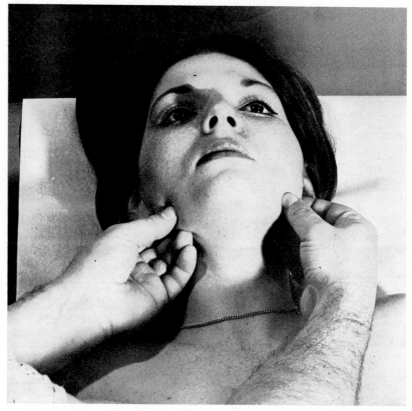

Figure 10-2.   Palpating the angles of the mandible for false motions.

unconscious patient an assistant is asked to open and close the patient's jaws.

The rami are difficult to palpate because they are covered by heavy muscles, but with a little experience the examiner can begin to appreciate subtle differences by palpating inside the mouth and the external surface simultaneously. Fractures of the ramus are relatively uncommon. When they are present there is usually an associated fracture of the contralateral ramus.

Subcondylar fractures are one of the most frequent injuries to the mandible. The narrow subcondylar neck is structurally weak. Bilateral subcondylar fractures produce a true anterior open bite by telescoping of the ascending rami on the condyles.

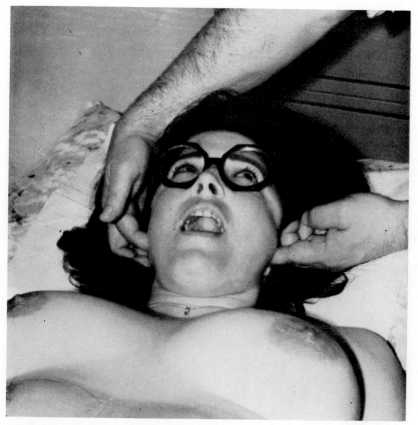

Figure 10-3.   Testing for fracture of the condyles of the mandible.

Maxilla

Injuries to the maxilla or segments of the maxillofacial structure are easy to diagnose. The key is false motion. It is true that there can be a simple linear fracture without false motion, but such fractures of the maxilla without false motion are clinically insignificant. Most injuries to this bone can be detected by grasping the teeth as illustrated in Figure 10-4 and attempting to move the maxilla in various directions. It is important that the patient be on a firm flat surface when this examination is done.

Malocclusion is a second sign of fracture of the maxilla. An

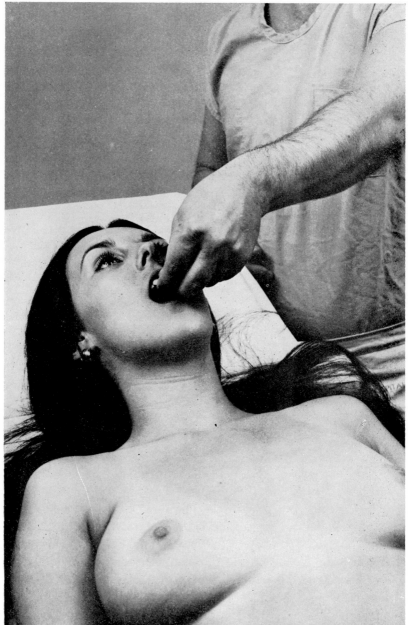

Figure 10-4.   The upper teeth are grasped between the thumb and index finger to test for fractures of the maxilla.

anterior open bite is a common finding but in itself is not sufficient evidence of a maxillary fracture. Fractures of the mandible must be excluded before malocclusion can be attributed to fracture of the maxilla.

Violent forces transmitted to the middle third of the face produce fractures of varying extent. Examination of the human skull in this region shows that fracture in more than one area is likely. The force can be transmitted entirely across the face causing a complete transverse fracture which can occur at any level and on the contralateral side produce separation at or near the maxillozygomatic suture line. Such extensive fractures can involve the floor of the orbit and sinuses. Severe lacerations, contusions and comminution of bone accompany such injuries.

These fractures of the maxilla and associated middle third of the face have been classified by LeFort into three groups.[4] His classification is so integral a part of understanding, detecting and treating maxillo facial fractures that every physician should become familiar with it. The three fracture planes described by Le Fort are transverse (Le Fort I), pyramidal (Le Fort II), and craniofacial disjunction (Le Fort III).

The Le Fort I (Figs. 10-5a and 10-5b) involves the alveolar process of the maxilla, the palate and pterygoid process in a single detached block. This kind of transverse maxillary fracture is evaluated by grasping the upper teeth and alveolar ridge with the fingers and lifting upward while the patient is lying flat as shown in Figure 10-4. The amount and location of false motion and crepitus outline the plane of fracture reliably.

The Le Forte II fracture is more complex. The whole central region of the face including the maxilla, half of the antrum, medial half of the infraorbital ridge, medial portion of the orbit and orbital floor, nasal fossa and nasal bones in violently torn from the cranial base (Figs. 10-6a and 10-6b). The upper teeth and alveolar ridge are again grasped and the amount of movement of the middle third of the face is appraised. There is considerably more false motion than in Le Fort I fractures. The false motion can be detected around the upper nose and over the zygoma. Edema is more extensive. When there is sufficient

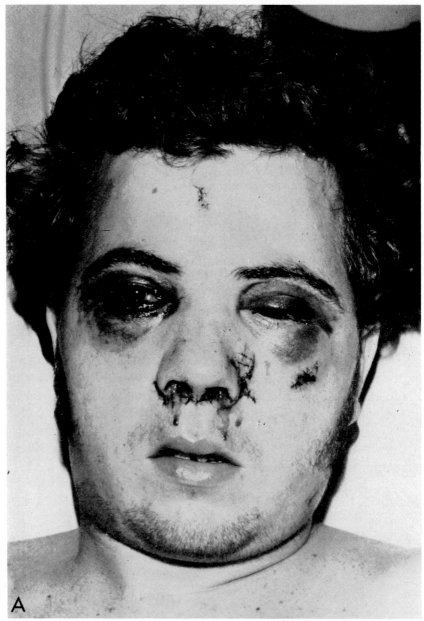

Figure 10-5. Twenty-three-year-old man with a LeFort 1 fracture of the maxilla (A). The line of fracture is illustrated (B).

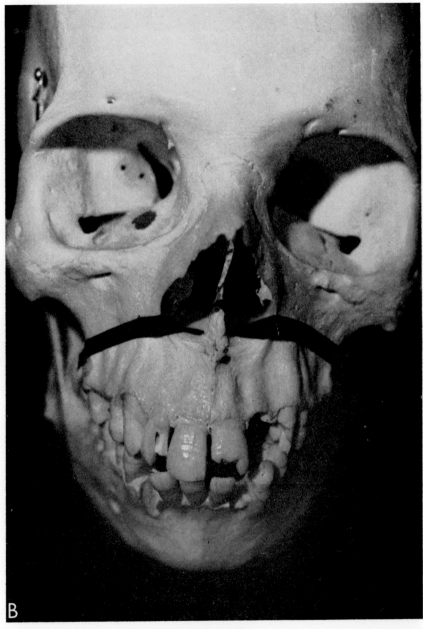

Figure 10-5b.

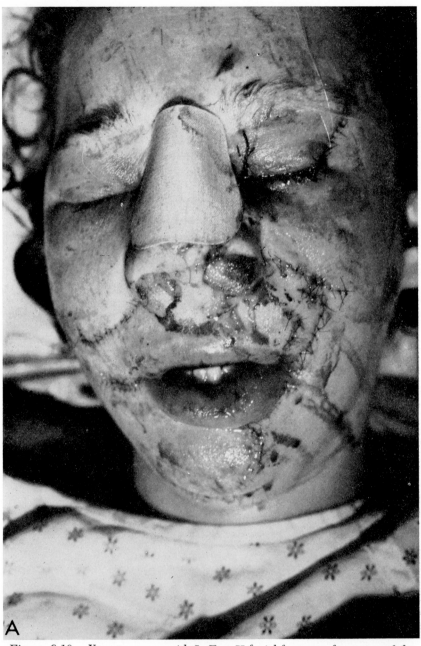

A

Figure 6-10. Young woman with LeFort II facial fracture after automobile accident (A). The fracture line is shown by the solid black line on the skull (B).

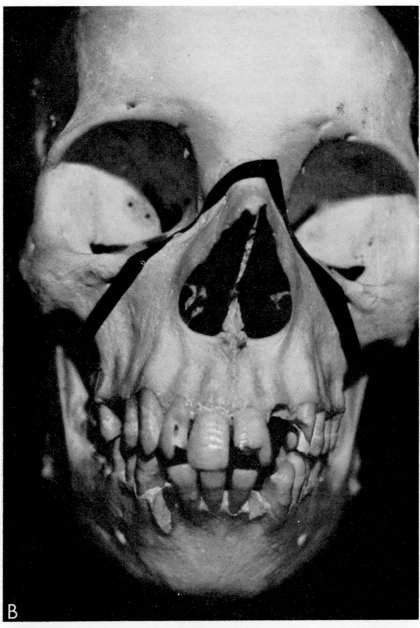

Figure 10-6b.

displacement of pyramidal fractures an anterior open bite is produced.

The extreme of facial skeletal injury is the total craniofacial disjunction (Le Fort III) the plane of fracture is at the junction of the facial bones with the cranium. The bones of the face are completely detached from the cranium, the face sags and presents an elongated appearance to inspection. It includes detachment of both zygomas, the maxillas, nasal bones, ethmoids, vomer and the lesser facial bones. The line of fractures run through the orbits, across the root of the nasal bones and through the zygomatic-frontal suture line (Figs. 10-7a and 10-7b). Many of the bones are comminuted and displaced. There can be unilateral or bilateral involvement and many various combinations producing segmental fracture patterns. The entire middle third of the face can be moved freely when the examiner grasps the maxilla and lifts. This section of the midface floats free. An integral part of evaluating this extensive craniofacial disjunction is occular support, malocclusion and spinal fluid leaks. These must be searched for and excluded as part of assessing Le Forte III injuries.

Nasal Bones

Fractures of these bones are usually classified: (1) depressed (2) laterally angulated (3) comminuted. Since the nose is the most prominent projection from the face it is the most frequently injured (see Table 10-II). Epistaxis is nearly always present and when present a nasal bone fracture must be considered. Periorbital ecchymosis, angulation swelling, tenderness, crepitus are additional signs of nasal bone fractures. Roentgenologic evaluation is unreliable and a patient should never be dismissed as not having a nasal fracture simply because it could not be seen on roentgenograms. Careful palpation of the nose must be done searching for crepitus and false motion.

Zygoma

The zygoma like the maxilla articulates with numerous other facial bones; injuries rarely involve the zygoma alone. A strong lateral buttress to the face is provided by the massiveness of the

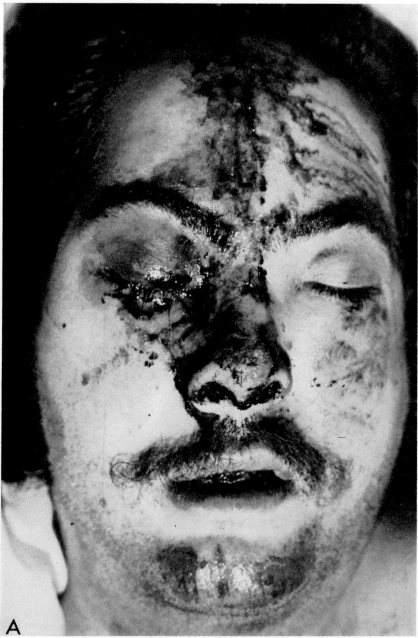

A

Figure 10-7. Craniofacial disjunction is present in this LeFort III fracture after the patient was involved in an automobile accident (A). The plane of the fracture is at the junction of the facial bones with the cranium and is illustrated on the skull by the hairy black line (B).

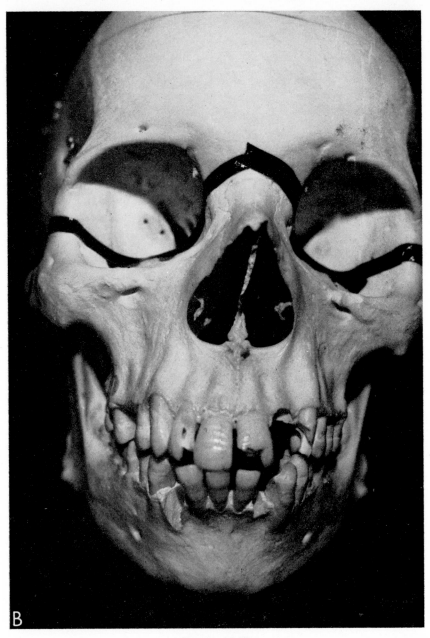

Figure 10-7b.

zygoma. Its articulations with the frontal bone and the maxilla provide a bridge between the upper and middle third of the facial skeleton. It also articulates with the sphenoid bone posteriorly and with the temporal bone through the zygomatic arch. Periorbital ecchymosis is an obvious visual sign of fracture of the zygoma. Reduction in the height of the malar eminence as viewed from above the patient's head points to fractures of this bone. This is caused by depression of the zygoma and this indicates three points of fracture separation: (1) along the infraorbital rim (2) at the zygomatic-frontal articulation (3) at the junction with the temporal bone in the zygomatic arch. Other findings in zygomatic fractures are: depression of the inferior orbital rim, tenderness at the zygomatic frontal suture line, and around the lateral and infraorbital rim. Hypesthesia of the nasolabial area and upper lip are present in severe fractures of the zygoma. Although fractures of the zygoma can occur independently, they are often associated with orbital fractures and occular function must always be evaluated.

The zygomatic arch may be fractured separately. In most people it is such a superficial structure that palpation is very effective in detecting (Fig. 10-8) these injuries. Swelling may be localized to the area of the arch. If edema and hematoma are not too severe, the careful observer can see depression or some degree of flatness over the arch area. Orbital ecchymosis is usually present on the side of the fracture. Occasionally with careful palpation crepitation can be discovered at the fracture site. If the fragments of the zygomatic arch are severely depressed they may impinge on the mandibular condyle or coronoid process and interfere with opening or closing of the mouth. Other fractures of the zygomatic arch are outbowing rather than depressions. The proper angle of force delivered to the body of the zygoma drives it backward producing a crumpling up effect which can be seen externally as a bowing outwardly. This raised and crumpled zygomatic arch can be palpated beneath the subcutaneous tissues.

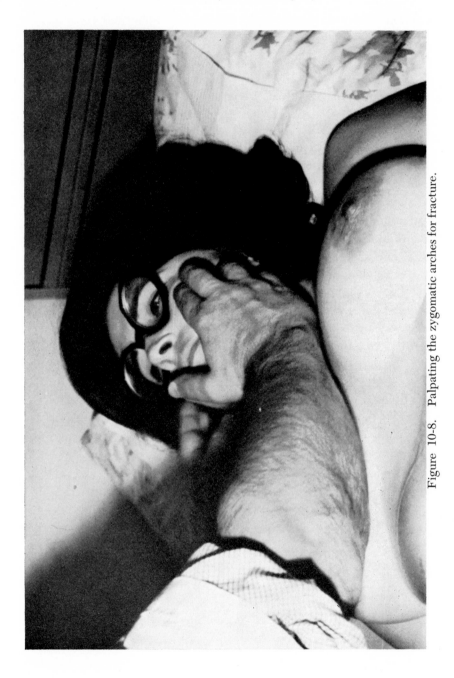

Figure 10-8.   Palpating the zygomatic arches for fracture.

Orbit

The discussion of eye and orbital injuries in critically injured patients is limited to those points of appraisal which can be done without specialized equipment, and which can be carried as far as limits of safety to the patient permit. It is also limited by the patient's co-operation. Most physicians equate the importance of an evaluating test with its complexity expense and sophisticated equipment. This is misleading. One of the most important screening test for eye injuries is visual acuity. A test as easy and cheap as visual acuity is usually discounted. But remember a sudden loss of visual acuity after an accident means a serious injury. Evaluation with specialized ophthalmic equipment must be done later for appropriate indications when the patients' conditions permits.

A bright well focused flashlight and a magnifying loupe (spectacles) are essential for adequate inspection of the eye. To find corneal abrasions the light is moved slowly from various oblique positions. Remember that a light directed straight into the eye alone the visual axis is often painful to the patient and it is certainly of less diagnostic help to the physician. As the light is moved slowly from an oblique direction, the examiner should look for irregularities in the corneal reflections of the light, and for shadows cast on the iris by otherwise invisible corneal lesions. Gauging the depth of the anterior chamber is critically important. Perforating injuries permit leakage of aqueous and the iris will come to lie against the cornea. Abrasions and ulcers cause irregularities and distortion of the light on the smooth mirror surface of the cornea. Shadows cast on the iris by abrasions and foreign bodies will move in the opposite direction in which the light is moving. These iris shadows can demonstrate very minute foreign bodies since their image is magnified. Remember also, corneal injuries hurt!

The eye should always be examined with the idea of a penetrating wound in mind. The classical "black eye" though usually harmless can hide a ruptured sclera or choroid, retinal detachment or dislocated lens. Physicians should always be

suspicious that the source of blood in subconjunctional hemorrhages may be hiding the rupture site.

Scleral rupture is frequently seen at the limbus (junction of
cornea and sclera) in the upper nasal quadrant. This usually
is due to trauma sustained most commonly at the inferior
temporal quadrant. Sclera rupture may also occur deep to any
rectus muscle. The examiner sets a standard opthalmoscope on 0
and observes the red reflex of the eye from in front of the patient
at a distance of about one foot. Then closing the lid over the
eye, the examiner gently palpates the globe. Finger tension is
important. Determine whether the globe is very soft or very
hard. If the eye is mushy soft there is a serious problem. Don't
push on it again and again. Don't ask multiple examiners to
feel the soft eye. More sophisticated assessment of pressures
should not be done when a ruptured globe is suspected. A poor
or absent red reflex, decreased vision and a soft globe suggests
complete or partial scleral rupture. Rupture of the choroid with
the retina and sclera remaining intact can occur. It is detected
by opthalmoscopic examination which shows a crescent shaped
white arc concentric to the disk. The visual field defect corre-
sponds to the white crescents. When the globe is ruptured the
evaluation ceases and the eye is protected with a large sterile
dressing. The dressing *must not* put pressure on the eye nor
compress it in any way. After other priorities are ascertained,
the opthalmologist is consulted.

If the globe is not ruptured, the evaluation progresses to
viewing the retina with an opthalmoscope. When the cause of
retinal detachment is traumatic in origin, an anterior defect in
the retina permits the vitreous to dissect into the potential space
between retina and pigment epithelium. The retinal detachment
begins peripherally at this defect. Viewing the defect which
precipitated the dissection is usually impossible because it is so
far anterior. Through the opthalmoscope the physician sees a
gray mound protruding into the eyes and disturbing varying
parts of the red fundus reflex. The surface of the elevated
retina may show ripple like striae. There may be varying sizes
of folds present in the retina. The vascular pattern of the choroid
is obscured in the section of the retina involved. The retinal

vessels in the detached retina are out of focus. They can be visualized by increasing the plus diopters of the opthalmoscope. The patient will have reduced vision in the quadrant opposite the detached retina. If the patient can cooperate and read from a newspaper or other visual acuity appraisal his macula probably remains intact and is not involved in the retinal detachment. When retinal detachment has been detected, the patient's eyes should be immobilized by patching and bed rest until definitive repair can be done.

After establishing there has been no penetration or rupture of the globe and no retinal detachment, fluroscein staining can be done to detect corneal pathology. Individually packed fluorescein-impregnanted paper strips are commercially available. Traumatic abrasions and ulcerations of the cornea concentrate the flurescent green stain.

The signs of perforation of the cornea include a faint gray ring of corneal edema around the laceration and blood in the anterior chamber of a soft eye. The leakage of aqueous allows the iris to bow forward and produce a shallow anterior chamber. If the amount of blood in the anterior chamber is scant this bowing of the iris can be seen on inspection with an oblique light source. The pupil contour may be distorted in the direction of the shallowest part of the anterior chamber. Very early after a penetrating wound uveal tissue appears brown or black. If several hours have elapsed before the patient is examined, the ischemic uveal tissue decolorizes and resembles mucous. If a transparent jelly protrudes this is likely lens or vitreous.

Other signs of corneal perforation include tremulousness and forward shift of the iris diaphragm. A black spot on the iris or a notch at the pupil margin may be a hole caused by a foreign body. These iris spots can be confirmed by observing the red reflex about a foot away from the patient, with an opthalmoscope at the 0 setting. The red reflex seen in the pupil would be joined by a red satellite spot corresponding to the suspected defect in the iris diaphragm.

Hemorrhage into the anterior chamber of the eye is known as hyphema. It occurs after moderately severe blunt trauma to the orbit or in association with a penetrating injury of the cornea and iris as described above. It can be seen frequently by simple inspection of the eye, but should also be searched for with an oblique light source as described previously. Even a small amount of blood in the eye must be considered serious because of other diagnostic implications and potentially grave consequences. When the entire anterior chamber is filled with blood it is called an eight ball hemorrhage. The lens is sometimes dislocated by trauma. If the iris trembles when the eye moves, the lens must be dislocated from its normal position behind the pupil. It may come to rest in front of the iris or far posterior free in the vitreous. The lens is recognized by its ovoid shape and clear mass of tissue approximated two thirds the size of the cornea. If a scleral rupture accompanies the lens dislocation, the lens may come to rest subconjunctivally.

The bones comprising the orbit are fractured in varying combinations. The orbital ridges are subcutaneous and fractures can be easily detected by skillful palpation. Although the supraorbital ridge is a substantial and massive structure it is sustaining trauma more and more frequently in motorcycle and auto accidents. The keystones in detecting supraorbital fractures are: flattened brow, downward displacement of the globe, anesthesia of the forehead, periorbital ecchymosis, mechanical restriction of upward gaze due to malfunctioning superior rectus muscle.

Blow Out Fracture of Orbit

The floor of the orbit is structurally unsound. The bones comprising the floor are eggshell thin and there is no underlying support. The air filled maxillary antrum beneath the orbital floor provides no substantial buttress to even minor traumatic forces. Blunt forces applied suddenly to the semi-solid contents of the orbit obey the basic laws of hydraulics exerting equal forces in all directions. The floor of the orbit which provides the weakest support gives way. Frequently the inferior rectus muscle is (Fig. 10-9) incarcerated in the bony defect and rendered nonfunctional. The fracture line sometimes extends over the infraorbital rim into the infraorbital foreamen injuring the infraorbital nerve. Such "blow out" fractures of the orbit produce a set of

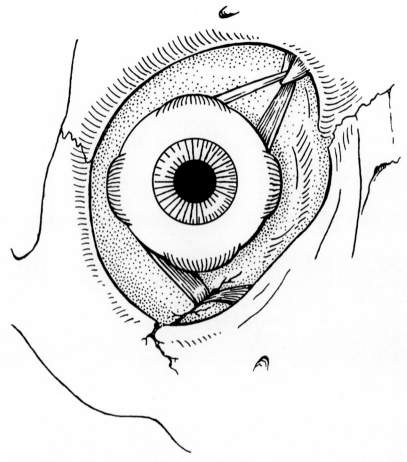

Figure 10-9. The inferior rectus muscle can be entrapped in the fracture line when the orbital floor is disrupted.

clinical findings easily recognized. They are: diplopia, extra-occular movement impairment, enopthalmos, infraorbital paresthesia, orbital ecchymosis. If the patient has double vision when he looks up, consider it a good indication of a blow-out fracture (Fig. 10-10).

In those variants not involving the infraorbital rim of the zygoma, the infraorbital nerve is not damaged and hypesthesia may not be a part of the overall picture.

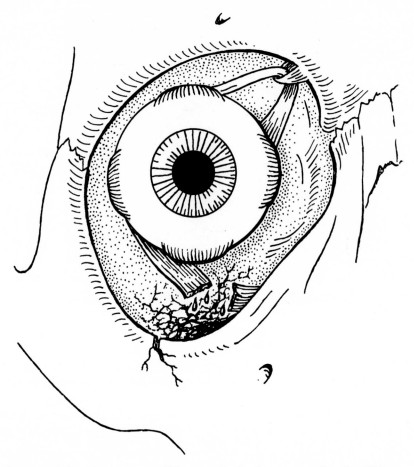

Figure 10-10. More severe "blow outs" of orbit may avulse the Obliquus inferior muscle allowing medial deviation of the globe on upward gaze and producing diplopia.

Air from the ruptured sinus may dissect into the orbit and become palpable around the globe and soft tissues. The patient is unable to move the eye up (Fig. 10-11). Depending upon the amount of descent of the globe into the floor the examiner should be able to detect this proptosis of the globe by holding a straight edge across the bridge of the nose and comparing the level of the pupils of each eye. The pupil on the side of the blowout fracture will usually be depressed a few millimeters

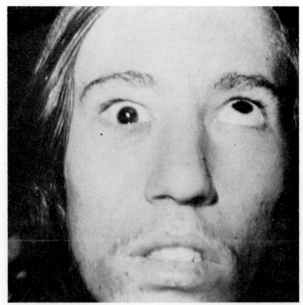

Figure 10-11. Blow out fracture of the orbital floor with incarceration of the inferior rectus muscle produced enopthalmous in this man and prevented his right eye from looking upward.

caudally, compared to the opposite pupil. Enopthalmos may be difficult to determine very soon after injury because of edema.

Another orbital injury which may produce diplopia is dislocation or fracture of the trochlea. This pulley for the superior oblique muscle is located at the upper nasal corner of the anterior orbit just under the rim. Occular movement for downward and lateralward gaze is impaired. The conscious patient tilts his head toward the contralateral side to compensate for the injury and maintain binocularity.

Fractures of the inferior rim of the orbit can involve two important structures. One is the nasolacrimal duct, avulsion, obstruction or transection of this duct can occur and should be evaluated by gently inserting a tiny polyethylene catheter into the duct to assess its patency. The infraorbital nerve is sometimes injured in severe trauma to the rim of the orbit. This can be detected by checking for sensory innervation around the nasolabial region on the injured side (Table 10-IV).

TABLE 10-IV

IMPORTANT DIAGNOSTIC SIGNS IN
FACIAL BONE FRACTURES

Visible fractures in open wounds
Bleeding from an orifice
Cerebrospinal fluid rhinorrhea
Malocclusion
Diminished mobility of jaw
Crepitation of bone
Infraorbital paresthesia
Subcutaneous emphysema
Dysfunction of occular movements
Diplopia
Enopthalmos
Facial Asymmetry

From *Facial Fractures* by Schults, R. C., Copyright 1970 by Year Book
Medical Publishers, Inc., Chicago. Used by permission.

Cerebrospinal Fliud Leakage

Severe trauma to the head and face frequently involves the
base of the skull. The dura is usually torn in these fractures and
this produces leakage of cerebrospinal fluid which gravitates to
the nearest external orifices: The nose and ears. All patients
sustaining severe head and facial trauma should have careful
inspection of both the ears and nose with appropriate specula
and light source. A thin clear discharge of fluid which floats on
top of the blood can usually be distinguished. Fractures of the
sphenoid sinus and the ethmoids cribriform plate frequently
produce cerebrospinal fluid leaks.[5] Rhinorrhea may also result
from fractures in the posterior wall of the frontal sinus.

REFERENCES

1. Schultz, R. C.: The nature of facial emergencies. *Surg Clin N Am,*
   5:299-106, 1972.
2. Mays, E. T.: Bursting injuries of the liver. *Arch Surg,* 93:92-106, 1966.
3. Rowe, N. L., and Killey, H. C.: Fractures of the facial skeleton.
   Baltimore, William and Wilkins Company, 1955.
4. Le Fort, R.: Etude experimentale sur les fractures de la machiore
   supérieure. *Rev Chir,* 23:208-360, 1901.
5. Lewin, W., and Carius, H.: Fractures of sphenoidal sinus with cerebrospinal fluid rhinorrhea. *Br Med J, 1*:16, 1951.

EVALUATION OF BURNS

───

T HE CLINICAL EVALUATION of severely burned patients is closely linked to their initial care. Appraisal of extent and depth of burn are integral part of managing "burn shock." The scope of this text does not cover the controversial aspects of resuscitation from burn shock but inherent within the idea of assessment of burn injuries is the idea of appropriate resuscitation.

The same priorities of airway and ventilation are essential in these injuries as in non-burned patients. Emphasis is again placed on Phase I care. Pre-hospital care in addition to correcting airway obstruction and assuring adequate ventilation must also arrest the burning process. In chemical burns flushing the surface with copious amounts of water is a high priority. Mechanical interruption of the burning process by removal of heavy smouldering clothing and covering the patient with moist sheets or blankets prevents evaporative water losses from extensive burns. Although definitive resuscitation from burn shock is usually considered within the realm of doctors inside hospitals it can be started in Phase I with a simple intravenous line and infusion of lactated Ringer's solution en route to the hospital.

PULMONARY BURNS

Obstruction of the upper airway by pharyngeal and laryngeal edema occurs soon after deep burns of the face and neck. Partial obstruction of either the trachea or the larynx produces pulmonary edema. In the past early tracheostomy was done in these patients. Now it is better to relieve the obstruction with an endotracheal tube and postpone tracheostomy until a later date. A recent study suggests that since there is a large early respiratory mortality among fire victims significant reduction of mortality could be achieved by making available resuscitative therapy for CO poisoning, smoke inhalation and asphyxia at the scene of the fire, enroute to the hospital and in the emergency department. Respiratory distress syndromes can also occur in patients with minimal body surface burns remote from the respiratory tract. This falls into the same category as post-traumatic pulmonary insufficiency and has already been discussed. Under this section we are evaluating the patient for direct thermal injury to the respiratory tract. Such appraisal is a high priority in burned patients and after establishing an airway evidence for respiratory burns should be evaluated first.

There are two major methods by which the respiratory tract is injured in burned victims: 1) inhalation of superheated gas, air or water vapor 2) inhalation of chemical gases. Inhalation of hot gases can directly burn the lung tissue. The greater the specific heat delivered to the lung tissue directly through the air passages, the more devastating the injury.[2] Because of the highly efficient heat-exchange mechanisms of the upper airways and the conscious patient reflexly closing his glottis and holding his breath this kind of respiratory burn is not common. Super-heated water vapors that can exceed the heat-exchange capacity of the upper airway can directly coagulate the protein in the bronchial mucosal cells. Another mechanism of direct burn of the tracheo-bronchial tree is when combustile vapors are inhaled and then completely oxidized deep within the respiratory tree.[1] Probably the most common mechanism of respiratory burn is when patients are trapped in a closed space with rapidly burning substances being vaporized into their various chemical components which are then inhaled into the respiratory tree. The injury is from the chemical gas inhaled rather than the actual amount of caloric heat in the inspired air. The burning of the many synthetic materials in buildings and in the furnishings of offices and domestic dwellings creates a variety of chemical compounds that can be vaporized releasing various chemicals for inhalation by the trapped victim. These noxious chemicals then interact with the mucosal lining of the respiratory tree and produce what is commonly referred to as "pulmonary burn."[1, 3] Such a burn produces a broad spectrum of pulmonary pathology ranging from pulmonary congestion edema and aveolar thickening, to parenchymal hemorrhage, epithelial desquamation, bronchopneumonia and pulmonary necrosis with abscess formation.

To evaluate a patient for possible pulmonary burn the examiner should look at the face and neck for any evidence of burn. Singed nasal hair, mucosal burns, a brassy cough or soot in the sputum are highly suggestive. Bronchospasm and audible wheezing may be present. The lungs should be ausculted for evidence of moist rales, or wheezes indicating early aveolar edema and bronchoconstriction. If these findings are present and the patient sustained his burn in a closed space and became unconscious before extrication then it may be assumed that a respiratory burn is present. Early bronchoscopy can confirm tracheo-bronchial trauma. Serial blood gas determinations disclose the pathophysiologic counterpart of this anatomic injury. Roentgenograms of the chest are rarely helpful.

Severe respiratory distress and hypoxemia with confusion, restlessness and respiratory rates greater than thirty to forty per minute develop rapidly and require immediate correction with tracheal intubation mechanical ventilation and regulation of F_1O_2. The criteria for detecting pulmonary burns are listed in Table 11-I. Carbon monoxide poisoning is always a possibility and

TABLE 11-I

CRITERIA FOR DETECTING PULMONARY BURNS

1. Patient burned in closed space
2. Patient lost consciousness before extrication
3. Brassy Cough
4. Soot in sputum
5. Singed nasal hair
6. Mucosal burns of nose, lips, mouth
7. Bronchospasm
8. Cyanosis
9. Labial and lingual edema
10. Tacypnea
11. Hypoxemia (Serial Blood Gas determination)

carboxy hemoglobin concentration should be done to confirm or exclude such a possibility.[1]

DEPTH OF BURN

Full thickness burns (third degree) are recognized by their charred, dry, coagulated appearance. They are also anesthetic and can be tested by pin pricks if some question arises in the mind of the examiner. Thermal burns are fairly accurately assessed but electrical burns are almost always underestimated in so far as their depth is concerned. Burns caused by electrical current extend deep coagulating bone, tendons and blood vessels. A pale greyish black eschar is the result of coagulation by heat or electricity and it has an easily recognizable appearance. Gross hemoglobin in the urine is an indication that the burn is deep.

Partial thickness burns retain tactile and superficial pain (pin pricks) and capillary pressure blanching. They appear moist and sometimes even wet. In some the surface is red smooth and glistening; in others the surface has hobnail appearance produced by the many islands of retained dermal tissues around hair follicles and sweat glands.

It is only possible by utilizing the above criteria to determine depth of burn in a few instances. In the majority of patients these will be combinations of both full-thickness and partial thickness and it is impossible to tell the difference on immediate examination. In most instances the depth of a burn cannot be accurately estimated for several days. If the burn heals without skin grafting it was a partial thickness injury; if after the eschar separates fat, muscle or bone is exposed it was a full-thickness injury. A partial-thickness burn can be converted to a full thickness burn by infection or pressure. Many patients are admitted to hospitals with partial thickness burns of the back and buttocks and, after several days in bed, pressure necrosis completes the job the initial injury failed to do.

The obsolete four category classification of depth of burn is no longer useful clinically (Table 11-II). It is shown for historical perspective only.

TABLE 11-II

DEPTH OF BURN CATEGORIES*

First degree	Erytherma (sunburn)
Second degree	Death of epidermis, ballae, epidermal appendages remain viable within the dermis
Third degree	Death of epidermis, dermis and all epidermal appendages within dermis
Fourth degree	Carbonification of the part

* Now of historical interest only. See text for present clinical classification.

EXTENT OF BURN

The percent of body surface burned is used in most volume repletion formulae to calculate the amount and kind of resuscitation fluids given. This will be discussed further in the next section. The mortality rate is inherently dependent upon the size of the burn. The estimate of percent of body burned is therefore a major part of evaluating burned patients.

The Vierdot Table[4] is one method of rapidly assessing extent of body burned. It is a fairly reliable and accurate method. One can see from the data in Table 11-III that a burn of both legs and both thighs with buttocks [2 x 14] + [2 x 6] = 40%) involves as much surface area as a burn covering the entire trunk, head, neck and one upper arm (28 + 5 + 2 + 5 = 40%). A burn of the entire lower torso extending up to the beltline (1/3 of the trunk) is calculated from the Vierdot Table to cover 55 percent of the body surface. While more frightening in appearance, a burn of the entire head, neck, and upper extremities and entire

TABLE 11-III

ESTIMATION OF PER CENT OF BODY BURN[4]

Area	Per Cent of Body Surface
Trunk	28
Thigh (with buttock)	14
Leg	6
Head	5
Upper Arm	5
Foot	3
Forearm	3
Neck	2
Hand	2

chest (1/2 trunk) actually is less serious to the extent it covers only 41 percent of the body surface area.

Age is a determining factor in the relationship of surface area to body mass (Table 11-IV). Any calculation of the surface area has to consider the patient's age. From the Vierdot Table one can appreciate that total surfaces are increased with age but the square centimeters of surface area per kilogram of body weight decreases.

A second method of estimating the percent of surface area involved in burned victims is the "Rule of Nines" (Table 11-V). The body surface is divided into regions (Fig. 11-1) and each region represents 9 percent or a multiple of nine (torso, front and back = 4 x 9 = 36%). When using the rule of nines in children there are relatively important differences. A greater percent of body surface is made up by the head and trunk in children with proportionately less surface area over the lower extremities.

TABLE 11-IV

AGE, SURFACE AREA, BODY MASS[4]

Age (Years)	Surface Area (Square Meters)	Surface Area/KG (Square Centimeters)
1/365	0.2599	812
1/2	0.4381	626
1	0.5181	575
2	0.6028	533
4	0.7020	495
7	0.8552	450
10	1,0092	312
12	1.1505	386
14	1.3676	354
25	1.8936	301

TABLE 11-V

RULE OF NINES

Area	Per Cent
Head and Neck	9
Upper Extremities	18 (2 x 9)
Lower Extremities	36 (2 x 18)
Anterior Trunk	18
Posterior Trunk	18
Perineium	1
	100

BURN FORMULAE

Although there is some contention about which body compartment is most depleted by burn trauma, all agree that hypovolemia is present. There is also universal agreement that a second important aspects of burns is the sequestration of large amounts of sodium into burned tissues. A variety of formulae to guide volume and sodium replacement (Table 11-VI) have been proposed. They differ primarily on the composition and quantities of fluids that best replace the fluid sequestered in the burn wound. It must be remembered that each is simply an estimate of volume and sodium requirements.

If one chooses to use any one of the three acceptable formulae he should periodically review his patients and analyze the type and amount of fluid given in relation to that predicted by the formula. Efficacy of resuscitation and complications due to utilization of the formulae must also be frequently assessed.

The Evans formula has been used since 1952 at the Medical College of Virginia Burn Unit.[5] Workers in that institute present data to show the Evans formula predicted accurately the fluid and electrolyte needs of burned patients.[6] They report their adult patients were well resuscitated and fluid overload was not a problem. In children they underestimated the sodium needs and suggest augmenting the predicted quantities by 50 percent to 100 percent.

The Brooke formula evolved from a group of clinicians working at the U.S. Army Surgical Research Unit of the Brooke Army Medical Center in the early 1950's.[7] They observed that a more appropriate urinary output could be maintained when additional quantities of electrolyte solution and lesser quantities of colloid were used.

Baxter[8] identified clinical signs of optimal resuscitation from burn shock to be a urine volume greater than 50 ml per hour, a pulse rate less than 120 per minute and a lucid calm patient. He found a balanced crystalloid solution to be as effective as colloid solution in maintaining these clinicial signs in the first eight to twenty-four hours after burn injury. Colloid given between eighteen and thirty hours after burn injury proved to be

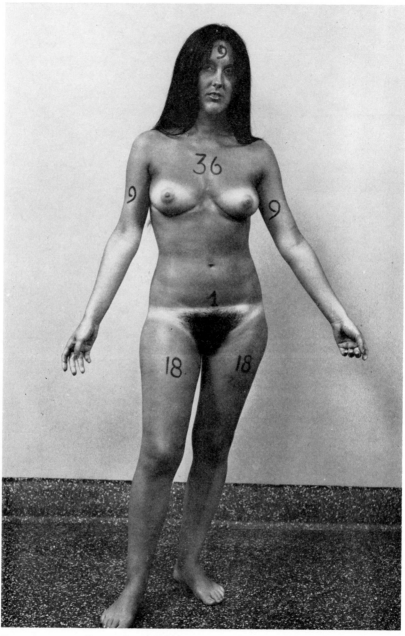

Figure 11-1. The body surface is divided into regions represented by nines or multiples of nine as a means of estimating percent of total body burn.

TABLE 11-VI
BURN FORMULAE

Evans

First 24 hours: Colloid 1 ml/kg/% burn, crystalloid 1 ml/kg/% burn maintenance water 2000 ml, half given over first eight hours
half given over next sixteen hours.

Second 24 hours: Colloid 0.5 ml/kg/% burn, crystalloid 0.5 ml/kg/% burn
crystalloid 0.5 ml/kg/% burn maintenance water 2000 ml 5%
dextrose in water.

Maximum calculated burn 50%

Brooke

First 24 hours: Colloid 0.5 ml/kg/% burn, crystalloid 1.5 ml/kg/% burn
maintenance water 2000 ml, half given during first eight
hours half given during next sixteen hours.

Second 24 hours: Colloid 0.25 ml/kg/% burn crystalloid 0.75 ml/kg/% burn
maintenance water 2000 ml 5% dextrose in water.

Maximum calculated burn 50%

Baxter

First 24 hours: 4 ml crystalloid/kg/% burn, half during first eight hours
half over next sixteen hours.

Second 24 hours: Maintain a normal serum sodium plus plasma 250 to 500 ml.

No maximum calculated burn

more effective in the correction of residual deficits in plasma volume.

The mere existence of several widely accepted formulae for replenishing volume and sodium in burned patients must not be allowed to become a source of confusion or frustration. Each physician should become generally acquainted with all the Burn Formulae but more specifically familiar with the pathophysiologic mechanisms producing the deficits. After years of interest in the subject Artz[9] placed them in proper perspective: "No mathematical formula exist by which all burns can be treated. A given formula should be regarded only as a means of providing the clinician with an order of magnitude of fluid requirements and not as a regimen that must be followed blindly." He particularly urges caution in children below two years of age. To prevent imposing too great a load on the infant kidney the salt solution should be given as a 1 to 3 or 1 to 4 dilution of lactated Ringer solution. The daily reqirement of 5 percent dextrose in water can be used as the diluent. This precaution prevents extreme flux in serum sodium concentrations. In burns over 30 percent in children it is wise to consider them as 30 percent burns thus avoiding acute fluid overloading. The fluids should be administered at a rate to keep the urinary output approximately 15 to 20 ml/hour. According to Artz colloids are of particular value for the support of the circulation in infants and children.

EVALUATION OF BURN SHOCK

Severe thirst, hypotension, collapsed veins, oliguria, and low central venous pressure denote a severe fluid deficit. On admission hemoglobin, hematocrit blood chemistries, blood gases and serum pH should be done. Specific gravity and osmolality of the urine should be determined. The pH of the urine and presence of hemoglobin or myoglobin in the urine should be determined.

The hemotocrit is a simple but very reliable means of assessing fluid deficits and change in hematocrit from hour to hour aid in determining the effectiveness of fluid therapy. Peripheral blood hematocrits are acceptable but if a central venous catheter is in place a central venous hematocrit is easily obtained and is much more reliable especially when peripheral perfusion is sluggish. Attempts to keep the hematocrit from rising by replenishing volume and sodium deficiencies must be vigorous. A falling hematocrit reflects adequate fluid replacement. As a general rule hematocrits above 50 percent in burn shock denote severe fluid deficits and the hematocrit must be lowered below 45 percent.

The volume of urine excreted each hour is perhaps the most reliable guide in evaluating degree of burn shock and effectiveness of replacement therapy. Most feel the urine output in burned patients should be somewhere between 40 to 70 ml per hour. If the urine output is in excess of 100 to 150 ml per hour the amount and rate of fluid administration is probably excessive. A small urine output (10 ml or less per hour) indicates severe fluid deficit or reduced cardiac output. Determining the specific gravity of the urine is helpful in differentiating between the two. Urinary hydrometers are available in all hospitals and any hospital attendant can be instructed in their use. Urine osmolarity gives the same information as specific gravity but requires special instruments* which permits determination of osmolarity on a very small quantity of urine. If the specific gravity of the urine is high (1.026 to 1.030) the oliguria is likely due to fluid deficits; if the specific gravity is low (1.010 to 1.012) the oliguria is probably tubular necrosis; if the specific gravity is fairly normal (1.015 to 1.020) the oliguria is most likely secondary to a reduced cardiac output. Myocardial depressant factors will be discussed later in this section.

Acute renal failure can be determined by measuring both the urine and plasma osmolarities and if they are almost equal acute tubular necrosis is present.

The determination of urine pH and presence of hemoglobin or myoglobin in the urine is important in evaluating the burned patient. The pH of the urine can be tested each hour along with the urine volume and specific gravity. This can easily be done with a piece of Nitrozine paper and recorded next to volume and specific gravity. When the pigment load of the urine is great as after deep burns and electrical burns the pH of the urine should be kept at 7.0 or above. The alkaline urine provides for greater hemoglobin and myoglobin solubility. Extra amounts of sodium bicarbonate can be added to the intravenous infusions to obtain the desired alkalinity to the urine.

These evaluations of renal function are much more reliable than determining vital signs. Reliable blood pressures are difficult to obtain in burn victims and the information gained is probably not worth the time and effort. If blood pressure is important in specific cases it can be more reliably obtained with a small indwelling arterial cannula attached to a pressure transducer and a continuous recorder.

Artz[9] feels that determination of central venous pressure is one of the best guides in evaluating burn shock and preventing over-infusion when attempting replenishment of fluid losses. Others voice concern that with infusions of lactated Ringers solution the pulmonary circulation can be over expanded with subsequent

---

* Goldberg Refractometer. American Optical Co. 1150 Avenue of the Americas, New York, N. Y.

pulmonary edema even in the face of an acceptably normal central venous pressure. As will be discussed in later chapters, when a physician feels that cardiac chamber pressures are important (cardiac lesions, decreased cardiac reserve, etc.) in assessing burn shock and subsequently evaluating adequacy of resuscitation it is probably best to utilize a balloon-tipped flow directed catheter to monitor right and left heart pressures. Measurements of cardiac output and cardiac index are important research tools but not available in the day to day evaluation of most burns.

MYOCARDIAL DEPRESSANT FACTOR

A decrease in the contractibility of cardiac muscle occurs in experimental burns.[10, 11] Dobson and co-workers showed that a decrease in cardiac output occurs before any change in plasma volume.[12] Cross perfusion experiments have disclosed substances circulating in the plasma of a burned member of a pair of experimental animals abruptly decreasing cardiac output in the non-burned parabiotic mate.[13] Dialyzed fluid from the serum or plasma of some large clinical burns exhibited depression of myocardial contractibility on isolated heart muscle preparations.[14] On the basis of such circulating factors in clinical burns, Baxter has postulated that direct myocardial depression may be the primary limiting factor in the effectiveness of fluid replacement restoring cardiac function in some severe burns.

In the chapter on physiologic concomitant we discussed lipid metabolism and the mobilization of fatty acids. In the absence of adequate serum albumin which is lost in massive amounts in burns these fatty acid anions may be free to exert their cytotoxic effect on the myocardium.

In evaluating burned patients the plasma concentrations of serum albumin and fatty acid anions should be determined. In the presence of fatty acid anions of greater than 1.0 meq/L sufficient serum albumin should be infused to bind excess fatty acids and obviate depression of myocardial contractibility.

PHYSIOLOGIC EVALUATION

Everyone is in general agreement that the "burn formulae" are meant to be flexible guides. All those responsible for taking care of burned patients have at one time or another been frustrated by the nearly impossible situation of supervising the hour to hour administration of fluids. This frustration peaks when supportive personnel do not understand the physician's concern in getting a calculated amount of fluid into patients on a calculated schedule. It is indeed rare that the calculated plan of resuscitation fluid infusion goes according to schedule. The actual achievement of fluid resuscitation of burns exactly on schedules calculated by any of the three formulae is at the most very difficult to accomplish except in very large specially staffed burn units.

Some authorities are aware of a tendency to determine volume and rate of fluid resuscitation of burned patients on a physiologic basis using each individual patient's responses as the basis of fluid needs. Obviously a physician needs some initial estimate of the kind and amount of fluid needed, but to rigidly adhere to any one of the formulae is not in keeping with developing trends in all areas of medicine to measure physiologic deficits, and correct these deficits while carefully monitoring the individual patient's response.

After initial assessment of ventilatory function, depth and extent of burn a central venous and urinary catheter are inserted. Blood samples are drawn for hematocrit, serum pH, blood gases, albumin, total protein, and electrolytes. The hourly urine output specific gravity, pH, sodium and urea content and osmolarity are monitored. Lactated Ringers solution is infused until the hourly urine output exceeds 50 ml per hour. The lungs are ausculted frequently for collection of aveolar fluid or evidence of broncho-constriction. If the urine pH is less than 7.4 additional sodium bicarbonate is infused until the urine is alkaline.

In this system the main determinant of kind of fluids and rates of administration is the hour to hour physiologic response of the patient rather than some pre-determined solution calculated by formulae.

All the burn formulae differ in several respects. There is lack of agreement as to which body compartment is most deprived of volume. There is lack of agreement as to how much colloid and timing of administration of colloid. The Evans and Brooke formulae give their colloid and crystalloid throughout the first forty-eight hours. In the Baxter formula the crystalloid is given rapidly in the first twenty-four hours and the colloid in the second twenty-four hours. The Evans and Brooke formulae calculate the fluid requirements initially for all burns greater than 50 percent of body surface as 50 percent burns whereas the Baxter formula calculates the requirements for all burns according to their actual size. The Evans and Brooke formulae differ in ratio of crystalloid to colloid. The one major feature common to all formulae is the administration of prescribed amounts of sodium. The Evans and Brooke formulae require similar amounts of sodium replacement. The Baxter formulae predicts the largest amount of sodium for adult burns, but agrees closely with the quantities of sodium the Evans and Brooke formulae predict for burned children.

These formulae have served a valuable service in the management of burns in the understanding of burn fluid and volume deficits. Today technology has made it possible for physiologic monitoring on a serial basis that has not been possible in past decades. With this newly recognized capability of determining on an hour to hour basis the physiologic response of burned victims it seems more rational to proceed along these lines utilizing the burn formula less and less.

In electrical burns the acidosis is much more severe than in thermal burns. Determining the degree of this acidosis and its rate of correction by sequential monitoring is just one area where physiologic indices are more valuable than formulae. Very deep burns with acute red cell destruction exceeding 15 percent of the total red cell mass presents a pathologic deficit not accounted for in the burn formulae. There is additional losses in red cell mass even after the initial onslaught. There is a striking increase in blood viscosity much greater than can be accounted for by high hematocrits. Platelet adhesiveness is increased, and there are tissue thromboplastic factors released from injured areas. Organ malfunction follows these various pathologic events. These are only a few of the physiologic indices that today can be determined and monitored in most hospitals. Such factors increase the tendency on the part of most physiicans to treat each individual patient on the basis of his physiologic function and the response in physiologic indices to resuscitation efforts, relying less and less on the various burn formulae.

BURN SEPSIS

This is a late complication of burns and is such a rapidly developing and complex field that it does not fall within the scope of a book on initial assessment of the patient. For interested readers who wish to pursue this subject an excellent text is available.[15]

REFERENCES

1. Zikria, B. A.; Weston, G. C.; Chodoff, M., and Ferrer, J. M.: Smoke and carbon monoxide poisoning in fire victims. *J Trauma, 12*:641-645, 1972.

2. Stone, H. H.; Rhame, D. W.; Corbitt, J. D.; Given, K. S., and Martin, J. D.: Respiratory burns: A correlation of clinical and laboratory results. *Ann Surg, 165*:157, 1967.

3. Thomas, D. M., and Couner, E. H.: Management of the patient "overcome by smoke." *J Ky Med Assoc, 66*:1051, 1968.

4. Vierordt, H.: Anatomische, Physiologische, und Physikalishe Dafen und Tabellen. Ed. 3, Jena, Fischer, 1906, p. 52.

5. Evans, E. I.; Purnell, O. J.; Robinette, P. W., et al.: Fluid and electrolyte requirements in severe burns. *Ann Surg, 135*:804-817, 1952.

6. Hutcher, N., and Haynes, B. W.: The Evans formula revised. *J Trauma, 12*:453-457, 1972.

7. Reiss, E;. Stirman, J. A.; Artz, C. P., et al.: Fluid and electrolyte balance in burns. *JAMA, 152*:1309-1313, 1953.

8. Baxter, C. R., and Shires, T.: Physiologic response to crystalloid resuscitation of severe burns. *Ann NY Acad Sci, 150*:874-894, 1968.

9. Artz, C. P.: The Brooke formula in *Contemporary Burn Management.* Boston, Little Brown Co., 1971.

10. Fozzard, H. A.: Myocardial injury in burn shock. *Ann Surg, 154*:113, 1961.

11. Merriman, T. W., and Jackson, R.: Myocardial function following thermal injury. *Circ Res, 11*:669, 1962.

12. Dobson, E. L.: Early circulatory disturbances following experimental thermal trauma. *US, AEC, UCRL,* 2987, 1955.
13. Baxter, C. R.; Cook, W. A., and Shires, G. T.: Serum myocardial dypressant factor of burn shock. *Surg Forum, 17*:1, 1966.
14. Baxter, C. R.: *Crystalloid Resuscitation of Burn Shock in Contemporary Burn Management. Ed. Polk and Stone,* Boston, Little, Brown and Co., 1971.
15. Polk, H. C., and Stone, H. H.: *Contemporary Burn Management.* Boston, Little, Brown and Co., 1971.

CHAPTER 12

EVALUATION BY OPERATION

AFTER MANY YEARS experience evaluating critically injured patients it is obvious to those who work closely in this field that there are a small number of patients who have serious injuries not detected by any of the methods we have outlined. It is these overlooked, undetected, or missed injuries that result in death. The actual management of the specific lesion by skilled specialists has reduced morbidity and mortality very impressively. With the knowledge now presently available in the total experience of medicine there are few injuries for which new research and new knowledge is needed. The critical area is detecting the lesions before deterioration of cell function has advanced to irreversible stages.

This section is devoted to the premise that even after meticulous evaluation by cautious alert physicians the three major body cavities may still conceal lethal injuries. These facts make the concept of operative exploration of such cavities a valid clinical tool. It is very rare that all three cavities will require exploration. We will deal with them on an individual basis. The terms exploratory laparotomy, exploratory thoractomy, exploratory craniotomy, have developed such connotative meanings to both the lay person and physician that they should be discarded. Regardless of how the physician-intellect tries to deal with these terms he still feels that an exploratory procedure is an admission of defeat or incompetence—that his ability and techniques to detect important injuries is so advanced he should not have to resort to exploring a cavity to find an injury. Patients and family often look upon the term "exploratory" as meaning they have an "inferior doctor" who isn't smart enough to know what's wrong without "cutting the patient open" or that they fell into the hands of a "knife-happy" surgeon. Reports by government and the lay-press have added to the confusion of this problem by emphasizing there are "too many unnecessary operations" done each year.

Such factors all interact in the physician-psyche to make him feel inept if he opens the abdomen for a ruptured spleen and doesn't find one or if he opens the cranium for an expidural hematoma and there is none. This thinking leads to procrastination, to the point of delaying the diagnosis until there is irreversible damage to cellular function. Such attitudes must be dispelled if death of critically injured patients from overlooked or missed injuries is to be prevented. The "negative craniotomy" or "negative thoracotomy" must not be looked upon as "negative." There is positive information gleaned from an operation of this kind even though no remedial situations are found. Operative procedures that find nothing requiring correction are usually alleged to be detrimental to the patients physiologic progress. This is not always true. Such positive information allows the physician to focus his attention fully on the patients remaining physiologic problems and manage them much more skillfully than he might have done were he spending frustrating hours rechecking the patient for suspected anatomic abnormalities.

LAPAROTOMY

Properly performed peritoneal lavage and careful physical examination as described in previous chapters detects most intraabdominal injuries sufficiently early so as not to adversely influence the outcome. There are a few patients in whom such initial evaluations are not specific. Such patients then fall into two general categories: 1. rapid progressive deterioration, 2. sufficiently stable to monitor sequentially.

Some patients may exsanguinate into the peritoneal cavity so rapidly that peritoneal lavage and multiple studies are unwarranted. These patients present a picture of severe shock progressing even while whole blood is rapidly infused into multiple veins. It is really not so difficult to recognize these patients as it may seem. There may be rapid distention of the abdomen and it becomes increasing clear that although blood is running in through two "14 gauge needles" blood is running out through four of five "10 gauge arteries." In these critically injured individuals immediate laparotomy must precede or parallel rather than follow restoration of blood volume. As Ravdin[1] stated, "Valuable time is all too frequently lost by attempting to restore blood loss before operation, for hemorrhage is often taking place faster than blood can be replaced. It is frequently impossible under certain of these conditions to get an adequate and effective blood volume." This perspicacious observation by Ravdin was confirmed by Mays[2] in a review of injured patients showing unnecessary delay and often death could be circumvented if the surgeon would not be so persistent in his efforts to restore blood volume before doing a laparotomy to control hemorrhage.

The second group of patients are those who have completed evaluation and/or operation for skeletal, cranial, thoracic, or facial injuries. They are hemodynamically stable and being monitored carefully. At this point in time it is obvious they are not bleeding to death from a ruptured liver or spleen. Other results of the initial appraisal are not so clear cut. There is also a question of retroperitoneal organ injury. The clinical pattern at this point can become very confusing. Physical signs are "comme ci comme ça," the peritoneal lavage did not show gross blood; should another be done? The patient is not getting well. There is enough question about his injury to suspect intra-abdominal injury; laparotomy is an excellent clinical tool for appraising these patients. It should not be withheld because of fear of a "negative abdomen" nor because a definite diagnosis is not yet established. Retroperitoneal rupture of the duodenum is an injury most difficult to detect by all known evaluating tests. Unless there is air dissection of the kidneys or pancreas showing on X-ray it is nearly impossible to detect this injury early in the patient's hospital course. The peritoneal lavage is negative because the injury is retroperitoneal. The physical findings are variable and changing. Blood loss is not great enough to give the picture of shock. It is only after several hours have elapsed that extra-cellular fluid loss and chemical irritation proclaim something bad is wrong. By this time anyone can propose exploration because it is obvious that the patient is in severe trouble. The morbidity and mortality are almost doubled by this delay. Laparotomy is the most efficacious method of detecting retro-peritoneal duodenal ruptures early enough to influence its deadly course.

Having elected laparotomy for his patient the surgeon is then obligated to a methodical evaluation of intra-abdominal and retroperitoneal organs. The same care that goes into assaying the total body injury must now be applied to intra-abdominal organs. A "negative laparotomy" in a severely injured patient should perturb no surgeon, but an overlooked intra-abdominal injury in an alleged "negative laparotomy" should disconcert everyone.

The vertical midline abdominal incision is excellent in trauma patients. It permits visualization of all abdominal organs at every operation. Should need arise it can be extended upward as a median sternotomy to gain access to the heart, lungs, great vessels diaphragm hepatic veins, etc. It can be extended down-ward to gain access to the pelvic organs, vessels and nerves. Every surgeon should have an organized method of exploring the abdomen. It doesn't matter what technique he devises so long as he does it in the same manner often enough to establish a pattern. In the perturbations of the operating room and emer-gency surgery it is only human to forget something at one time or the other. Repetition for the purpose of organization is no crime. The small bowel should always be examined from the ligament of treitz to the ileocecal valve. The duodenal region should be inspected for "bile staining" or retroperitoneal air then mobilized for direct inspection. The colon should be examined from cecum to rectum. Any hematomas must be un-roofed down to serosa before perforation can be excluded. The liver can be palpated over most of its surface. When indicated it can be extensively mobilized by cutting the supporting ligaments. The gallbladder and stomach, espohageal and aortic hiatus can be inspected directly. Retroperitoneal organs should be palpated for consistency and areas of softening. Any suspicious feeling organ such as the kidney, pancreas, ureter, etc., should be unroofed and inspected directly. Retroperitoneal hematomas present a dilemma. Because they are so striking they are usually noted soon after opening the abdomen. This gives an opportunity to allow time to pass while systematically examining all other organs, then coming back and assessing the change in the retroperitoneal hematoma.

An unquestioned enlargement of the hematoma over important organs or vessels usually dictates unroofing the hematoma and inspecting the underlying vein, artery or organ directly. Most unchanging hematomas are best left undisturbed.

THORACOTOMY

The use of operative thoracotomy as an evaluating tool is generally unacceptable. Even though the abdomen is readily opened to exclude intra-abdominal problems in a deteriorating patient opening the thoracic cage appears too formidable to most surgeons. Reasons making thoracotomy as an evaluating technic unacceptable are many. Some were predicted on battlefield conditions.[3] A quick glance back to Chapter 2 at the wounding capability of military rifles compared to civilian weapons, confronts us with the fact that in wartime if a soldier survives a high velocity missile wound long enough to be evacuated to a field hospital he most likely does not have a major vessel or heart injury. The wounding capacity of the military rifle is so great that it immediately divides the victims into two groups; those who die quickly from major vascular or heart injury and those with only pulmonary parenchymal involvement.

Because of this selectivity it was quickly noted that those patients who had placement of intercostal tubes and closed water seal drainage fared better than those who had thoracotomy. The evacuation of blood and air from the pleural space permits rapid pulmonary re-expansion, when injury is limited to pulmonary parenchyma this lung re-expansion is an excellent method of achieving hemostasis in the low pressure system existing in the lungs.

This same selection of patients on the basis of those with pulmonary parenchymal injury surviving while those with pulmonary, great vessels, or heart injury dying before hospitalization can also exist in civilian practice in some referral centers. But in many hospitals throughout the land rapid transportation of seriously injured patients brings both groups of patients under the physician's survelliance. Those principles gleaned from patients surviving the M-1, M-14 or M-16 and evacuated sometime later to a field hospital cannot possibly pertain to an individual shot in the chest in a metropolitan barroom and transported immediately to a civilian operating room where a surgeon must evaluate his injury five to ten minutes after the injury was afflicted. For this civilian surgeon must be capable of selecting those patients who have only pulmonary parenchymal injury and will do well with an intercostal chest tube alone from those who need immediate thoracotomy for a wound of the heart, aorta, pulmonary artery, etc. This selection has been made for the military surgeon by the extreme energy of the wounding force.

The indications for thoracotomy have been outlined in a previous chapter. Just as laparotomy is occasionally indicated as a resuscitative measure so in some instances thoracotomy also is indicated for resuscitation. This operative procedure may be necessary before extensive evaluating procedures have been done. DeMuth[4] had the courage to voice what many surgeons have thought, "I wonder how many people with severe intrathoracic arterial injuries have literally been studied to death." A major pitfall I have seen in patients with thoracic trauma who have cardiac arrest while being evaluated is the conclusion that their cardiac arrest is from blood loss elsewhere and that blood volume must be restored in order to permit the physician in charge to proceed with his test to detect intrathoracic injury. This leads to efforts at external cardiac massage, volume expanders and cardiac stimulants. A patient with evidence of chest trauma either blunt or penetrating who develops cardiac arrest needs a resuscitative thoracotomy. The concept of immediate resuscitative thoractotomy is only valid in civilian practice where injured patients are on the operating table within five to ten minutes after sustaining injury. In most other situations the kinds of injuries requiring immediate exploratory thoracotomy will have selectively been excluded by death of the patient.

An early delayed thoracotomy is sometimes necessary as an evaluating tool. After intercostal tube placement and re-expension of the lung there are some few patients who continue to deteriorate. It is difficult to define exact rates of intrapleural hemorrhage indicative of thoracotomy. Each center has usually established its own arbitrary figure. But borderline situations always exist. It is these indefinite zones where clinical data and sequential monitoring are indecisive that early thoracotomy for evaluation is helpful. It must be emphasized that the patients for early thoracotomy differ from patients requiring an immediate or resuscitative thoracotomy. In the early thoracotomy patients all the evaluating technics described in previous chapters have been done. Intercostal tubes are in place, circulating blood volume is restored, pericardiocentesis or echocardiography has been completed, BA swallow done, chest X-ray and EKG, completed. But even though the patient has been thoroughly evaluated there is still some question. Several of the tests were borderline. There is suspicion of diaphragm injury or esophageal injury. In some there is persistent air leak or clotted hemothorax. In all these situations there remain questions. These questions are best answered to the benefit of the patient by an evaluating thoracotomy.

CRANIOTOMY

Most patients with craniocerebral trauma do not require surgery. Raaf[5] reported 76.2 percent of 2,024 patients with acute craniocerebral injury were treated without surgery. This gives some idea of the small group of patients who are candidates for any kind of surgical procedures. In the 23.8 percent of operated patients, there were eight various operative procedures done: 1. elevation of simple depressed skull fracture, 2. debridement of compound skull fracture, 3. internal decompression, 4. drainage of meningeal effusions, 5. drainage of internal hydrocephalus, 6. decompression by bone removal, 7. burr hole exploration with negative findings, 8. evacuation of intracranial hematomas. This brief review of a very large group of patients with head injuries shows the number of victims to whom the concept of an assessing cranitomy is small indeed. The utilization of cerebral arteriography described in preceding chapters reduced this group to even smaller numbers.

There are a few deeply comatose patients with increased intracranial pressure after trauma who cannot be transported to facilities for arteriography or if arteriography is available the patient is deteriorating so rapidly that the delay for arteriograms may result in irreversible changes.

In these few patients brain decompression is essential prior to study just as described under immediate resuscitative thoracotomy and laparotomy. Percival Pott stated, "the reason for applying the trepan springs from the nature of the mischief which the parts within the cranium have sustained and not from accidental division of the bone."

Burton and Blacker[6] admit that burr holes are preferable in these situations, but admonish us that there are circumstances where the burr may not be quickly available. They recommend twist drill decompression of the intracranial cavity as a prelude to formal surgery, and report its use at Johns Hopkins and Baltimore City Hospitals has converted moribund patients into candidates for definitive therapeutic procedures.

The twist drill is four inches, the bit is type 316 stainless steel with a Rockwell hardness of approximately C34 and a diameter of 0.155 inches. It is used in patients whose survival could be measured in minutes. After the scalp has been shaved, prepped, draped and infiltrated with local anesthesia, a 4 mm skin incision is made to the bone. Handle design of the drill is such that a maximum amount of force can be applied alternately pronating and supinating the hand with the wrist in neutral position.

When the drill bit has penetrated the diploic space the drill will hold its position without support. At this point clockwise turning will allow the bit to emerge from the inner table of the skull. This is felt as a definite end point by the operator. The average time to place a twist drill hole in clinical conditions has been thirty seconds. After placement of the hole the operator has access to the epidural, subdural and ventricular areas with suitable needles and can further evaluate the patient's injury.

The hand drill used in this manner serves as both an evaluating tool as well as therapeutic instrument. They have found it particularly beneficial in evaluating deeply comatose patients suspected of having chronic subdural hematomas. In these patients twist drill holes allow access to the subdural space. The presence or absence of a chronic subdural collection can be determined by passing an appropriate needle through the dura and removing enough liquefied material to reduce intracranial pressure. They report there is often an immediate and dramatic improvement in the level of consciousness following decompression by this technic.

Under conditions where arteriography cannot be done a twist drill hole provides a convenient appraisal of the ventricular system. By exchanging a small amount of cerebrospinal fluid with air and then exposing an anteroposterior skull X-ray, the ventricles can be delineated and shifts across the midline disclosed.

The use of a twist drill under these circumstances is not without risk. Subdural, subarachnoid and intraventricular hemorrhage have been found in some patients. The risk entailed in the procedure must be balanced against the possible good achieved.

Such small openings are only temporarily effective and should not be misconstrued as definitive treatment. Harvey Cushing[7] pointed out many years ago in regard to burr holes that such openings rapidly become filled with bulging brain and drainage cannot be effective. He advocated an intermusculotemporal operation. The temporal muscle is split in line with its fibers and the thin squamous wing of the temporal and adjoining sphenoid are rongeured away exposing the region overlying meningeal vessels. The dura is opened and usually there is escape of bloody cerebrospinal fluid. In patients where this craniectomy on one side is ineffective the opposite side is explored at the same or a subsequent operation. Cushing points out such an exploration is not attended by shock and lists the following advantages: 1. the exposure of the meningeal territory and ease of determining the presence of an extradural hemorrhage, 2. draining through a split muscle instead of through the scalp, 3. protective action of the muscle in case a hernia tends to form in consequence of traumatic edema.

The emergency decompression of the brain in rapidly deteriorating patients is only one area in which craniectomy may be a necessary evaluating tool. The second group are those patients who have been studied by cerebral arteriography brain scans, echoencephalography and observed closely with the neurologic flow sheet described in earlier chapters. These evaluating technics are not always black and white. There are gray zones. Arteriography was not available to Harvey Cushing[7] but his statement is still timely, "an exploration may often be necessary before it can be determined whether there is an extradural or intradural hemorrhage." It is often difficult to determine upon which side of the head the hemorrhage has occurred. Dilatation of the pupil may be of cortical origin or due to peripheral involvement of the motor oculi.

The effect of extensive brain decompression on physiologic function was strikingly illustrated in two victims of the 1974 April tornado in Kentucky and Indiana. Two patients arrived simultaneously; one an elderly female had the entire right hemicranium explosively ripped from her head and the right cerebral cortex massively extruded; the other patient a boy of twelve had a severe basilar skull fracture extending upward in the coronal plane. Both were unconscious. Because of the continued arrival of multiple other victims the female patient with extruded cortex was triaged to low priority. Later the wound was debrided, cleaned, and dura and soft tissue closed. The young boy with the closed head injury deteriorated rapidly in spite of attempts to reduce intracranial pressure with fluid restriction, steroids, and osmotic diuretics, and died the night of admission. The elderly female with a right hemi-craniectomy supported her own respiration spontaneously and was still alive five days later. She had a left hemiplegia as expected by the nature of the injury.

Such patients provide important information and should help the surgeon who does adequate craniectomies as evaluating procedures and finds no surgically correctable lesion (negative) avoid mental self-flagellation.

EXPLORATION OF NECK AND GROIN WOUNDS

The anatomical structure of the neck is compact. In a very small area there are components of the digestive, respiratory, vascular, neurologic and skeletal systems which influence regulation and function of the entire organism. Any injury to the neck is a potential threat to the continued function of all these systems.

Wounds of the neck are deceptive and difficult to evaluate. Blunt trauma frequently produces no wound but are most difficult to evaluate. The neurologic deficits are usually obvious and the skeletal aspects can usually be detected by roentgen examination. But soft tissue injuries are frequently overlooked. Penetrating wounds are much more frequent and often appear innocuous. After initial evaluation has been completed most of these wounds dictate operative exploration.

In three large series,[8, 9, 10] thirty-six of fifty-seven deaths (63.1%) were the direct result of blood vessel injury and twenty-one (36.9%) deaths were due to complications of laryngeal, tracheal or esophageal injury. Proper and early application of arteriography as described in Chapter 14 should reduce the large number of deaths due to blood vessel disruption. In most instances arteriography gives precise location of the site of injury. But arteriography has its limitations; every physician has encountered a major arterial laceration in patients with normal arteriograms. In some patients with multiple injuries arteriography is prohibited by the patient's condition.

Such facts create an urgent need to explore most neck wounds soon after injury. Jones and associates[11] reported on 274 wounds of the neck. They describe fifteen patients with clinically negative neck wounds, i.e. no external bleeding, no shock or hypovolemia, no visible hematoma. In this group of clinically negative wounds there were thirteen injuries to major vessels, two thoracic duct injuries. They emphasize that these patients would not have had surgical exploration at some hospitals. Even more informing are 103 patients whom they explored but found no significant injury. These patients were discharged to outpatient status within seventy-two hours and there were no deaths or serious complications.

Fogelman and Stewart[10] found the mortality in patients promptly explored was 6 percent while in those where operative exploration was omitted or postponed the mortality rate was 35 percent. In Shirkey's study six of twenty-two deaths occurred in patients in which exploration was delayed beyond six hours or omitted entirely.

Procrastination in accurate evaluation of neck wounds by operative exploration results in delayed and sometimes uncontrolled hemorrhage in septic wounds, airway compromise, fatal or crippling brain damage, fistulae, lethal sepsis, false aneurysms or arteriovenous fistulae. These experiences make exploration of neck wounds a desirable evaluating method to be employed in most wounds of the neck.

The entire chest should be prepared and draped. A transverse neck incision can be extended in various directions to achieve exposure of most cervical structures. When needed this primary incision can be extended in T fashion through the midsternum to expose the origin of the great vessels and the heart. In some patients a unilateral cervical incision anterior to the sternocleido-mastoid muscle is appropriate. This incision can also be extended into the mediasternum in hockey stick fashion by sternotomy. Either of these incisions allow anatomic exposure of most neck structures. The sternotomy component should not be avoided nor delayed because immediate proximal control of the great vessels frequently will mean the difference between death and life in these individuals.

Those patients who require immediate surgery to resuscitate may be only a small portion of the total number of neck wounds encountered. In other patients who are stable, evaluation by angiograms, laryngoscopy, bronchoscopy, esophagoscopy, BA swallow, etc. should be done. As before negative results in these preliminary appraisals do not contradict operative exploration.

Although the femoral area does not contain the same number

of vital structures as the neck, groin wounds can often be devastating. Arteriography has again contributed greatly to the evaluation of these wounds, but once again it is not the final answer. The major risk in groin wounds is exsanguination from large arteries, but in addition to hemorrhage these wounds may also extend into the peritoneal cavity, urinary bladder, uretha, vagina and rectum.

The exploration of groin wounds is comparatively minor surgery yet many surgeons are hesitant to commit themselves to such an exploration unless there are positive findings on arteriograms or absence of pulses distal to the injury. Every clinician has encountered patients with peripheral pulses and a laceration of a major artery proximally.

Operative evaluation of patients with critical injuries must not be looked upon as an admission of defeat, nor lack of ability on the part of physicians. Neither should it be reserved for desperate situations or delayed until forced upon an unwilling surgeon. Conversely operative evaluation must take its rightful place alongside other universally acceptable methods of evaluating critically injured patients.

REFERENCES

1. Ravdin, I. S.: In discussion of Shaftan, G. W.: Gliedman, M. L., and Capelletti, R. R.: Injuries of the liver: A review of 111 cases. *J Trauma, 3:*72, 1963.
2. Mays, E. T.: Bursting injuries of the liver. *Arch Surg, 93:*92-106, 1966.
3. DeBakey, M. E.: The management of chest wounds, collective review. *Int Abst Surg, 74:*203-237, 1942.
4. DeMuth, W. E.: Discussion of Keller, T. W., et al.: Thoracic injuries due to blunt trauma. *J Trauma, 7:*549, 1967.
5. Raaf, J.: Treatment of the patient with acute head injury. *J Trauma, 4:*168-179, 1964.
6. Burton, C., and Blacker, H. M.: A compact hand drill for emergency brain decompression. *J Trauma, 5:*643-646, 1965.
7. Cushing, H.: *Surgery of the Head. Keen's Surgery.* III Philadelphia, London, W. B. Saunders, 1916.
8. Stove, H. H., and Callahan, G. S.: Soft tissue injuries of the neck. *Surg Gynecol Obstet, 117:*745-752, 1963.

9. Shirkey, A. L.; Beall, A. C., and DeBakey, M. E.: Surgical management of penetrating wounds of the neck. *Arch Surg*, 86:955-963, 1963.

10. Fogelman, M. J., and Stewart, R. D.: Penetrating wounds of the neck. *Am J Surg*, 91:581-593, 1956.

11. Jones, R. F.; Terrell, J. C., and Salyer, K. E.: Penetrating wounds of the neck: An analysis of 274 cases. *J Trauma*, 7:228-237, 1967.

CHAPTER 13 ――――――――――――――――――――――――――――――――

EVALUATION BY
SEQUENTIAL MONITORING

―――――――――――――――――――――――――――――――――――

AFTER THE PRECEEDING initial methodical assessment is completed there cannot be a total cessation of additional observation. A common reason for overlooking serious injuries is the knowledge that the patient has already been examined. In critically injured patients evaluation is a continuing process rather than an event which has a final completion point. Even though all the appraisals described in preceding chapters have been done there is still an imperative need for a concerned "team captain" to return to the patient's bedside at frequent and regular intervals and feel, look, and listen. Airways have a way of becoming obstructed—chest tubes occluded—intravenous fluids and blood running onto the sheet instead of into the patient. Aside from these "mishaps," human error must never be discounted. Regardless of how carefully our initial examination may have been done even the most competent and experienced physician can miss a significant injury particularly in the excitement and confusion that frequently accompanies admission of a critically injured patient.

It is failure of continued and sequential monitoring of injured patients that causes such tragedies as anoxic necrosis of the brain in a young girl having a minor hand injury repaired, death from a missed tension pneumothorax in a young man whose femoral fracture was immobolized and the patient transferred to the intensive care unit for the remainder of the night, death from exsanguination due to an undetected ruptured liver in a

367

twenty-four-year-old man having a scalp laceration sutured, brain necrosis in an eighteen-year-old man due to anoxia while a minor soft tissue laceration was repaired in the operating room. The geographic area of the patient in the hospital is unimportant. Sequential monitoring must be a progressive careful and constant factor whether the patient is in the recovery room, on the operating table, in X-ray, in the intensive care unit or on the ward. A physician team captain must be responsible in seeing that such monitoring is being done. Although he may choose to delegate such responsibility to the anesthesiologist, a nurse, junior residents, recovery room personnel, or paramedical personnel, he has a moral obligation to the patient to guarantee meticulous sequential monitoring.

Many injuries are treacherous. They have insidious sequelae which sometimes are not detectable until many hours after the injury. Some of these injuries cannot be detected at the initial examination by even the most senior or experienced physician. In other patients the initial examination is sometimes equivocal. The experience of medicine is not all black or white. There are many grey zones. It is especially important in such patients to repeat examinations at intervals to avoid overlooking an injury. Other injuries are strongly suspected from the initial assessment but the objective findings just do not support the suspicion. Every student of medicine is admonished by his mentors to have a "high index of suspicion" and nearly every physician makes this a part of his mental makeup. But something more is needed than just a "high index of suspicion." Frequent anatomic and physiologic sequential monitoring divulges nearly all injuries, grey zones, insidious, suspicious, equivocal or otherwise. A small number will reqiure operative evaluation as discussed in the last chapter.

The geographic area in which sequential monitoring is done is not nearly so important as the imperative to get it done. Those medical centers with Trauma Research Units are ideal and perhaps in Utopia all hospitals will have such units. But realities of the present proclaim that most critically injured patients are cared for in community hospitals which are not blessed with $400,000 Trauma Research Units. But most of the practical means of monitoring patients can be available in most hospitals regardless how small or how far removed from the large medical centers. In the discussion that follows methods that appear too sophisticated or expensive for some hospitals have been added only for completeness. The practical, reliable and significant methods are available in most hospitals.

HEMODYNAMIC MONITORING

A real tragedy in the education of students of medicine today is emphasizing sophisticated and complex testing and under-emphasing the significance of blood pressure, pulse and respiration. The consequences of such spreading philosophy is to separate the physician and nurse from the patient. In evaluating critically injured patients new emphasis must be placed on the heart rate. The nature of pulsations in peripheral arteries and the pattern and rate of respiratory movements. An alert physician by careful observation over a period of years, can tell a great deal about the hemodynamic status of his patient simply by palpation of the femoral, carotid, or radial arteries.

Once blood volume has been replaced in a severely injured patient, the physician must observe him closely for indications of his once again losing effective circulating volume. An increased heart rate, reduced blood pressure with air hunger and cold clammy skin developing after adequate initial replacement of blood volume indicate recurrence of bleeding or overlooked sites of exsanguination. An immediate response after further volume replacement confirms the suspicion of additional hemorrhage and immediate steps must be taken to locate and control the site of continued blood volume reduction.

Not only is blood pressure and pulse important in monitoring flux in blood volume they also reflect intracranial pressure. A forty-two-year-old man recently focused on the value of sequential monitoring of blood pressure and pulse. He was admitted because of cranio-cerebral trauma. An arteriogram failed to disclose any evidence of space occupying lesions. During the following hours he was sequentially monitored. His blood pressure began to increase. The heart rate also increased, but the patient was febrile with a co-existing pneumonia. An alert house officer noted the increasing blood pressure and correctly discounted the absence of bradycardia in a febrile patient. Even though cerebral angiography had been normal, the patient was taken to the operating theatre and a large frontal extradural hematoma removed. Two principles are emphasized by this patient. 1) Cerebral arteriography has "blind spots," notoriously the intermediate frontal and the posterior parietal. 2) Sequential monitoring of the blood pressure and pulse are valid appraisals of intracranial pressure changes.

The microcirculation evaluated by observing the nailbeds and the rapidity with which they fill after being blanched out by pressure is an important observation to add to the blood pressure and pulse. In discussing pulse it must emphasized that it is not only the rate of cardiac systole that should be observed. The complete expansion of a progressive unobstructed pulse wave with good "crescendo" and normal progressive decrescendo indicate adequate circulating volume. The observer should look for the reduced "water hammer" type pulse usually discussed in association with aortic insufficiency but in the injured patient may denote marked reduction in circulating blood volume with a young, completely normal heart.

The importance of measuring central venous pressure was discussed in previous chapters. It is essential, however, to understand that a single determination of central venous pressure provides little information. Because the zero point is an approximation on the external topography of the level of the right atrium. The sequential changes in venous pressure are more critical than the initial determination. Monitoring the central venous pressure on an hour to hour basis gives useful information that when combined with blood pressure, pulse and the peripheral microcirculation give fairly accurate patterns of the hemodynamic status. In most patients the pressures in the right heart reflect the pressures in the left and are reliable in assessing the seriously injured patient. This is not true in patients with significant cardiopulmonary disease. These latter patients are better monitored with the flow-directed Balloon-tipped catheter proposed by Swan and associates.[1] This catheter is produced by Edwards

Laboratories, 624 Dyer Road, Santa Ana, California. It is a No. 5 French double lumen catheter with a balloon just proximal to the tip of the catheter. The catheter is inserted into the basilic cephalic subclavian or jugular veins and advanced to the right atruim. Monitoring pressure as the catheter moves toward the heart signifies the location of the catheter tip to that point. The balloon is inflated with 0.8 ml air and carried by the flow of blood through the right heart and into the pulmonary artery. In that position mean pulmonary artery pressure can be monitored. Inflating the balloon and allowing the catheter and balloon to wedge themselves in a pulmonary artery makes it possible to monitor the wedge-pulmonary pressure. This pressure is significant because it reflects the pressure in the left atruim. This left atrial pressure and flux in response to replacement therapy is the information needed in hemodynamic monitoring. As I noted previously many critically injured patients are young and have normal cardiac and pulmonary systems. It is not necessary to use the flow-directed balloon-tipped catheter in these individuals because in such patients the right atrial pressures adequately reflect left atrial pressure changes.

The Swan-Ganz catheter is not needed in every critically injured patient. There are serious pulmonary complications associated with use of the catheter. Foote and colleagues[2] report a 15.2 percent pulmonary infarction or hemorrhage from using the catheter. Scott and associates[3] noted a tendency for the catheter to slip into the persistent wedge position.

In the original description of the balloon-tipped catheter Swan and his associates suggested advancing the catheter 1 to 3 cm farther after the initial wedge pressure had been obtained. This method of positioning may lead to rupture of pulmonary vessel and is undesirable particularly if a satisfactory wedge pressure is obtained in the first instance.

To prevent pulmonary complications from these catheters Foote and his colleagues emphasize that. (1) meticulous attention must be paid to their insertion and maintenance, (2) repeated evaluations of the character of the pulse tracing enables prompt recognition of unintentional catheter wedging, (3) frequent chest roentgenograms for catheter position should be done (4) constant infusion through the catheter lumen be maintained at all times and heparin (10 IU/ml) added to the infusing solution.

There are many technics and numerous catheters designed for monitoring central venous pressure. It is not within the scope of this text to describe all of them. They have been well described by Bower.[4] Certain pitfalls in technic must be mentioned. In order that the pressure measurements be reliable in evaluating the critically injured they must reflect as nearly as possible true atrial pressures. Venous catheters lying in peripheral veins cannot give this information. Unusually long catheters inserted into peripheral veins and threaded into central veins introduce factors of resistance, viscosity and flow within rigid narrow tubes. Peripherally placed catheters also have a high incidence of thrombotic and necrotic complications and are colonized by pathogenic bacteria frequently.

Percutaneous placement of catheters into large central veins reduces many of the complications and achieves an increased duration of their use.[5] Although the ultimate goal is monitoring the pressure changes in the right atruim, these catheters should never be placed in the right atruim. Cardiac perforation is a frequent and lethal complication if these cannulae are allowed to remain in the heart chambers. Roentgenograms of the chest to determine exact catheter position is extremely important if a physician chooses this method of monitoring his patient.

Other complications of inserting and maintaining catheters for monitoring patients hemodynamically are: hemothorax, pneumothorax subcutaneous emphysema, brachial plexus injury, septicemia, intrapleural administration of fluids producing hydrothorax, subclavian artery injury, hematomas, "fibrin sleeve" formation around catheter and catheter emboli. The incidence of all these complications have been shown to be inversely related to the training and experience of the physician inserting the catheter. Central venous pressure monitoring is a valuable clinical tool but should not be delegated to the most junior or inexperienced physician. It is a technic that should be taught by supervision just as we teach a cholecystectomy, hysterectomy or cardiac valve replacement. Any physician desiring to master the technics should review the anatomy of the region, dissect a cadaver or participate in several necropsies to acquaint himself with the anatomic relationships of the central veins of the upper torso.

Some authorities have questioned the value of central venous pressure measurements and emphasize that left ventricular overload and pulmonary edema can occur while right ventricular function as monitored by central venous pressure remains acceptably adequate.[7] This is particularly true as I mentioned above in patients with pre-existing cardiac lesions. In these patients pulmonary wedge pressures are needed. Most patients involved in trauma, however, are young and have normal cardiac reserves. Changes in central venous pressure from hour to hour and in response to fluid infusion *do* indicate the ability of the myocardium to pump the volume presented to it.[8] It is also extremely useful in evaluating not just the total volume of replacement but the *rate* of repletion.

This is a bedside measurement and not an exact reading. The normal central venous pressure ranges from —2 to +5 mm Hg[9-10] (Table 13-I). A mistake propagated in the past was to accept values up to 15 mm Hg as normal. But such values were obtained from peripheral, not central, veins. The level of the right atrium is taken as the zero baseline. Unfortunately, it is at best only an estimate. A distance 10 cm from the dorsal spine is used by some clinicians as the level of the right atrium.[11] Weil and his associates[8] use the mid-lateral position of the chest, and yet others favor the anterior third of the chest in a patient lying on a firm surface.[12]

Interpreting the changes in central venous pressure can be misleading. The central venous pressure does not indicate total blood volume. Prout[13] found the blood volume needed to be 40 percent above the predicted normal value to maintain a normal

TABLE 13-I

NORMAL PRESSURES IN THE RIGHT AND PULMONARY ARTERY

Site	Presure (mm Hg)
Right Atrium	—2 to +5
Right Ventricle	—0.5 to +7
Pulmonary Artery	8 to 19
Pulmonary Capillary (wedge)	5 to 13

central venous pressure. The sequential changes in CVP simply reflect the relationship between superior vena caval pressure and right heart function. This is an important relationship because the end-diastolic volume of the right ventricle depends upon caval volume and pressure. Failure of the right ventricle to eject the end-diastolic volume causes a progressive increase in caval pressure in normovolemic patients. In hypovolemic patients who have normal cardiac action stroke volume is reduced and caval pressures are reduced to zero or below. As stroke volume falls off cardiac output is reduced and urine output decreases.

The presence of increased caval pressure or caval pressures that increases with rapid infusion of fluid or blood yet there is either no change or a reduction in cardiac output indicates impairment of cardiac function. Usually this is primary myocardial deficiency but the physician must also remember that in severely injured patients the defect in the pumping mechanism may be mechanical obstruction as occurs in cardiac tramponade, shifted mediastinum from tension pneumothorax, or mediastinal compression from a hemothorax or a positive pressure ventilator. These are correctable lesions and must be kept in mind when interpreting central venous pressure determinations.

There is a peculiar variant that sometimes occurs after severe injuries which render the patient extremely hypovolemic. As the situation worsens coronary artery perfusion decreases to such a degree that primary myocardial decompensation ensues. The central venous pressure is about 10 to 12 cm H_2O when repletion starts, but because of previously reduced coronary artery perfusion with cardiac decompensation, the central venous pressures go very high (25 to 35 cm). This is usually an indication to restrict fluids but in this case additional volume must be given in quantities sufficient to perfuse the coronary arteries. Once coronary artery perfusion is normal the failing myocardium recovers and the central venous pressure falls back to 0 to $+5$ cm H_2O.

Thus far I have outlined methods of sequential monitoring that are available in most hospitals. Other helpful hemodynamic measurements when available are cardiac output and total peripheral resistance. Resistance to the flow of blood through distal vessels cannot be measured directly and must be calculated:

$$\text{Total peripheral resistance} = \frac{\text{Mean arterial pressure-central venous pressure}}{\text{cardiac index}} \quad \text{L/min/m}^2$$

The *mean arterial pressure* is a systolic and diastolic mean of the arterial blood pressure taken from a pressure type transducer recorder. It normally is approximately 95 mm Hg. The *central venous pressure* normally measured in cm H_2O or saline must be converted to mm Hg before inserting it into the equation.

The *cardiac index* is determined by:

$$\text{Cardiac index} = \frac{\text{Cardiac output (L/min)}}{\text{Surface area (sq m)}}$$

$$\text{Surface Area} = 1.73 \text{ sq m average}$$
$$\text{normal man}$$

$$\text{Cardiac output} = \frac{\text{Oxygen consumption (ml/min)}}{\text{arterio venous oxygen difference ml/L}}$$

Wilson[14] has described the method of determining cardiac output using the arteriovenous oxygen difference but more rapid and direct measurements of cardiac output are now available. These require only intra-arterial cannulation in addition to the central venous catheter discussed above. Indocyanine green can be injected through the central venous catheter and the time of injection recorded electrically. Arterial blood is withdrawn from the indwelling intra-arterial cannula and the blood passed through a densitometer. In this fashion a dye curve is recorded. Computers have now made analysis of the dye curve rapid and automatic dealing also with the problem of recirculation of the dye and extrapolation of the exponential decrease in dye concentration. The normal cardiac output in healthy young men is 4 L/min. This inserted into the above equation gives normal cardiac index in an average 1.73 sq m patient of 3.12 L/min/m². The stroke volume is the cardiac output divided by the pulse rate:

$$\text{Stroke volume} = \frac{\text{Cardiac output}}{\text{Heart rate}}$$

Physicians evaluating patients in hospitals without the more sophisticated computers and equipment for obtaining the above data should not forget there are simple and reliable methods of assessing total peripheral resistance and cardiac output. Increased total peripheral resistance is disclosed by pale cold skin, and nailbeds whose capillary filling is very slow after pressure blanching. Low total peripheral resistance is manifested by warm dry skin and plethoric capillaries. Reduced cardiac output is disclosed by decreased urine output and impaired cerebration. Normal cardiac output results in normal glomerular filtration and improved mental alertness.

RESPIRATORY MONITORING

Much information can be gleaned by repeated auscultation of the lung fields. Occasionally a pneumothorax develops slowly. Breath sounds may have been normal upon admission but after several hours tension increases in the pleural space and serious ventilatory problems may develop. Patients supported with positive pressure may rupture a bleb or puncture a lung against a sharp segment of broken rib. These changes are sometimes insidious and can only be detected by careful repeated auscultation of the chest.

Observing the nature and pattern of respiratory excursions after the patient has been resuscitated gives valuable information. The loss of lung compliance or severe bronchoconstriction increase the work of breathing and prolongs the expiratory phase. And, if one looks closely, he can notice an added forceful effort at the end of expiration. The diaphragm, abdominal muscles and accessory muscles of respiration have to push a little harder to clear air from the lungs.

If this is due primarily to bronchoconstriction instead of "stiff lungs" there will be audible wheezing.

Endotracheal tubes have a way of migrating to one mainstem bronchus and precluding the aeration of the opposite lung. About the only way such "mishaps" can be detected in time to obviate serious anoxia and subsequent brain necrosis is sequential monitoring of the patient by ascultation of the lungs and observing the respiratory excursions. The hemothorax not aerated will lag behind the normal ventilated one and will never expand to the same degree as the side with normal ventilation. Other things which produce the same findings in critically injured patients are aspirated dental prosthetics, aspirated foreign bodies and mucous plugs.

Reliable and simple to use blood gas and pH analyzers are commercially available. Their acquisition by most hospitals has suddenly placed sequential monitoring of the respiratory system on a practical basis. In these instruments oxygen tension is measured directly by a polarographic electrode consisting of a platinum cathode and silver anode. A thin plastic membrane permeable to oxygen separates the cathode from the blood. The number of electrons that pass through the membrane when a constant polarizing current (0.6 volt) is applied is proportional to the number of oxygen molecules present (partial pressure of oxygen). Small samples of heparinized arterial and venous blood are obtained anerobically then immediately analyzed. If the samples must be stored the syringe should be firmly stoppered after making an effort to remove all air bubbles.

Carbon dioxide is determined directly by the Clark electrode, which measures the pH of a solution of bicarbonate. A Teflon membrane separates the gas or blood sample from the solution of bicarbonate but it is freely permeable to carbon dioxide. The carbon dioxide in whatever sample is being tested diffuses across the membrane producing flux in the pH of the bicarbonate solution. The electrode records resistance changes as a function of hydrogen ion changes across the tip of the electrode. Samples containing known partial pressures of carbon dioxide are used to calibrate the instrument. The unknown samples of blood should be read immediately upon withdrawal from the patient.

An instrument with a platinum unicell electrode can be purchased to determine blood pH. Blood samples can be placed in the electrode and the tip of the electrode immersed in a solution of supersaturated potassium chloride. The potassium chloride provides an electron bridge and pH is read directly from the calibrated instrument panel.

Arterial samples for blood gases and pH determination can

be obtained from any peripheral artery. Sequential samples can be safely obtained by carefully using small No. 22 or 25 sterile disposable needles. In some patients sequential arterial sampling can be done with an indwelling Teflon or Siliastic catheter inserted into a radial or femoral artery. The blood samples are withdrawn into plastic or glass heparinized syringes. Very little heparin is needed. Only the barrel of the syringe need be wet; any more Heparin than this is excessive and dilutes the samples giving errors in the determinations.

To interpret the results and evaluate the patient with data collected by sequential monitoring of the respiratory system the reader must acquaint himself with the terminology of pulmonary physiology. The Federal Proceedings Report of 1950[15] has standardized the symbols and abbreviations that are universally applicable. The following conventions were adopted by the Federations for symbols denoting location and molecular species:

1. Localization in the gas phase is represented by a small capital letter immediately following the principal variable. Thus pressure in alveolar gas is represented by P_A.

2. Localization in the blood phase is represented by a lower case letter immediately following the principal variable. Thus pressure in arterial blood is represented P_a.

3. Molecular species is denoted by the full chemical symbol to be printed in small capital letters immediately following the principal variable. Thus pressure of carbon dioxide is represented by $P\,CO_2$.

4. When specifications of both location and molecular species is required then the first modifying letter will be used for localization and the second for species. Thus the pressure of carbon dioxide in aveolar gas in represented by P_ACO_2 in this case the chemical symbol appears as a subscript.

Table 13-II shows common abbreviations and symbols used in describing respiratory physiology. Recognition and comprehension of the more commonly employed terms will greatly benefit the physician who is assessing sequential respiratory responses in seriously injured patients. Figure 13-1 shows the various segments of lung ventilation.

TABLE 13-II

STANDARD SYMBOLS AND ABBREVIATIONS IN
RESPIRATORY PHYSIOLOGY

ABBREVIATIONS

STPD = Standard temperature, pressure dry
       (0°C, 760 mm Hg)
BTPS = Body temperature, pressure, saturated with water
ATPD = Ambient temperature, pressure dry
ATPS = Ambient temperature, pressure, saturated with water

SYMBOLS

$\overline{X}$ Dash above any symbol indicates a mean value

$\dot{X}$ Dot above any symbol indicates a time derivative

CAPITAL LETTERS

P =   gas pressure in general
V =   gas volume in general

$\dot{V}$ =   gas volume per unit time

$\dot{Q}$ = volume flow of blood
F =   fractional concentration in dry gas phase
C =   concentration in blood phase
R =   respiratory exchange ratio in general $\left(\dfrac{\text{vol } CO_2}{\text{vol } O_2}\right)$

D =   diffusing capacity in general (vol/unit time/pressure difference)

LOWER CASE

f =   respiratory frequency (breaths/min)
b =   blood in general
a =   arterial blood
v =   venous blood
c =   capillary blood

SMALL CAPITALS

ɪ = Inspired gas
ᴇ = Expired gas
ᴀ = Alveolar gas
ᴅ = Dead Space
ʙ = Barometric
ᴛ = Tidal gas

TABLE 13-II

COMMON TERMS

F_IO_2 = fraction of inspired oxygen

F_ECO_2 = fraction of expired carbon dioxide

P_AO_2 = partial pressure of alveolar oxygen

P_aO_2 = partial pressure of arterial oxygen

P_B = barometric pressure

$\dot{V}_A$ = alveolar ventilation (liters/min)

$\dot{V}_A/\dot{Q}$ = ratio of alveolar ventilation to cardiac output

V_DV_T = ratio of deadspace to tidal volume

$\dot{Q}s/Qt$ = ratio pulmonary shunt flow to total blood flow

A-aDO$_2$ = alveolar-arterial oxygen difference

$S\text{-}_vO_2$ = percentage saturation of mixed venous blood

C_aO_2 = content of oxygen (ml O_2 per 100 ml of arterial blood)

Boyd[16] has delineated common pathophysiologic relationships important in the patient after trauma. He recommends using the Wright respirometer and Sierra low resistance nonrebreathing valve for sequential monitoring of respiratory function. The Sierra valve can be attached to a mouthpiece or tracheostomy tube. It is connected by an anesthesia flex tube with the Wright respirometer and then to a three way directional valve. A noseplug should be used to block the nostrils when the mouthpiece is used. When using a tracheostomy the endotracheal cuff must be inflated to ensure against air leaks while collecting gas samples. A 5 liter anesthesia bag is used for collecting expired gas.

Individual tidal volumes may be measured directly. It is better however, to measure the total amount of expired gas over a one minute period (Minute Ventilation) and divide this volume by the number of breaths taken (f) this gives the mean expired tidal volume (MEV). A special precaution in this test is to ensure a closed system without air leaks.

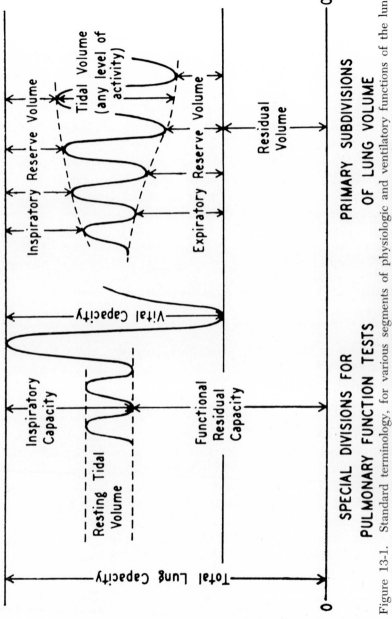

Figure 13-1. Standard terminology, for various segments of physiologic and ventilatory functions of the lung proposed by the Federation Proceedings Report. Reprinted from Federation Proceedings, 9:602-605, 1950.

Usually patients are tested initially breathing room air. The F_1O_2 must always be determined to enable correct interpretations of the responses. After completing initial testing the F_1O_2 is is increased to 1.0 and a nitrogen washout test done. The necessary precaution is to be certain that 100 percent oxygen ($F_1O_2 = 1.0$) is delivered without air leaks. This can be doublechecked by incorporating a rapid responding nitrogen analyzer to the expired gas line. When the expired nitrogen falls below one percent the F_1O_2 has completely replaced all alveolar gas except carbon dioxide and water vapor. At this point arterial blood oxygen tensions correctly reflect the aveolar - arterial gradient (A-aDO_2) and pulmonary shunt for oxygen. Paramagnetic oxygen analysis of the inspired gas to determine the F_1O_2 is always necessary, if the collected data is to be accepted as reliable.

The maintenance of normal blood gases is dependent on the relationship of pulmonary blood flow ($\dot{Q}$) and effective alveolar ventilation ($\dot{V}_A$) Normal alveolar ventilation is about 4 liters per minute and normal cardiac output ($\dot{Q}$) is approximately 5 liters per minute. The normal ventilation perfusion ratio $\dot{V}_A / \dot{Q}$ is around 0.80.[17] In alveolar hypoventilation, alveolar gas exchange is reduced, sometimes as much as by half. If this were the case $\dot{V}_A / \dot{Q}$ would drop to 0.40 and half the blood perfusing the lungs would not contact effective alveolar gas units. In such an imbalanced situation gaseous exchange cannot occur normally, and venous blood returning to the heart from these gas units is hypoxemic. It is then ejected from the heart into the systemic circulation. The prolonged stay in the supine position by patients who are not ambulated produces this same imbalance between perfusion and ventilation. This inequality of ventilation and perfusion is also an indication of chest wall injury, pulmonary trauma or hypovolemia.

The Alveolar-arterial gradient (A-aD) indicates the maximal quantity of oxygen that can be made available to perfusing capillaries after nitrogen has been completely displaced from every alveolus. Usually the "nitrogen washout" curve becomes completely flat after breathing 100 percent oxygen for 7 to 10 minutes; after 15 minutes all patent alveoli contain only oxygen carbon dioxide and water. Under these circumstances the P_AO_2 should approximate 673 mm Hg (760-47-40=673). Direct measurement of the PaO_2 at this time should define the alveolar-arterial gradient:

$$A\text{-}aDO_2 = P_AO_2 - P_aO_2 + P_ACO_2 + P_AH_2O$$
$$P_AO_2 = \text{alveolar oxygen tension}$$
$$PaO_2 = \text{measured directly}$$
$$P_ACO_2 = PaCO_2 \text{ (assumption)}$$
$$P_AH_2O = 47 \text{ mm Hg at } 37° \text{ C.}$$

Significant intrapulmonary shunting is present if there are discrepancies between alveolar and arterial oxygen tensions. About 3 percent of the cardiac output normally goes through anatomic shunts from the right to left heart by way of bronchial pleural and thesbian veins. Increases beyond this indicate pathology. After trauma such pathologic shunting occurs and sequential monitoring of the A-aDO$_2$ should indicate improvement or a worsening of the situation.

When the $F_IO_2 = 1.0$ the shunt equation (Chapter 3) is modified.

$$\dot{Q}s/\dot{Q}t = \frac{0.0031\,(P_A - P_a)}{[Ca + P_A - P_a)\,0.0031] - C_V}$$
$$P_A = P_B - PH_2O - Pa\,CO_2$$

The equation compares the observed arterial (C_aO_2) and venous ($C_v\,O_2$) oxygen contents to the theoretical maximal oxygen content that would be present in pulmonary veins after complete nitrogen displacement.

As discussed in the chapter on physiologic response to trauma, there is a 12 to 15 percent physiologic shunt almost consistently present after severe trauma. If in the process of sequential monitoring this physiologic shunting increases to 35 or 40 percent, the responsible "team captain" must search for overlooked causes of such increased shunting. Undetected hypovolemia is the most frequent cause if retained bronchial secretions and prolonged immobilization in supine position are excluded. The hypovolemia is not always due to overt hemorrhage. It can also be caused by: sequestration of extracellular fluid in tissues by trauma, a missed retroperitoneal injury to the duodenum with extravasation of bile and pancreatic juices into the area, chemical peritonitis, bile peritonitis, or sequestration into thermal burns.

Wilson and associates[18] found that patients with shunt fractions greater than 50 percent rarely survive. Such an observation makes it imperative that we find and correct the cause of shunting before it reaches 50 percent. This is the role of careful sequential monitoring. They also reported that patients with shunts 40 percent or below can survive when recognized early and appropriately treated.

After major trauma the ventilatory effort usually is increased but the effectiveness is decreased.[19] They show significant decreases in tidal volume with increased respiratory frequency. Such a situation usually increases the V_D/VT ratio. The Bohr Equation delineates the respiratory deadspace for any gas x and explains why the above described patients have less effective, less efficient breathing even though ventilatory effort is increased.

$$V_{DX} = \frac{(FE_X - FA_X)}{(FI_X - F_{AX})} \cdot V_T$$

The Bohr equation can be modified to the standard terms outlined in Table 13-I and CO_2 substituted for gas x.

$$V_D = \frac{PaCO_2 - P_ECO_2}{PaCO_2} \cdot V_T$$

Tidal volume (V_T) is measured directly and arterial partial pressure (P_aCO_2) has been substituted for alveolar carbon dioxide tension (P_ACO_2) because there is complete equilibration between the alveolar and pulmonary end-capillary carbon dioxide. The expired carbon dioxide tension (P_E-CO_2) of the timed sample (3 min) is measured directly. After proper substitution the respiratory deadspace for CO_2 is calculated. These assumptions and calculations are not valid in advanced pulmonary insufficiency when CO_2 is being retained in abnormal amounts.

After the deadspace V_D been calculated by the Bohr equation the ratio V_D/V_T is obtained. It normally does not exceed 0.3. Usually deadspace volume is 150 ml and Tidal volume 450 ml.

$$\frac{V_D}{V_T} = \frac{150}{450} = 0.3$$

After serious trauma rapid shallow breathing usually occurs. This can reduce V_T moderately, but changes the ratio of wasted deadspace to tidal volume significantly (0.5). Increasing the V_D/V_T ratio means less effective ventilation. If this occurs during sequential monitoring the physician should look for problems that reduce tidal volume such as undetected hemothorax, ruptured diaphragm, flail or unstable segments of chest wall. In doing so he must also assure himself that deadspace (V_D) has not been increased.

Not all these measurements need be done in every critically injured patient. The physician must use his sense of practical judgement in sequential monitoring of his patient's respiratory function. Blood gases and pH are becoming universally available in most hospitals and these should be obtained early to give a baseline. Sequential blood gas determinations can then give valuable information in evaluating the critically injured patient. Sequential blood gas determinations are also important in monitoring cranio-cerebral injuries as discussed in the next section.

NEUROLOGIC MONITORING

There are no clinical signs, pictures or patterns of neurologic findings that are pathognomonic of epidural, subdural or intra-cerebral hematoma. This fact underlies most of the frustration involved in evaluating patients with head injuries. It is the progression of neurologic signs that are important. This is why sequential monitoring of the neurologic system becomes the most important factor in assessing these patients. The clinical pattern of a patient receiving head trauma severe enough to cause concussion, having a lucid interval and then relapsing into unconsciousness has been established in past medical communications as a classic history. This is uncommon.

TABLE 13-III

NEUROLOGICAL EXAMINATION RECORD

Instructions: Record vital signs in Unit I. If the patient can talk, check (x) one subdivision in Units II, III, and IV. An orientated patient should know his name, age, etc. A moan can be checked as "garbled" speech. If unable to talk, check "none" in Unit III and one block in Unit V. In an "inappropriate" response the patient is not effective in removing the painful stimulus; when "decerebrate," the extremities reflexly extend and/or hyperpronate. In Unit VI, draw the size and shape of each pupil and (x) for a reaction to light. Under Unit VII, normal strength (4); slight weakness (3); a 5 percent reduction in strength (2); marked weakness and without spontaneous movement (1); total paralysis (o).

UNIT		TIME
I Vital signs	Blood pressure	
	Pulse	
	Respiration	
	Temperature	
II Conscious and	Oriented	
	Disoriented	
	Restless	
	Combative	
III Speech	Clear	
	Rambling	
	Garbled	
	None	
IV Will awaken to	Name	
	Shaking	
	Light pain	
	Strong pain	
V Non-verbal reaction to pain	Appropriate	
	Inappropriate	
	"Decerebrate"	
	None	
VI pupils	Size on right	
	Size on left	
	Reacts on right	
	Reacts on left	
VII Ability to move	Right arm	
	Left arm	
	Right leg	
	Left leg	
	Time:	

Reproduced by permission Bouzarth, W. F.: *J Trauma*, vol. 8, 1968, p. 30.
TIME

Cerebral angiography has played an important role in definitive diagnosis of head injuries. But even the most experienced will readily admit that there are borderline problems; problems solved only by carefully observing the progression of neurologic signs. Depending upon the degree and nature of these neurologic observations, repeat cerebral angiography or craniotomy are done.

The changes in level of consciousness are extremely important in monitoring the patient who has experienced cranio-cerebral trauma. Abnormalities in pupil equality and reaction to light as well as changes in strength of the extremities are additional observations that need to be followed in a sequential fashion. Harvey Cushing[20] promulgated the importance of vital signs in patients with increased intracranial pressure. The Cushing Triad (increased blood pressure, decreased pulse rate and slowing respirations) indicate increased intracranial pressure. As these different appraisals of the patient's condition are observed they should be recorded in a systematic fashion. A "neurologic watch" should be done on every patient who has sustained cranio cerebral trauma. This information can be forwarded to more definitive tertiary case centers and if carefully and clearly done can make a valuable contribution to the patient's overall management. An example of a good neurologic monitoring record that can be utilized for both the initial examination and sequential evaluation is shown in Table 13-III. With adequate instruction paramedical personnel, nurses and medical students can rapidly and accurately contribute to sequential monitoring of these patients.[21]

The last unit (VII) records the strength of the extremities and helps in detection of localizing muscle weakness. This is judged by asking the patient to demonstrate the power of his bicep muscle or hand grip. For the lower extremity, the ability to flex the knee against the examiner's hand or to dorsiflex the foot is usually sufficient. Uncooperative patients are stimulated with pin pricks and an adequate response to pain is graded normal. When there is no response to pain by any movement a zero grade is recorded. In comatose or unconscious patients the response in extremity movement is again listed, although the grading of strength of muscle power is not so accurate as in the conscious cooperative patient.

The signs of increasing intracranial pressure are bradycardia, hypertension, bradypnea, vomiting, headache, restlessness, decreasing level of consciousness and increasing neurologic deficit. When intracerebral pressure has become great enough to produce unilateral herniation of the uncal gyrus decerebrate posturing, motor hemiparesis contralateral to the herniation and ipsilateral oculomotor nerve paresis develops. When a dilated pupil and a hemiparesis are found on the same side of the body the dilated pupil has the greater importance in localizing the herniation. A frequent concomitant of uncal herniation is loss of consciousness.

Lumbar punctures are not routinely done for assessing head injuries. The results are ordinarily not pathognomic of any specific injury. Busch[22] found a correlation with serious head injuries and high cerebrospinal fluid pressure associated with bloody fluid. This correlation may be helpful as to prognosis. Because lumbar punctures offer so little information that can aid in evaluating head injuries, they should not be used in sequential monitoring of the patient.

Although the electroencephalogram is not very helpful as part of the initial evaluation, it can be a very useful sequential monitoring tool. A single electroencephalogram is not pathognomonic of any specific injury but serial electroencephalograms can give a progressive pattern of the development or resolution of focal brain damage. In comatose patients caused by concussion high voltage but slow and irregular activity is present in the delta band in tracings obtained soon after injury. As consciousness returns the alpha rhythm reappears. Over epidural or subdural hematomas either a delta wave focus or a focal reduction in the amplitude of all potentials is present.[23]

When available echoencephalography is helpful in detecting shifts of midline structures of the brain. In experienced hands the accuracy of echoencephalography approaches that of cerebral angiography. It is a noninvasive technic and can be effectively utilized on a sequential basis with no risk to the patients.

Some authorities advocate direct and continuous monitoring of intracranial pressure. Vries and associates[24] have developed a special subarachnoid screw for monitoring intracranial pressures. These procedures require skilled specialists and are not always available in every situation.

RENAL FUNCTION MONITORING

Monitoring the hourly urine output is basic in each critically injured patient. If the kidneys have responded to initial volume repletion by producing 30 to 50 ml per hour, then suddenly the urine output falls to 10 ml/hr or less, there is almost certainly undetected hemorrhage somewhere. Cardiac decompensation can have the same effect on the formation of urine but there are generally additional signs of reduced cardiac output such as high right atrial pressure, tachycardia dyspnea, "stiff lungs" and difficult respirations.

Detection of the more critically injured patient early after injury can be accomplished by serial evaluation of the renal metabolism of urea or sodium. As described in earlier chapters, the kidneys reflect changes in renal plasma flow quickly. This in turn is reflected in glomeular filtration rate and urine formation, when urine flow is adequate. The team captain can feel confident that the brain, heart, lungs and liver are perfused (unless there are defects in the arteries supplying these organs). Contrawise if hourly urine output is less than 10 ml/hr he can be assured that major organ failure will follow shortly.

Urine output as low as 400 ml/24 hrs requires active investigation. It is usually due to one of three causes: dehydration, renal failure or low renal plasma flow. Renal plasma flow is increased by repletion of blood volume, control of hemorrhage and improved cardiac output. Dehydration can be evaluated by giving a test infusion of 5 percent Dextrose in water rapidly. After 500 to 1,000 ml are infused the hourly urine output should increase, if on the other hand the oliguria is due to renal insufficiency the hourly urine output will increase only minimally if at all. If renal insufficiency is the cause of oliguria the urine sodium will be less than 15 meq/L and the urine urea and blood urea ratio is less than 14:1; while the urine to plasma osmolality ratio is less than 1.5.

An entire spectrum of secondary renal injury may be present after severe trauma. It can vary from oliguric renal failure to transient depression of glomerular filtration and tubular function to high output renal failure.

The diagnosis of renal failure is generally first suspicioned by reduction in the hourly urine output followed by chemical evidence of azotemia. A variant of renal insufficiency has been observed after burns, head injury and soft tissue trauma. These patients are characterized by normal or increased urine volumes but increasing retention of urea nitrogen. The clinical course of these patients has been shown to be qualitatively the same as that in oliguric renal insufficiency. Quantitatively, however, these patients retain a limited ability to excrete products of metabolism, potassium and urea. This particular variant of renal insufficiency of itself did not cause death in one major series of patients.[25]

A mild metabolic acidosis occurs. This can be controlled by using sodium lactate infusions to restore extracellular fluid volumes and sustain serum sodium concentrations. The normal or high daily outputs of urine allow administration of large quantities of water. Blood Urea Nitrogen, Serum electrolytes, urine specific gravity and when available urine and serum osmolality should be sequentially monitored. The chief dangers of high output renal failure are: (1) failure to detect the existence of the renal insufficiency. The normal output of urine is misleading. (2) the repeated administration of potassium salts intravenously. Five of nine patients reported by Shires and associates required therapy for hyperkalemia. Both these pitfalls can be avoided by careful sequential monitoring of renal function after trauma. The serum level of potassium should be determined daily after trauma in addition to blood and urine urea nitrogen.

Most available evidence suggest that high output renal failure represents the renal response to a less severe or modified episode of renal injury than that required to produce classic oliguric renal insufficiency.

HEPATIC MONITORING

The complexity of hepatic function makes it impossible to discuss all the various methods of evaluating hepatic function. We have already dealt with the bilirubinemia and hyperenzymnemia in a diagnostic role of detecting hepatic contusions not requiring operative intervention. In this section we will limit our discussion to monitoring a few limited aspects of hepatic function which can be done in most hospital laboratories.

Hepatic ischemia causes "glucose dumping." This sudden outpouring of glucose from the liver causes an initial hyperglycemia. This hyperglycemia is misleading because if the cause of hepatic ischemia is undetected and uncorrected glycogen stores are quickly depleted and profound hypoglycemia ensues. The depletion of hepatic glycogen reflects depletion of tissue glycogen and this is usually of such severity that death is the final outcome. A careful monitoring of blood glucose should detect these changes in time to correct both the cause of hepatic ischemia and the "glucose dumping."

Other features of severe hepatic ischemia are hypnatremia, hypotension and profound acidosis. The reader will quickly recognize that such a combination of chemical abnormalities also occurs in "Addisonian Crises." Indeed the syndrome of acute hepatic ischemia mimics an acute Addisonian crisis.

Hepatic ischemia of sufficient degree to produce the above clinical pattern is usually due to reduced portal vein flow or oxygenation. As discussed in the chapter dealing with physiologic concomitants the splanchic blood flow is one of the first to be severely reduced after serious hemorrhaging trauma. Ordinarily a replenishing of blood volume corrects the low flow state in the portal venous system and nothing further is needed. However, in some instances when sequential monitoring of serum sodium, blood glucose, serum pH and blood pressure show significant reductions in all these, additional efforts to improve portal blood flow must be taken. Glucagon which has been shown to improve splanchic blood flow by 100 percent is given in a 5 or 10 mg bolus intravenously and repeated at intervals until there is objective improvement in hepatic function.

The methods of monitoring chronic hepatic insufficiency are so well known to interested students of medical physiology that we will not outline them except to point out that biosynthesis of proteins, lipids, and carbohydrates are severely curtailed as are the excretory and secretory functions of the liver. These can be sequentially monitored by standard laboratory test.

CONCATENATING MONITORING DATA

In an effort to achieve completeness I have discussed the organ systems separately to emphasize the various technics of monitoring that particular system. In the critically injured patient the different organ systems cannot be so neatly divided into separate units. The failure of one organ system influences the function of other systems and their decompensation prevents the initial system from full recovery. This "multiple organ failure" is an important concept in detecting injuries and assessing the efficacy of the treatment initiated.

Early in the management of critically injured patients the most common causes of multiple organ failure is underestimated or undetected hypovolemia producing a low flow state. The sequential monitoring of multiple organs can also reflect continued or concealed blood loss. For example if extracellular fluid deficits and blood losses have been replaced, the pH of the blood, vital signs, urine output and blood gases should approach normal ranges and become reasonably stable. The patient should become mentally alert (in the absence of brain stem contusions). If while monitoring the multiple organ systems hypoxemia, acidosis, hypotension, oliguria develop it is very likely that additional blood loss or extracellular fluid loss from an undetected source is occurring and all the efforts described in the preceeding chapters should be repeated in an effort to discover concealed losses from the vascular space.

By the same reasoning if a stable period in which organ systems seem to be recovering never occurs then it is incumbent upon the evaluating physician to increase the rate and volume of his replacement therapy even though by all calculations his first efforts should have been enough. A persisting arterial acidosis frequently is the first early sign of incomplete volume repletion. I am using the term "volume repletion" to include extracellular deficits as well as actual exsanguination. In isolated injuries to the retroperitoneal duodenum blood loss is minimal and abdominal tenderness is not impressive. After a few hours these patients began to show multiple organ failure due to extracellular fluid sequestration in the retroperitoneal space. This injury frequently is not detected until multiple organ failure from hypovolemia catches the attention of an alert physician who is meticulously monitoring his patient.

A second cause of early organ failure is the presence of devitalized tissue. Sometimes this ischemic tissue is clearly visible such as an ischemic extremity, crushed skeletal muscle, or soft tissue destruction by a shot gun blast. At other times the necrotic tissue may be concealed (segment of dead bowel or devitalized liver inside the peritoneal cavity). Should monitoring data indicate an adequate circulating blood volume and perfusion of most tissue, but a recalcitrant acidosis is present, the team captain must instigate a search for dead or dying tissue.

Whereas hypovolemia is the leading cause of multiple organ failure early in the care of critically injured patients sepsis is the most frequent cause later. The source of sepsis is often an undetected injury somewhere in the gastrointestinal tract or collections of blood, feces, or succus entericus in tissue spaces. Thus progressive hypoxemia, azotemia, oliguria, acidosis, mental confusion point to multiple organ failure and if late in the course of the patient's injury the site of sepsis must be detected by whatever methods necessary. This often means re-exploration of a body cavity that may have already been opened previously. Such a decision is hard to make in an already seriously ill patient. If putting together all the data from sequential monitoring discloses multiple organ failure exploration of indicated body cavities is justified.

Isolated organ failure or decompensation of two closely interrelated systems such as heart and kidneys has a different meaning particularly if other organ system function is acceptable. Assessing the data from sequential monitoring may disclose loss of lung compliance, early moist rales, increased central venous pressure, tachycardia and oliguria. The data point to the heart with failure of "pump mechanics" as the precipitating cause of reduced urine output. In this situation every effort should be made to improve the cardiac output.

By carefully evaluating all the data collected from sequential monitoring it is usually possible to delineate whether multiple organ or isolated organ failure is predominant. This is the true value of sequential monitoring after severe injury.

REFERENCES

1. Swan, H. J. C.; Ganz, W.; Forrester, J., et al.: Catheterization of the heart in man with the use of a flow-directed balloon-tipped catheter. *N Eng J Med, 283*:447-451, 1970.
2. Foote, G. A.; Schabel, S. I., and Hodges, M.: Pulmonary complications of the flow-directed balloon-tipped catheter. *N Eng J Med, 290*: 927-931, 1974.
3. Scott, M. L.; Webre, D. R.; Arens, J. F., et al.: Clinical application of a flow-directed balloon-tipped cardiac catheter. *Am Surg, 38*:690-696, 1972.
4. Bower, E. B.: Choosing a catheter for central venous catheterization. *Surg Clin North Am, 53*:639-647, 1973.
5. Mays, E. T.: A microbiologic investigation of percutaneous central venous catheters. *South Med J, 65*:830-832, 1972.
6. Weakley, S. D., and Mays, E. T.: Percutaneous catheterization of the subclavian vein. *J Ky Med Assoc, 67*:902-906, 1969.
7. Forrester, J. S.; Diamond, G.; McHugh, T. J., and Swan, H. J. C.: Filling pressures in the right and left sides of the heart in acute myocardial infarction. A reappraisal of central-venous pressure monitoring. *N Eng J Med, 285*:190, 1971.
8. Weil, M. H.; Shubin, H., and Rosoff, L.: Fluid repletion in circulatory shock. *JAMA, 192*:669-674, 1965.
9. Fowler, N. O.; Westcott, R. N., and Scott, R. C.: Normal pressures in the right heart and pulmonary artery. *Am Heart J, 46*:264-267, 1953.
10. Guyton, A. C.: *Circulatory Physiology.* Philadelphia, W. B. Saunders Co., 1963.
11. Longerbeam, J. K.; Vannix, R.; Wagner, W., et al.: Venous pressure monitoring. *Am J Surg, 110*:220, 1965.
12. Gowen, G. F.: Interpretation of central venous pressure. *Surg Clin North Am, 53*:649-651, 1973.

13. Prout, W. G.: Relative value of central venous pressure monitoring and blood-volume measurement in management of shock. *Lancet, 1*:611, 1968.

14. Wilson, J. N.: Rational approach to management of clinical shock. *Arch Surg, 91*:92, 1965.

15. Federation Proceedings, Report. *Fed. Proc., 9*:602-605, 1950.

16. Boyd, D. R.: Monitoring patients with posttraumatic insufficiency. *Surg Clin North Am, 52*:31-46, 1972.

17. Comroe, J. H.; Forster, R. E.; Dubois, A. B., et al.: *The Lung: Clinical Physiology and Pulmonary Function Tests.* Chicago, Year Book Med. Publ., 1965.

18. Wilson, R. F.; Suncion, Z.; Carrasquilla, C.. and Lucas, C.: Respiratory failure in clinical shock and trauma. In: Zuidema, G. D., and Skinner, D. B. (Eds.): Current topics in surgical research. New York, Academic Press, Vol. 1, 1969, pp. 361-374.

19. Proctor, H. J.; Ballantine, T. V. N., and Broussard, N. D.: An analysis of pulmonary function following non thoracic trauma, with recommendations for therapy. *Am Surg, 172*:180-189, 1970.

20. Cushing, H.: Some experimental and clinical observations concerning states of increased intracranial tension. *Am J Med Sci, 124*:375-400, 1902.

21. Bouzarth, W. F.: Neurosurgical watch sheet for craniocerebral trauma. *J Trauma, 8*:29-31, 1968.

22. Busch, E. A. V.: Brain stem contusions: Differential diagnosis, therapy and progrions. *Clin Neurosurg, 9*:18, 1963.

23. Jasper, H.; Kershman, J., and Elvidey, A.: Electroencephalography in head injury in "Trauma of the Central Nervous System" Res. Publ. *Assoc Nerv Ment Dis, 24*:388, 1945.

24. Vries, J. K.; Becker, D. P., and Young, H. F.: A subarachnoid screw for monitoring intracranial pressure. *J Neurosurg, 39*:416-418, 1973.

25. Shires, G. T.; Carrico, C. J., and Carrizaro, P. C.: *Shock.* Philadelphia, W. B. Saunders.

CHAPTER 14

EVALUATION BY ANGIOGRAPHY

T HE DEVELOPMENT OF improved contrast material and catheters for selectively cannulating the vascular system have made angiology clinically applicable in critically injured patients. Some early critics raised the question as to whether it would delay definitive surgery and adversely influence the patient's recovery. Just the opposite proved to be true. Frequently the information obtained from angiography has hastened the decision of the responsible surgeon to operate.

Although Rich and his associates[1] found pre-operative angiography of little value in combat zones it is proving to be of inestimable value in civilian experience. Some very obvious facts reconcile these differences. Civilian trauma has many closed injuries in which blunt injury to vessels is entirely unexpected. When the wounding forces produce a penetrating wound in civilian life it is usually made by a very low velocity missile compared to the high velocity penetrating wounds of military trauma.

The effective use of angiography in evaluating injured patients is again dependent upon the team approach. The angiologist is a valuable and active member of the team. He is consulted in the same manner as the orthopedist, neurosurgeon or plastic surgeon. Any hospital that seriously intends to receive and treat critically injured patients must provide twenty-four angiographic capability. If the hospital governing board feels such extensive service is unreasonable or beyond their economic planning, they should inform the appropriate emergency medical transport systems in their region not to bring these seriously injured patients to their hospital.

Since angiography is a newly developing science a considerable discussion of technic is appropriate before proceeding to definitive kinds of injuries where angiography is most helpful.

CATHETERS

Catheters are generally of two (2) types: catheters used for midstream study and catheters used for selective work. Midstream catheters are teflon and range in size from French 4 —French 8. The selective catheters are of two types primarily the blue polyurothane catheters ranging also in size from French 4—French 8 and the polyethylene catheters. The polyurothane catheters have excellent memory and torque control primarily because of the fine wire that is woven within the catheter material. The polyurothane catheters must use a teflon coated guidewire to avoid scratching the inner surface of the catheter. These catheters, although having a superior memory, cannot be reformed at the table because of the stability of the catheter material. The polyethylene catheter material is the green, red, yellow, these catheters have less torque control and a poor memory, however these can be reformed during the procedure. The polyethylene catheters can utilize either teflon or stainless steel guide. If the softer selective catheter is used prior to the midstream teflon catheter, the vessel dilator will probably be necessary. Inserting the midstream catheter is rarely a problem. Catheters are always inserted with the finger tips at the most distal end of the catheter and the catheter is pushed into the artery with a screw type of motion. A general rule is that the largest possible guidewire should be used to fit the catheter to avoid the possibility of coring the artery.

Selective catheters used to follow the midstream catheter must be of the same French size or larger. If a smaller selective catheter is utilized, there will be an unacceptable amount of leakage around the selective catheter at the femoral puncture site. Always use the smallest possible catheter that will perform a given study allowing injection of an adequate amount of contrast material in a short enough period of time. If a large catheter, particular #8F catheter is utilized, it is wise to monitor the pulse distal to the catheter site to avoid complete occlusion of the artery. If there appears to be a significant diminution in the arterial pulse following the use of the catheter, the catheter should be withdrawn to the level of the iliacs and a hand injection made at fluoroscopy. If there appears to be a great deal of spasm as if the catheter is essentially occluding the artery, interarterial Xylocaine® up to 10 to 15 cc's may be of value. In unusual circumstances a vasodilator such as Priscoline®, 25 mg can be utilized. While Xylocaine can be used with relatively little systemic affect in the artery, Priscoline does have a cardiac affect which must be taken into consideration. Xylocaine given into the venous circulation has a significant cardiac affect!

Injection rates of the midstream catheters: for a #4 French catheter, approximately 8 to 10 cc's per second, for a #5, approximately 10 to 14 cc's per second, for a #6, approximately 15 to 18 cc's per second, a #7 short can take an injection rate up to 30 cc's per second, the long #7 catheters, approximately 22 to 24 cc's per second, the long #8 catheters, 30 cc's per second. In the #7 and #8 catheter, the injection rates are governed to a significant extent by the ability of the clear connector to withstand the pressure. The connector should be examined particularly at the base where it has a tendency to bend and become weak and this is usually the point of blowout. It is unlikely that the Viamonte Injector will allow a catheter to be disrupted inside the patient as the Viamonte itself is programmed to discontinue injecting at a pressure of 1,200 PSI. Always examine the catheter tip and the catheter itself prior to insertion. A catheter tip will sometimes become bent and conceivably could break off inside the patient and embolize.

Injection rates for selective catheters are not a problem as far as the total contrast that the catheter can withstand. The governing factor with injection of the selective catheters is the position of the catheter in the selective vessel and how much the catheter will accept prior to being displaced from the vessel. A feel for this can be obtained while injecting at fluoroscopy.

GUIDEWIRES

Guidewires are available in both teflon and stainless steel varieties in sizes ranging from .025-.032, .035, .038 and .045. As mentioned above the general rule is the largest possible guidewire to fit the catheter. There are three varieties of the teflon guidewire; there is a movable core "J" which is the guidewire of choice in patients with severe atherosclerotic disease, as the floppy tip can be varied in length to provide maximum flexibility. This will enable you to navigate through severe arterial plaquing that is dangerous with other forms of guidewires. The straight teflon guidewire is more limited in its usefulness. The straight guidewire can be used in young people where the possibility of hooking the tip under a plaque is not a significant danger. This guidewire can also be used for catheter exchange as it has less of a tendency to go out the side holes of the catheter than some of the "J" shape wires. The straight teflon wire can also be used in children. A third variety of the teflon wire is the fixed "J." This is a teflon wire that has a curve tip but does not have a movable core. This is a relatively safe wire although it does not have the versatility of the movable core "J" and that the latter has a variable floppy tip. All stainless steel wires have "J" shapes. There is generally no indication for using a straight stainless steel wire. The stainless steel can be used in most young and middle aged patients. Occasionally in the older age group the lack of the movable core and inability to vary the floppy tip may make the "J" teflon a superior guidewire.

Prior to beginning the examination, you should always see that the guidewires, needles and catheters are compatible with each other in regard to size with snug fitting guidewire and catheter.

NEEDLES

A variety of needle types are available. The general needle used for adult patients is the four part teflon sleeve needle. This needle allows the seating of a teflon sleeve and assures the needle is positioned well inside the lumen of the vessel. The teflon sleeve can also be used for injections in femoral studies. This is an 18 gauge needle that is also available in 20 gauge pediatric needle with a three part assembly. The axillary needle is a four part teflon sleeve needle but is 2.5 inches as opposed to the longer 4 inch femoral needle. The needle should be examined prior to usage to insure that the teflon sleeve does not project beyond the needle tip and that the tip is not unduly damaged by previous use. Another needle that is available is the pencil point which is sharper and smaller in external diameter than the teflon sleeve needle and is particularly of value in infants. The sharper needles may be of value in arteries that are heavily plaqued as the broader teflon sleeve needle has more of a tendency to roll off the vessel particularly when it becomes dull by usage. The disadvantage of a pencil point is that you may have to utilize smaller guidewires and gradually workup to a larger guidewire-catheter combination. The Seldinger needle is a four part metal cannula needle that is widely used in angiography. A needle that has been utilized recently is the disposable Cournand needle which is of particular value in arteries that are heavily plaqued. This needle has an extremely sharp point and is a smaller external diameter than the teflon needle; it is an 18 gauge thin wall needle. Finally, there is a special translumbar needle consisting of a long teflon sheath needle and a specially designed safety trans-lumbar guidewire.

In puncturing the femoral artery the usual landmark is to palpate the anterosuperior iliac spine and the pubic symphysis as this delineates the inguinal ligament. Usually two fingers below the inguinal ligament is the spot to make the skin nick. The needle is then directed in an angle of 30 to 45 degrees and the artery entered through both walls. The needle is withdrawn and following good pulsatile flow the teflon sleeve is advanced for several millimeters into the lumen of the artery. The blunt obturator is placed in the teflon sleeve and with a very minimal amount of pressure the needle is seated to the hub. At that point the blunt obturator is removed and there should be excellent arterial flow. If at any time there is not satisfactory arterial flow, the needle is malpositioned and the guidewire will not enter the vessel lumen. It is important initially to take the time to locate the proper position to make the needle puncture. Never do the percutaneous puncture of the artery too high. This makes compression of the artery difficult or impossible. If the needle stick is made too low in the superficial femoral artery or the profunda femoral artery, there will be much difficulty inserting the guidewire. If the needle cannot be seated properly and good arterial flow is not obtained, it is easier to withdraw the needle, compress the artery four to five minutes and begin again. As long as a hematoma is not formed in the groin, the artery can be entered several times without difficulty.

Attention should be paid to the groin during the entire procedure to insure that no hematoma is formed. Particular attention has to be paid to the groin during exchange of catheters. In general the number of catheter exchanges should be kept to the minimum that enables a good diagnostic study. Many complications are related to hematoma formation and excessive hematomas should be avoided.

At the termination of the procedure attention is paid to compressing the artery. This is the most significant aspect of the entire case. The distal pulses should be examined at this time to insure that the artery is not occluded. When necessary, interarterial Xylocaine and/or fluoroscopic observation of the iliofemoral system is recommended. The catheter is withdrawn with two fingers placed on the artery above the punctured site. The compression should done with a gloved hand and not with gauze sponges. The artery must be held for a minimum of ten minutes; with hypertensive patients it should be compressed a minimum of fifteen to twenty minutes. Initially the peripheral pulse should be nearly or completely obliterated. During the remainder of time only the systolic thrust should be dampened since it is conceivable a vessel could be thrombosed from too diligent compression. Following a ten to fifteen minute interval, pressure should be gradually released and the groin observed to assure that there is no continued bleeding. The groin is uncovered and the patient should remain in the vascular room under constant observation for the next ten to fifteen minutes. The patient should always be examined following his removal to the stretcher as this may cause rebleeding in the groin. The patient must also be seen on the afternoon of the study to re-evaluate the groin for possible bleeding and to determine that the peripheral pulses have not diminished in intensity since the angiography.

CONTRAST MATERIAL

Renografin®, 76 and 60 percent, is high in methylglucamine and low in sodium. Pure methylglucamine contrast agents can be utilized. The exception is angiography of the ascending aorta. Here the injection of pure methylglucamine salts can produce arrhythmias if injected into the coronary arteries. Seventy-six percent Renografin is used for all midstream studies. Sixty percent Renografin is used for selective work and always in the carotid system. For studies in the subclavian vessels, a 60 percent solution is generally utilized. Selective innominate injections can utilize either 60 or 76 percent solutions. The renal artery will also accept either 60 or 76 percent solution. If a large volume of 76 percent Renografin is injected into a relatively small vessel such as the renal artery, it should be thoroughly flushed with heparinized saline following the injection. If one is in doubt about injecting excessive volume of high percentage contrast material into a particular organ, the organ should be examined at fluoroscopy. When a persistent effect is present, the vessel should be thoroughly irrigated with heparinized saline. A general note on irrigation is that the selective catheters, particularly those with side holes, should be watched carefully and irrigated frequently. The side holes have a greater tendency to form thrombi. A general rule in the carotid system is that the catheter should be irrigated as necessary but not excessively. If catheter placement was done without difficulty, an additional safety factor is to withdraw the catheter into the midstream aorta for flushing.

There is always a danger of injecting either a bubble or foreign material into the carotid system particularly when a closed system is not utilized. A closed system is preferable.

There are multiple articles on the toxic facts of contrast media. In general the minimal amount of contrast material possible to provide a diagnostic study is used. A general rule is approximately 2 cc of contrast material per pound total. The patient should have good renal function and must be *well hydrated*. Total contrast injected into the head should be kept to an absolute minimum and several minutes should elapse between injections.

CONING AND TECHNIQUE

Scout films should be examined prior to injection and any changes at technique should be decided upon. A constant rule in filming is the tightest possible coning, particularly on selective and subselective studies. Coning is of particular value in selective work, however care must be taken not to cone excessively.

HEAD AND NECK

Aortic arch study constitutes a large percentage of examinations for trauma. The routine arch study can be done as part of an evaluation of the carotid vessels. It consists of a right posterior oblique position with the patient turned approximately 35 to 40 degrees. Usually the #8F catheter is utilized as a large bolus of contrast material is highly desirable in the ascending aorta. This consists of a total 30 cc injection for 1.8 to 2 seconds. The patient is positioned so that the bottom of the film contains the top of the aortic arch and the origins of the great vessel and the top of the film includes the base of the skull. The primary interest of course is in the area of the carotid bifurcation and this may require either multiple oblique views or combination of a standard right posterior oblique and selective injections. Film sequence in the carotid system is three per second for two seconds, two per second for two seconds and 1 per second for four or five seconds, or if the technique is such that filming cannot be carried out at three films per second, two per second for three seconds, one per second for three seconds and every other for three to four seconds. It is desirable to obtain the three films per second if the technique allows this in the carotid system.

It is not uncommon that the carotids cannot be evaluated

adequately in the oblique projection and a selective study is indicated. The most commonly used catheter is the headhunter or Hincks catheter. The latter comes in 7 and 8 French sizes and the size selected depends on the arch catheter that was utilized. Generally, this will require an 8 catheter. The selective headhunter catheter is an end hole only catheter and comes in a variety of configurations. The Hincks #1 is utilized in a great majority of cases. This catheter should be inserted to the ascending aorta and then torqued into the selective vessel of interest. The catheter should be positioned in the mid common carotid so that an injection rate of approximately 5 to 10 cc per second will not cause the catheter to be whipped back into the aorta. Injection rates in the head of the Hincks catheter vary from 5 ml per second for 2 seconds, to 10 ml per second for 1.2 seconds. Approximately 10 ml of total contrast material (60%) is injected. Injection rate will depend on the catheter position and the apparent stability of the catheter. A special technique is necessary when the left carotid originates from the base of the innominate artery. This occurs in 15 to 30 percent of all cases.

Filming in the head consists of two films per second for three seconds and one every other second for three or four seconds. The selective injection consist of an AP study of the head and a lateral view with the latter including the head and neck. These bi-plane studies with films alternately loaded give good results.

Selective subclavian studies are not infrequent. Again the #7 and #8 headhunter catheter is utilized. The catheter is usually positioned just distal to the vertebral artery and 60 percent Renografin is the contrast material of choice. A primary consideration in this study is to be sure that the catheter is not in the vertebral artery. After pressure injection, the catheter sometimes whips into the vertebral artery. The patient should be examined fluoroscopically after injections to determine catheter location. There will be some reflux into the vertebral from the injections, but the total volume will be acceptable. Thyrocervical trunk injections and internal mammary studies can also be done with the same Hincks catheter. An arch study may be indicated prior to selective work in the subclavians. In the subclavian an injection rate of 5 to 6 cc per second for two to three seconds is usually adequate. Filming can be done at two films per second generally and need not be carried out for a long period of time.

Chest

Thoracic Aortograms are performed with centering over the chest to see the entire thoracic aorta and the origins of the great vessels. Again, a 7 or 8 French teflon catheter can be utilized. The catheter should be positioned close to the aortic valves particularly for post traumatic transections to insure the competency of the valves and lack of involvement of the coronary arteries (see Chapter 5). The catheter position is different than in an arch study. For the latter a catheter is positioned with the tip just proximal to the innominate artery. Filming for transection of the aorta is usually done in the lateral and right posterior oblique positions with the latter view unfolding the thoracic aorta.

Pulmonary Angiography

These studies are done with a #7 and a #8 NIH catheter. There is a right angle bend at the tip and a side hole only catheter. There is no end hole in the NIH catheter, therefore the catheter must be inserted through a myelar sheath percutaneously or through a venous cutdown. The same catheter that is used for injection in the main pulmonary artery is utilized for selective injections. Injection rates are about 25 to 30 cc of Renografin 76 for 2.5 sec in the main pulmonary artery and 25 to 30 cc for 1.5 sec in the selective vessels. Filming is carried out over approximately sixteen to twenty seconds with the initial film at three films per second. An EKG monitor must be utilized with all pulmonary angiography and any work above the diaphragm where the patient has a significant cardiac problem.

Abdominal Studies

Midstream abdominal studies are generally done with a short 7 F teflon catheter with multiple side holes. Injection rates are usually 25 cc for 2 to 2.5 seconds the catheter is positioned about T12 to insure filling of all branches including the celiac axis. If the study is primarily done for the renal arteries, then the centering is somewhat lower with the side holes opposite the renal arteries. Filming of the abdomen is generally two films per second for three seconds and one per second for three seconds, then every other second for three to four seconds. Delays are not necessary in midstream work since it is unusual to see a significant venous phase. If the study is done primarily for the renal arteries, then take three films per second in order to see the origin of the renal arteries prior to filling of the remainder of the vessels of the abdominal aorta.

Selective Celiac Study

A variety of catheters are available for catheterizing the celiac trunk. Generally these are end hole catheters although in some instances the side hole catheter may be superior. The most utilized catheter is the #7 yellow Squibb catheter or the #7 Ducor cobra catheter. There is also visceral shape catheter that we perform prior to examination; this is a green polyethylene catheter material. The advantage of the Squibb catheter is that it seats well and will usually accept the desired rate of 8 to 12 cc per second, without being displaced from the artery. The cobra or the visceral catheters are used for supra-selective studies in that this catheter can be advanced into the splenic or hepatic. The stiffer Squibb catheter cannot be advanced beyond the celiac axis. Total volume of contrast material injected into the celiac axis is usually 50 cc. There are instances for portography workups when a larger amount of contrast material is required. This is usually optimally injected into the splenic artery itself. Filming is usually two films per second for three seconds, one per second for three seconds and every other for eight to ten seconds. Usually in the range of twenty to thirty seconds is required to insure visualization of the venous phase and to evaluate the flow into the portal system and of filling of collateral veins. On occasion catheterization of the celiac axis may be difficult and stable catheter position may not be possible. In this instance, a lower injection rate of perhaps 6 to 8 cc per second for a longer period of time may give a diagnostic study.

Superior Mesenteric

Usually any catheter will be adequate for the superior mesenteric artery. Injection rates here are usually 30 to 50 cc total of Renografin 76. Renografin 76 can be used for all the major aortic branches. Film sequence is the same as for the celiac.

Inferior Mesenteric

The vessel is highly variable in size and often not well seen on the midstream study. A simple acute angle bend catheter is the configuration of choice. Injection volumes will lie in the 12 to 20 cc range. Film sequence is shorter than the celiac or superior mesenteric artery.

Splenic

As mentioned the preferred catheter for the selective catheterization of the splenic artery is the Ducor cobra catheter. Primary indications for selective splenic catheterization are in patients with suspected splenic trauma. Unsually in cases of splenic trauma, a volume of 30 to 50 cc will be quite adequate. In case of trauma to the spleen, oblique views may frequently be of advantage. Another indication for selective splenic angiography is in evaluating the pancreas for more concentrated filling of the pancreatic vessels arising from the splenic artery.

Hepatic Studies

The common hepatic injections are done when evaluating the liver and for looking in detail at the head of the pancreas. Usually 20 to 30 cc of contrast material is injected. The catheter may be positioned selectively in the gastroduodenal artery to visualize the head of the pancreas. Also, it is occasionally possible to selectively catheterize the dorsal pancreatic vessel. This latter vessel may arise either from the hepatic or more commonly from the splenic artery. Generally, the gastroduodenal artery will take 8 to 16 cc total contrast material and the dorsopancreatic 6 to 12 cc total. Some feel for the required volume of contrast material or how much the vessel will take without the catheter being displaced can be obtained during the fluoroscopic injection.

Renal Study

Three catheters are used primarily for studying the renal artery. The yellow #7 Squibb catheter, the cobra catheter and the double curve Ducor catheter. Squibb now makes the cobra type catheter and the torcon catheter also comes in the cobra configuration. Either an end hole catheter or a side hole catheter is acceptable. If reflux into the aorta is desirable to see the origin of the renal artery, the side hole is of value. With the end hole catheter, it is easy to place the catheter beyond early bifurcating branches or beyond the origin of the inferior adrenal artery. The selection of the Squibb versus the cobra or double curve Ducor is based on the angle at which the renal artery originates from the aorta. Generally, the Squibb catheter is quite satisfactory and the position is quite stable during injection. The renal artery will take approximately 5 cc per second for two seconds with a single renal artery present. If there are several renal arteries, injection rate is reduced in each vessel. Again, the renal artery should be noted on the midstream study and if stenotic, should not be selectively catheterized. *No significantly stenosed artery should be selectively catheterized.*

Filming is usually at two per second for three seconds, one per second for three seconds and every other for four. One likes to see the renal vein and this usually takes from nine to fourteen seconds. Again if the possibility of an A-V fistula exists, film speed is more rapid.

Aorto-Iliofemoral Studies

The usual study is performed with the femoral percutaneous approach utilizing a #5 or #6 French teflon catheter with multiple side holes. Injection rates are usually 10 to 12 cc per second for four to five seconds. Film sequence is usually at three, six, nine, twelve and eighteen seconds. A more delayed film may be necessary if there is a significant block and delayed reconstitution. This is done on a 51 inch cassette with a long leg changer. The usual contrast material used is 76 percent Renografin, although this procedure can be done with 60 percent Renografin with less pain to the patient. The catheter is positioned with the tip above the aortic bifurcation.

If a unilateral study of the femoral artery is indicated, then a teflon sleeve needle can be utilized. Another alternative in the selective injection of one side is to use the contralateral femoral artery and hook a catheter over the iliac bifurcation.

When aortic rupture or thrombosis is suspected the trans-axillary approach is used. This utilizes a 2.5 inch teflon axillary needle with the "J" teflon safety movable core guidewire. A #6 long catheter is used. The difficulty in transaxillary study is primarily in getting the guidewire down the descending aorta. This may require the use of a selective catheter to turn the guide to the descending aorta and then replacing this with a long midstream teflon catheter. A defector system has also been utilized in this approach. The radial pulse should be monitored during the axillary study and particular attention must be paid to the axilla with regard to compression at the end of the study. It is possible to obtain a large hematoma in the axilla that is not immediately apparent. Whereas Xylocaine can be used with relative impunity in the femoral artery, complications have been described utilizing Xylocaine in the axillary artery. There may be situations when the configuration of the aorta is such that the innominate arises relatively high on the arch and there is generally straight shot across from the innominate to the descending aorta. However, negotiating the guidewire down the descending aorta is easier from the left side.

Finally, the translumbar approach is the last alterative in defining the distal aorta and runoff. The special translumbar needle and guidewire are utilized for this purpose. Injection rate through the teflon sleeve is again approximately 40 to 50 cc total. Filming is at the same rate. Preferably the teflon sleeve can be directed downstream in the translumbar study so as not to fill primarily the celiac, mesenteric and renal vessels.

Inferior Vena Cavography

This can generally be done with the sleeve or catheter in the femoral vein or in the iliac vein or the low inferior vena cava. On occasion teflon sleeves can be placed in both femoral veins and the inferior vena cavogram obtained without the artifact of nonopacified blood coming from the opposite iliac system.

Superior Vena Cavography

Superior vena cava injections can usually be satisfactorily performed by placing a large bore needle in both antecubital veins and injecting approximately 50 cc of contrast material on each side. If this produces too much artifact from nonopacifying blood flowing into the system, a catheter can be selectively placed from the arm as in doing a pulmonary angiogram.

CEREBRAL ANGIOGRAPHY

The problems in differentiating intracranial hematomas has been discussed in Chapter 7. Unless the patient's condition is deteriorating so rapidly that craniotomy must be done without delay cerebral angiography offers the most reliable method of evaluating for intracranial space consuming lesions. Clark and Grossman[2] recommended the following criteria for timing and selection of cases for cerebral angiography:

1. Focal Neurologic Deficits: These patients are usually unconscious with either a hemiparesis or evidence of herniation of the uncal gyrus. In this group of patients cerebral angiography is done on admission to the hospital.

2. Decerebrate Posturing: In this group of patients the localizing signs of cerebral hemisphere compression have been completely replaced by the signs of brain stem compression. Cerebral angiography is done on admission to delineate the cause of the compression.

3. Unconscious Patients: This group has no focal or lateralizing neurologic signs. Cerebral angiography is done three to five days after admission if the patient shows no improvement in neurologic status.

4. Progressive Neurologic Deficit: These patients should have cerebral angiography at some time during the course of hospitalization.

Normally the cerebral arteries extend out to the inner table of the cranium. Displacement of the cerebral vessels away from the inner table indicates a space occupying lesion between the cerebral arteries and cranial bones (Fig. 14-1). A "bowing" or stretching out of the vessels over the cerebral hemisphere

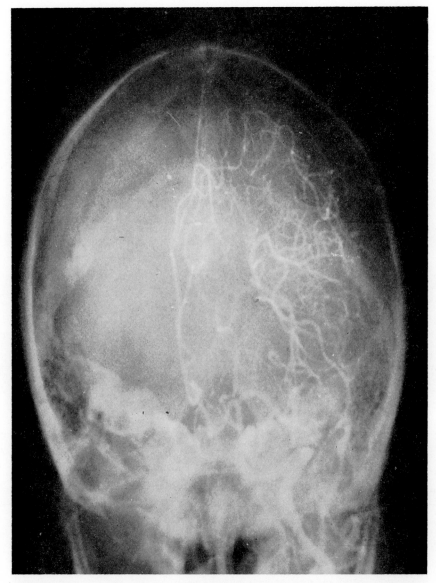

Figure 14-1. Left carotid arteriogram in thirty-year-old lady after a serious head injury. Note space between cerebral arteries and inner table of the skull also displacement of anterior cerebral artery across the midline. Craniotomy relieved the massive subdural hematoma covering the entire left cerebral hemisphere.

suggest intracerebral space consuming lesions. The arteries are pushed outward against the inner table of the skull by the hematoma thus giving the appearance of stretching.

Under duress it is sometimes necessary to do a quick "single shot" cerebral arteriogram. These are often helpful but can be misleading. A bi-plane study is more accurate when time permits.

SPLENIC TRAUMA

Rupture of the spleen after blunt trauma is an easily recognized event in most patients, presenting classic clinical finding (Chapter 6). However, in approximately 15 percent of injuries the diagnosis is doubtful and added dimensions of detecting splenic trauma are necessary. Norell[3] first showed a ruptured spleen could be detected by abdominal aortography in 1957. Freeark and associates[4] confirmed the efficacy of abdominal aortography in blunt trauma and reported its greatest accuracy to be detecting injuries to the spleen.

Villareal-Rio and Mays[5] found radiologic definition of splenic trauma could be enhanced by selective splenic arteriography. Percutaneous retrograde femoral access as described in the preceding section was used in our study. The primary indications for selective splenic arteriography are:

1. Clinical assessment precipitates doubt
2. Craniocerebral trauma with clinical hypovolemia
3. Palpable mass in left upper quadrant
4. Abnormal roentgenograms (plain) of the abdomen
5. Unexplained reduction in hematocrit or hemoglobin concentration

Salient abnormal roentgenographic features of splenic trauma disclosed by selective splenic arteriography are:

1. Disruption of intrasplenic arterial pattern
2. Stretching out or "bowing" of vessels
3. Extravasation of contrast material (Fig. 14-2)
4. Arteriovenous shunting

Ballinger and Ersher[6] reported approximately 15 percent of nonpenetrating injuries of the spleen result in delayed or occult

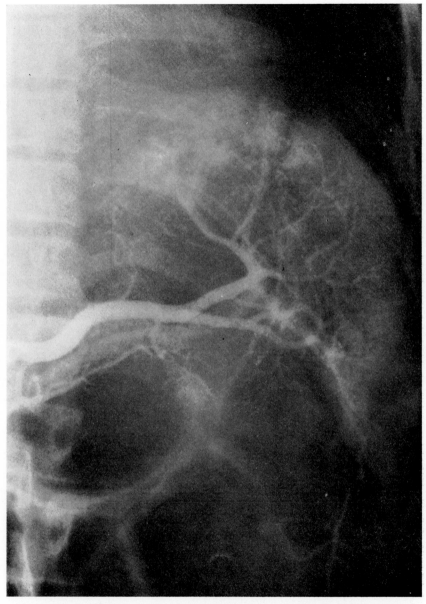

Figure 14-2. Selective splenic arteriogram in a patient who sustained blunt trauma to chest and abdomen shows rupture of splenic pulp with extravasation of contrast material.

splenic rupture. In actuality both delayed and occult rupture are likely due to missed or overlooked splenic trauma which finally manifests itself at a later date. An undetected splenic disruption could organize to form hematomas or pseudocysts which at some later date undergoes secondary hemorrhage and rupture. Such patients are very difficult to manage because they have usually been discharged from the hospital and the initial trauma forgotten. When the secondary problem arises they often are seen by another physician in another hospital or even another city.

Prevention of these two extremely confusing clinical entities makes selective splenic arteriography a very worthwhile procedure to use in evaluating critically injured patients. The absence of false normal or abnormal angiographic patterns make this technic a useful clinical tool with great reliability.

Vascular Injury

Angiography is obviously the most definitive clinical tool for evaluating trauma of the vascular system. As stated in earlier chapters a palpable distal pulse is unreliable when there is strong suspicion of vascular involvement. At one time it was thought that a perforating injury involving an artery or vein was the most treacherous situation possible pertaining to vascular trauma. But gradually we are awakening to the reality that blunt forces produce vascular damage in such an unexpected and insidious manner that most physicians are completely thrown off guard.

One such injury is thrombosis of the abdominal aorta after blunt trauma. A patient encountered at the Louisville General Hospital is briefly reviewed to illustrate the need for increased use of angiography after blunt trauma.

> A sixty-eight-year-old man complained of pain and tenderness in both legs after an automobile accident. Roentgenograms of the extremity failed to show any skeletal injuries. Additional examination disclosed a soft and completely nontender abdomen a normal chest and heart and peripheral pulses.
>
> Because of progressive difficulty in moving his legs neurosurgical consultation was sought. The absence of vertebral fractures on roentgenographic assessment led to the conclusion that this was probably a spinal cord contusion.

A peritoneal lavage returned clear fluid, but because of suspicion of occult intra-abdominal injury a laparotomy was done and nothing abnormal found.

The next day a percutaneous transaxillary aortogram was done because of the unrelenting pain and paralysis of the lower extremities. The aortogram showed complete thrombosis of the terminal abdominal aorta up to but not including the renal arteries. (Fig 14-3a and 14-3b) There was increased collateral circulation with good distal run-off in both lower extremities.

A repeat laparotomy was done and thrombectomy of the terminal aorta achieved. Pain and paralysis subsided; the patient was later discharged to be followed in the outpatient clinic.

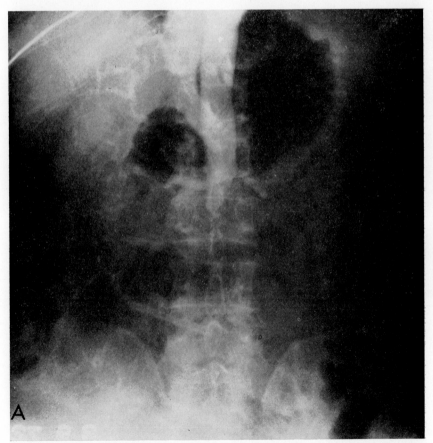

Figure 14-3. Abdominal aortogram in a man who sustained blunt abdominal trauma shows complete thrombosis just below the renal arteries: (a) AP view (b) lateral.

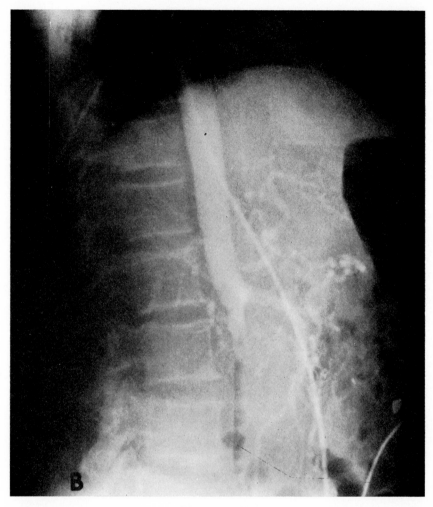

Figure 14-3b.

Thrombosis of the abdominal aorta after blunt trauma is rare but has also been reported by others.[7, 8] Thrombosis of the external iliac artery is reported by Edwards and Lyans.[9] Their patient was a worker struck in the abdomen by a swinging load of steel. Usually the cyanosis, coldness, numbness paralysis and absence of lower extremity pulses alert the physician to problems in the vascular tree But occasionally the findings may be related to spinal cord dysfunction as described in the patient above. In any event, angiography is an invaluable technic for detecting vascular injuries after blunt trauma.

Approximately 95 percent of aortic ruptures are in the thoracic segment and as described in Chapter 5 most of these are just beyond the left subclavian artery at the juncture of the ligamentum arteriosum. If the patient's condition is not rapidly deteriorating an aortagram is extremely helpful in detecting injuries at this point as well as injuries more proximal.

When aortic injury is a possibility, it is wise to use the percutaneous approach through the axillary artery. This gives an antegrade aortogram rather than the retrograde aortogram obtained when using the femoral route.

Angiography is again a valuable clinical means of evaluating the status of renal circulation after blunt trauma. Renal arteries can also be thrombosed by blunt trauma (Figs. 14-5a and 14-5b).

The subclavian artery is only one of many peripheral arteries thrombosed by blunt trauma (Fig. 14-6). Angiography can be useful in delineating the site and extent of the injury as well as detecting the problems. The superficial palmar arch in the hand is particularly suspectible to thrombosis after blunt trauma.[10, 11] Intimal disruption with thrombosis of the arteries can occur in skeletal fractures as well as tears, perforations and avulsions of these vessels. In some fractures assessment of the vascular system takes priority over the evaluation of the fracture itself.

In addition to thrombosis, arteriovenous fistulae, aneurysms and pseudoneurysms result from injury. True aneurysm include all layers of the vessel wall and result from blunt trauma. False aneurysms and arteriovenous fistulae result from undetected or overlooked penetrating trauma. False aneurysms do not include the original vessel wall but consist of a fibrous membrane organized from the hematoma developing around an injured artery as the hematoma communicates with the lumen of the vessel pulsatile flow causes gradually enlargement of the fibrous membrane (Figs. 14-7a and 14-7b).

Arteriovenous fistulae are well delineated by angiography (Fig. 14-8). They are rarely diagnosed until six to eight weeks

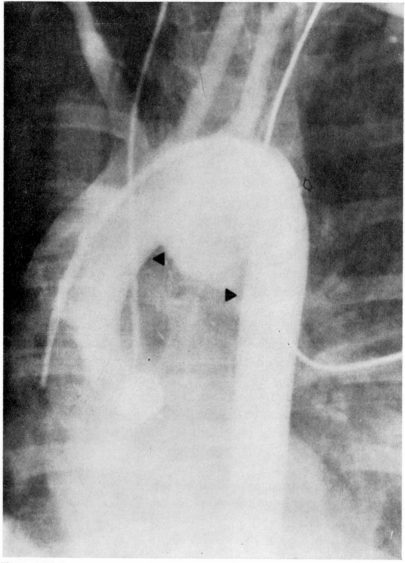

Figure 14-4. Aortogram after blunt thoracic trauma showing rupture at level of ligamentum arteriosum (plain arrow) and extravasation of contrast material into the mediastinal tissue (solid arrows).

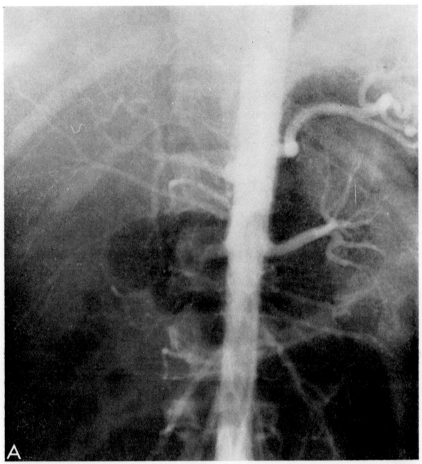

Figure 14-5. Aortogram after blunt abdominal trauma shows thrombosis of right renal artery (a) selective catheterization of the renal artery delineates the intimal tear in the artery which precipitated the thrombosis (b).

after the initial trauma. At that time operative repair can be very difficult. The ultimate goal is detection of vascular defects by angiography at the time of injury and immediate angioplasty to establish normal flow.

Miscellaneous Injuries

Angiography has also been proposed to have merit in detecting ruptured livers,[12] kidneys, pancreas and duodenum.[4] The

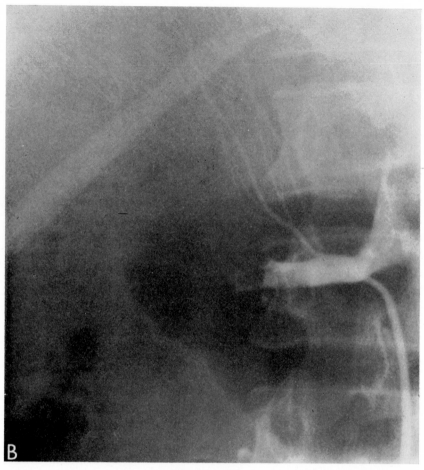

Figure 14-5b.

extremely serious hepatic injuries exsanguate so quickly that I do not believe it is wise to delay laparotomy for any diagnostic tests. The patients are usually in profound shock with massive hemoperitoneums. In patients with stable hemodynamics and questionable liver involvement selective hepatic arteriography can be helpful in detecting the presence of liver injury. Hepatic angiography is particularly helpful in evaluating subcapsular hematomas of the liver and patients who develop hemobilia after hepatic injury.[13] The merit of angiography in abdominal visceral injuries must be determined by additional experience.

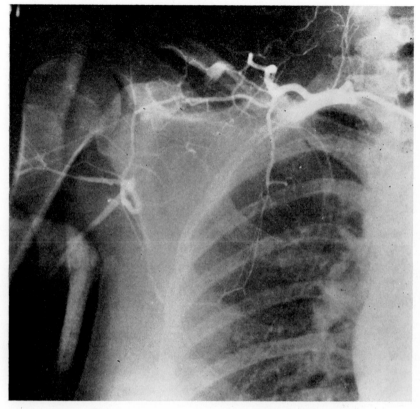

Figure 14-6. Selective arteriogram of the right subclavian artery after blunt trauma which fractured the clavicle shows complete thrombosis of this vessel.

REFERENCES

1. Rich, N. M.: Vascular trauma. *Surg Clin North Am,* 53:1367-1391, 1973.
2. Clark, K., and Grossman, R. G.: Trauma to nervous system. *Care of the Trauma Patient.* New York, McGraw-Hill, p. 273.
3. Norell, H. B.: Traumatic rupture of the spleen diagnosed by abdominal aortography. *Acta Radial,* 48:449, 1957.
4. Freeard, R. J.; Love, L., and Baker, B. J.: The role of angiography in the management of blunt trauma. *J Trauma,* 8:557, 1968.
5. Villarreal-Rios, A., and Mays, E. T.: Efficiacy of clinical evaluation

and selective splenic arteriography in splenic trauma. *Am J Surg,* *127*:310-313, 1974.

6. Ballinger, W. F., and Ersler, A. J.: Splenectomy: indications, technic and complications. *Curr Probl Surg,* 1965, p. 1051.
7. Walker, A. G., and Walker, R. M.: Traumatic thrombosis of the aorta. *Br Med J, 1*:1514, 1961.
8. Borja, A. R., and Lansing, A. M.: Thrombosis of the abdominal aorta caused by blunt trauma. *J Trauma, 10*:499, 1970.
9. Edwards, W. S., and Lyon, C.: Traumatic arterial spasm and thrombosis. *Ann Surg, 140*:318-323, 1954.
10. Kleinert, H. E., and Volianitis, G. J.: Thrombosis of the palmar arterial arch and its tributaries. Etiology and newer concepts in treatment. *J Trauma, 5*:447-455, 1965.
11. Mays, E .T.: Traumatic aneurysm of the hand. *Am J Surg, 36*:552-557, 1970.
12. Boijsen, E.; Judkins, M. P., and Simay, A.: Angiographic diagnosis of hepatic rupture. *Radiology. 86*:66-72, 1966.
13. Gundersen, A. E., and Green, R. M.: Traumatic hemiobilia: accurate pre-operative diagnosis by hepatic artery angiogram. *Surgery, 62*: 862-864, 1967.

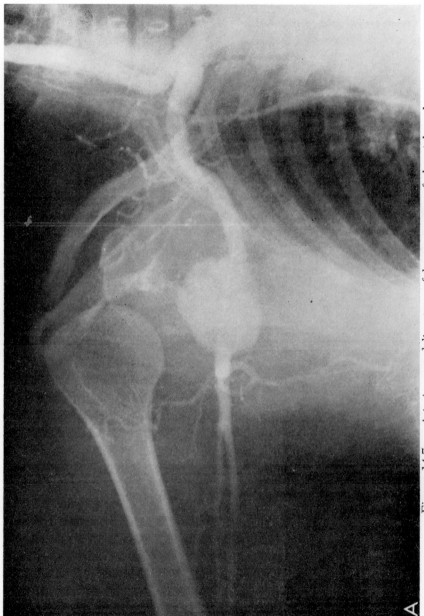

Figure 14-7a. Arteriogram delineates a false aneurysm of the right subclavian artery ten days after the patient was shot with a .38 cal. revolver.

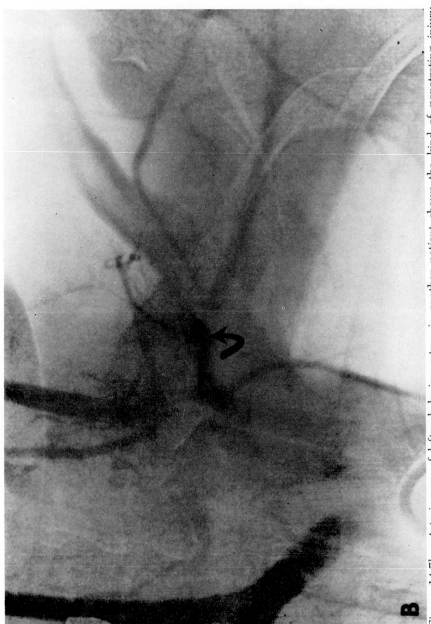

Figure 14-7b. Arteriogram of left subclavian artery in another patient shows the kind of penetrating injury (arrow) leading to later development of false aneurysm. The anteriogram was done at the time of admission and the artery repaired thus preventing the late complication illustrated in Fig. 14-7a.

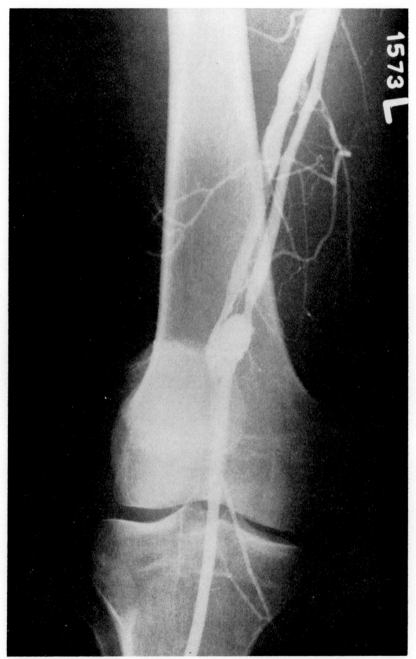

Figure 14-8. After a gunshot wound of the leg this arteriogram of the popliteal artery showed immediate filling of the popliteal vein through a large arteriovenous communication.

────────────────────────────────

CHAPTER 15

PSYCHOLOGICAL ASSESSMENT

────────────────────────────────

INDIVIDUALS REACT DIFFERENTLY to external stress. The critically injured patient is hurled into the operating room or accident ward unconscious or against his will without choice on his part of geography, hospital or doctor.

There has been no previous mental preparation on the part of the patient for such an unexpected disaster. It is difficult enough for a patient to prepare himself over a period of days or weeks for a bout of elective surgery but to be suddenly and unexpectedly thrust on the operating table under emergency circumstances is psychologically catastrophic.

The physician who is alert to this extreme psychic trauma will recognize psychological assessment requires the same expertise and attention as the technical problems of operative repair. A disregard or non-recognizance of the role of psychologic derangements in the critically injured patient regularly produces unnecessary suffering, prolonged hospitalization, bizarre complications and a general resistance to the overall plan of management adopted by the physician.

The quality of life when survival has finally been insured by modern operative technique is often determined more by proper psychological assessment and support than any other factor.

Every physician has observed the different responses of patients to the unexpected but necessary amputation of an extremity. Amputations from the standpoint of operative technique do not vary that much, but patient responses to the loss of a leg or arm are protean.

Application and evaluation of psychometric methods of personality testing are tasks for the trained clinical psychologist. The surgeon neither has the time nor the interest to become skilled in these techniques. But such sophisticated testing does not necessarily yield valid predictions of personality when applied to situations outside the laboratory.[1] The mature, alert, experienced surgeon must learn to assess the seriously injured patient who has a real threat to life, limb, job and social relationships. The psychological evaluation appropriate to this situation is an intuitive, not an experimental one.

Relying upon this initial assessment, the physician must decide which is an appropriate problem for the psychiatrist-clinical psychologist, the medical sociologist, or the chaplain, and utilize these ancillary personnel for specific indications. He must decide the ethical question of which patients need be subjected to psychological testing.

Hetherington[2] defined areas of cooperation in which the clinical psychologists can aid in these situations, listing rehabilitation of brain damaged patients, problems of communication and modification of the environment of prolonged hospitalized patients.

Just as the priority of airway obstruction is primordial in the physical evaluation, so priority is given in psychological assessment to what a person aims for in the future not his experiences in the past. The critically injured patient who has lost a leg or close relative in a severe automobile crash is evaluated on the basis of his projected plans for the future and his determination to overcome his losses no matter how great.

The accurate evaluation by the surgeon of the protean personality responses in these critical areas will determine the type of consultation his patient needs just as decreasing level of consciousness and localizing signs suggests consultative aid from a neurosurgeon.

DENIAL

This patient reacts with the common, "Oh no! This couldn't happen to me!" attitude. Past experiences have congealed this attitude that plane crashes, skyjacking, and automobile accidents are all things that happen to other people. His loss of a leg, a wife or child, or even sometimes a combination of these is one of purest disbelief.

In his recovery room bed he anticipates the lost relative suddenly walking up to the bedside and inquiring as to how he is getting along. Many patients are amnesiac regarding the accident and others regard it as a horrendous nightmare that never really happened.

This type individual looks at his amputated stump or feels the eye patch and compensates by believing that his leg will be placed back on by some form of modern surgical miracle, or that he could never really lose an eye so quickly.

These individuals are trying hard to keep the image of "self intact." These defense mechanisms are operating to maintain integrity and identity of the personality.

This problem is particularly difficult in a patient if the particular part of his body is a major factor in his identity, e.g. an amputated hand of a concert pianist, an eye of an artist, a leg of a cross-country olympic champion. In some instances another person may be so related that his loss disrupts unity of the image of self in the surviving patient, e.g. a brother who is also a business partner, a wife as a part of a man-wife duet, a son who drives his invalid father to the office each day.

This patient is recognized by his overly solicitous treatment of recovery room and intensive care unit nurses and personnel, his inappropriate response to his serious condition, and general denial that this is actually "himself" caught up in such a sequence of events.

As the physician informs the patient of his losses or amputations he must watch for these responses. The hospital chaplain and psychiatrists are the immediate consultants.

LOSS-DEPRESSION

Most individuals perceiving significant separation with a part of their body or death of a loved one live through a process of mourning as described by Freud. The symptoms involve temporary withdrawal and internalization of behavioral characteristics, often maintaining their loss on a symbolic level (phantom limb pain).

These patients do not have the problem of accepting reality of their loss of a part or a loved one but, rather, they accept their losses too readily and enter into profound depression and mourning. This response to serious injury primarily affects survival itself and not to such a great extent the quality of life after survival as in the first instance.

This mental depression influences the patient's physical recovery from his injury in numerous ways. He is ineffective in coughing and clearing his airway of retained secretions and is, therefore, more susceptible to atlectasis and pneumonia. He may become hostile toward nurses and physicians trying to clear his airway and improve his condition. He refuses to co-operate with pulmonary therapists and in extreme cases, will even be abusive to such individuals.

Their chief attitude is "Why did this happen to me?" Many times an individual in this group suffers from deep feelings of guilt,[3] especially so if alcohol was involved in the accident or if he was the driver of the car in which his wife or loved one was killed. He may imagine the affection of the rest of the family being withdrawn. If he was the chief supporter financially of the family he becomes depressed at the thoughts of a prolonged or enforced period of invalidism or loss of his occupation, because without his leg or arm he cannot continue to work on a plant assembly line.

This combination of loss-depression, guilt, and fear can influence the overall recovery of this group of patients in a real way.[3] The alert, experienced physician must recognize these psychological factors and request consultation. The patients in this depression group can be aided by consultation from the medical sociologists, hospital chaplain, physiotherapists and rehabilitation personnel.

EGO-DEFENSE

This critically injured group is not faced with loss of a loved one nor loss of a portion of their body through amputation, but their injuries may threaten the ego-defense mechanism.

The quality of this individual's life after recovery from his severe injury is greatly dependent upon the continued existence of ego-defense mechanism.

The coping processes of the patient may have been impaired or totally destroyed by the critical injury. The physician must assess these factors and request consultation from his psychiatric colleagues. This particular type of personality is so complex and may have precursors in the dynamics of early experience; hence, the clinical psychologists may also render service with psychometric testing and give valuable information in the rehabilitation of this patient.

REFERENCES

1. Semeneoff, B.: Personality assessment: Prediction or description. *Adv Sci, 26*:161-171, 1969.
2. Hetherington, R.: Psychology in the general hospital. *Br Psychol Soc Bull, 20*:7-10, 1967.
3. Gruneberg, R.: Psychological assessment in trauma. *J Trauma, 12*:364, 1972.

APPENDIX A

CURRICULUM FOR TRAINING EMERGENCY MEDICAL TECHNICIANS

24 three-hour sessions plus four in-hospital training sessions

Session	Topic	Content and objectives
		These Sessions Are Designed to—
1.	General information and orientation	Describe ambulance and equipment; objectives of training; responsibilities to patient, family, religion; police and
2.	General information and orientation	news media; public relations; control of scene; handling of the deceased; sorting multiple casualties; defensive and emergency driving°; communications; reports and records.
3.	Anatomy and physiology	Describe, using visual aids, anatomical structures as they should be understood by emergency medical technicians;
4.	Anatomy and physiology	physiology of respiration, circulation, nervous, osseous and muscular systems; and how to evaluate diagnostic signs.
5.	Review, questions and evaluation session	Make certain students have assimilated material presented in previous sessions and are prepared for those to follow.
6.	Life-threatening problem—pulmonary	Emphasize necessity to establish and maintain airway. Describe artificial ventilation such as mouth-to-mouth and other methods (bag-mask resuscitation units and manually triggered units). Demonstrate use of suction equipment and airways.
7.	Life-threatening problem—cardiac arrest	Teach how to recognize arrest and perform external cardiac compression, using inflatable mannequins, and film "Pulse of Life."
8.	Practice session— cardiopulmonary resuscitation	Review techniques of providing and maintaining an open airway, using equipment; artificial ventilation; use of oxygen and external cardiac compression. (Students are separated into groups depending on number of inflatable mannequins available but never in a group of more than ten per instructor and mannequin.)
9.	Review, questions and evaluation session	Make certain students have assimilated material in lessons 6, 7, and 8; re-instruct them in techniques covered in those sessions.
10.	Life-threatening problem—bleeding and shock	Teach how to recognize and control bleeding, using pressure dressings; explain limited use of tourniquet; give measures to overcome shock, including intravenous fluids; conduct general discussion and demonstration using training arm (actual performance during training in hospital sessions).

431

Session	Topic	Content and objectives
11.	Acute medical problems	Instruct on heart attack, stroke, diabetes, contagious disease, allergic reactions, convulsive disorders, unruly patient,
12.	Acute medical problems	nosebleed, poisonings, exposure to heat and cold; heart failure; pulmonary edema; emphysema and unconscious states.
13.	Review, questions and evaluation session	Make certain students have assimilated material in lessons 10, 11 and 12; and re-instruct them in techniques covered in those sessions.
14a.	Emergency obstetrics and care of infants	Instruct on physiology of childbirth; how to deliver infant, protecting it and mother; ligation of the cord; afterbirth; care of infant, including transportation of the premature infant. Film "Medical Self Help," Lesson 11 (page 4) is excellent for teaching.
14b.	Eye, body cavity and genitalia injuries	Instruct on care of eye injuries; protective dressings; care of thoracic cage injuries, including fractures, crushed chest, flail chest and sucking wounds; care for evisceration and blast injuries of the abdomen; protect genitalia and transport avulsed genital parts.
15.	Wounds, burns, and environmental injuries	Instruct on soft tissue injuries, including thermal, electrical and radiation injuries.
16.	Fractures and dislocations of long bones and pelvis	Instruct on anatomy and terminology of fractures; how to suspect fractures; reasons for splinting; splinting equipment and its use. Demonstration.
17.	Spinal fractures and head injuries	Instruct on danger of spinal fractures; reasons for protecting spine against movements; extrication, including use of backboards; dressings and splinting prior to movement; significance of head injuries and handling the unconscious accident victim.
18.	Practice session	Apply dressings, bandages, and splints.
19.	Movement of patients	Describe lifts and carries; use of litters and stretchers, including movement of patients under difficult circumstances; presentation of slides and demonstration of lifts and carries by instructors.
20.	Extrication	Describe surgical principles—presentation and demonstration by instructors.
21.	Practice session	Practice use of lifts and carries, litters and stretchers, including movement of patients under difficult circumstances.
22.	Practice session	Practice extrication, including care of patient, dressing, bandaging and splinting prior to movement.
23.	Practice session	
24.	Written and practical examination	Determine proficiency of technicians.

The four supplemental sessions are designed to —supply in-hospital training with exposure to cardiopulmonary resuscitation, obstetrical problems, general care of patient, intravenous fluids and blood pressure monitoring.

°In this course, defensive and emergency driving are discussed in general terms. It is highly desirable that emergency medical technicians avail themselves of the present courses given in each state in defensive and emergency driving.

Reprinted courtesy of Farrington, J. D., and Hampton, O. S., Jr.: A curriculum for training emergency medical technicians. *Bull Am Coll Surg,* Sept-Oct, 1969.

AIDS FOR INSTRUCTORS

Printed Material for Instructors

Curriculum for Training Emergency Medical Technicians, Division of Emergency Health Services, Public Health Service (First Report under American College of Surgeons–Public Health Service Contract No. 110-69-10).

Cardiopulmonary Resuscitation, A Manual for Instructors. Published by the American Heart Association, Catalogue #EM408. One for each course.

Reference Material for Instructors

Emergency Medical Guide, Second Edition. John Henderson. New York, Blakiston Division, McGraw-Hill Book Co., Inc., 1969.

First Aid, Diagnosis and Management. Edited by Warren H. Cole and Charles B. Puestow. New York, Appleton-Century and Crofts, sixth edition, 1965. One for each course.

Emergency Victim Care and Rescue Textbook for Squadmen, 1965. Ohio Trade and Industrial Education Service, Division of Vocational Education, State Department of Education. Published by Instructional Materials Laboratory, Ohio State University, Columbus.

REFERENCES FOR STUDENTS

Printed Material for Students

Topics	Session
Wonderful Human Machine, The. Published by American Medical Association, Catalogue No. OP9. One for each student	3-5
Training of Ambulance Personnel in Cardiopulmonary Resuscitation. Discussion guide published by American Heart Association,	

Catalogue No. EM386A. One for each student.   6-9
Emergency Measures in Cardiopulmonary Resuscitation. Discussion guide published by American Heart Association, Catalogue No. EM376A. One for each student.   6-9
Minimal Equipment for Ambulances. Committee on Trauma, American College of Surgeons. Bulletin, A.C.S. March-April, 1967. One for each student.   10, 14b, 15-17
First Aid for Laryngectomees. International Association of Laryngectomees-American Cancer Society, 219 East 42 Street, New York 10017. One for each student.   6-9

Reference Material for Students

Emergency Care of the Sick and Injured. Edited by Robert H. Kennedy, and sponsored by the Committee on Trauma, American College of Surgeons. Philadelphia, W. B. Saunders Co., 1966.   1-23
First Aid for Emergency Crews: A Manual on Emergency First Aid Procedures for Ambulance Crews, Law Enforcement Officers, Fire Service Personnel, Wrecker Drivers, Hospital Staffs, Industry, Nurses. Carl B. Young, Jr. Springfield, Thomas, 1966.   1-23
Pennsylvania Ambulance Attendant Training Manual. Edited by Dan D. Gowings, Pennsylvania Department of Health, Harrisburg.   1-23

AUDIO-VISUAL AIDS

Topics   *Session*
A.C.S. slides set: Series A (Sessions 1, 2); C (3, 4); F (6, 7); G (10); M (11, 12); N (14a, 14b); H (15); J and K (16); L (17); B (20). One set (560) slides for each course.
Training of Ambulance Personnel in Cardiopulmonary Resuscitation. American Heart Association. Slide set, Catalogue No. EM386. One set for each course.   6-9
Emergency Measures in Cardiopulmonary Resuscitation. American Heart Association. Slide set, Catalogue No. EM376. One set for each course.   6-9
Medical Self-Help. Lessons 1-11 (motion pictures). U.S. Public Health Service. Available through: Regional Program Director, P.H.S.   1-23
Breath of Life, motion picture. American Heart Association   6-9
Pulse of Life, motion picture. American Heart Association.   6-9
Cry for Help, motion picture. U.S. Public Health Service Audio-Visual Facility, Atlanta, Georgia. Code MIS 682   12

EQUIPMENT

Topics   *Session*
Blackboard, chalk and eraser   1-23
Mannequins
   Resusci-Anne of equivalent   6-9
   Thoracic cut-away or equivalent   6-9
   Anatomic-Anne of equivalent   6-9
   Clothes mannequin and moulages provided locally for simulated injuries   10, 13-17, 20-23
Simulated or outdated blood (simulated blood made with liquid starch and food coloring) to pour on rugs, carpet, car seats, clothes, etc., to simulate injuries and aid in instruction in esti-

mating blood loss.   10, 13-15
Long and short spine boards (use of a scoop-type stretcher
optional).   16-18, 20-23
Automobile front seat affixed to table to demonstrate proper appli-
cation of short board to sitting injured and application of long
board.   20-23
Minimal Equipment for Ambulances. Committee on Trauma,
American College of Surgeons.   10, 13-17, 20-23
(Bulletin, A.C.S., March-April, 1967). One of each item listed,
and in addition, inflatable splint, blood pressure manometer, two-
way teaching stethoscope.
Aluminum foil, roll eighteen inches wide, for wrapping premature infants, except for face, when ambulance does not carry
incubator, and also for covering eviscerations and sucking wounds
of the chest.   14a, 15
Doll, approximately seventeen to twenty inches long, for practice
of above.   14a

APPENDIX B

ESSENTIALS OF A RESIDENCY TRAINING
PROGRAM FOR EMERGENCY PHYSICIANS*

PROPOSED ESSENTIALS OF A RESIDENCY TRAINING
PROGRAM FOR EMERGENCY PHYSICIANS*

I. The provisions of the General Requirements (Section 1-10) as stated in the "Essentials of Approved Residencies" must be met.

II. *Special Requirements* for Residency Training for an Emergency Physician Residency training for Emergency Physicians should be specifically designed to meet the needs of graduates intending to become Emergency Physicians. An Emergency Physician is defined as one who

   a. Provides first contact emergent, urgent, and immediate health services to patients of all ages;

   b. Evaluates the patient's emergent, urgent, and immediate health needs and provides such services as are immediately indicated, and refers the patient to appropriate other physicians for further definitive care when indicated; and

   c. Insures that the patient will have available to him appropriate follow-up care in or out of the hospital as may be required.

   He will be a physician trained in all phases of evaluation and treatment of emergent, urgent, and immediate problems.

III. *Duration of Training*

   The duration of training should be a total of thirty-six months following graduation from an accredited medical school. The training may be organized as a two-year residency to

---

* Taken from *Directory of Approved Internships and Residencies*. American Medical Association, 1969-1970.

* *Directory of Approved Internships and Residencies*, American Medical Association, 1969-1970.

follow a year of an approved internship. As an alternative, it may be organized as a three-year graduate training program without an internship.

IV. *Principles*

1. Since the Emergency Physician will utilize the skills, techniques, and knowledge of all other disciplines, it will be necessary that the resident spend a considerable portion of his residency learning each of the traditional specialties. He must not, however, lose his identity as an Emergency Physician Resident, and his training should be designed with emphasis on the recognition and treatment of acute problems.

2. The hospital and the Emergency Department responsible for the administration of the residency program must meet with the following minimal requirements:

    a. There must be a patient load of approximately 36,000 patients visits per year in the Emergency Department.

    b. There must be a full-time Director of the Emergency Department.

    c. The Emergency Department must be constituted as a full and equal department within the hospital organization.

    d. The Emergency Department Director must assume responsibility for the entire training program.

    e. The hospital must provide inservice beds and residency training programs in at least four of the following specialties:

    > Medicine
    > Surgery
    > Ob-Gyn
    > Pediatrics
    > Family Practice

    f. University affiliation is to be strongly encouraged.

3. Training need not take place in one geographical location nor in one institution, provided 80 percent of training time is spent in the parent institution and that the train-

ing is coordinated to insure completeness and that the department director retains administrative control of the resident.

4. At least every six months, an evaluation of the resident's experiences will be conducted. In addition, the resident will provide for the Director, a critique of the program. The program should provide enough flexibility that possible deficiencies may be corrected. Evaluations and critiques must be written and a copy kept in the departmental files for inspection.

5. Periodic in-training examination of the resident (written, oral, and practical) is required in order to evaluate the program and the resident and to provide experience in taking future certification examinations. Copies of both the examination and results must be kept in departmental files for inspection.

6. Prerequisites for a two-year residency program shall include successful completion of at least one year of formal, postgraduate training.

7. Financing shall be the same as other graduate training programs of the institution providing that residency.

8. The residency program examinations of ACEP will make the final recommendations to ABEP for approval of a particular residency program.

V. Content

1. The Emergency Physician Resident shall be trained in the emergency aspects of the other disciplines. He should be made familiar with the principles of continuity of care in the other disciplines in order that he may more properly initiate emergency treatment.

2. A portion of the residency shall include training in Intensive Care and Coronary Care Units supervised by attending physicians.

3. Since much emergency care is provided for ambulatory patients, a certain amount of out-patient care training is desirable. This may be provided in multi-disciplinary setting of a hospital out-patient department, or it may, in some instances, be provided in physician's offices.

4. The following proposals are made as approximate allotments of time to be spent (a) in a two-year program with an internship, and (b) in a three-year program without an internship. In either case, emphasis in the major areas of those aspects which relate to emergency medicine should be made.

	2-year Program	*3-year Program*
Medicine and Subspecialties (especially Infections, Endocrine, Cardiology, Metabolic, Drug Reactions, and Dermatology)	4 mo. (11%)*	6 mo. (16%)**
Surgery and Subspecialties (especially Acute Abdomen, Chest Injuries Projectile Wounds, Burns, G.I. Hemorrhage, Cut-Downs, Plastic Closure, Tracheostomy, Shock)	4 mo. (11%)*	4 mo. (11%)**
Pediatrics (especially Infections, Poisoning, Convulsions)	2 mo. (5.5%)* 2 mo. (5.5%)**	
Ob-Gyn (especially Deliveries, Pelvic Infections, Vaginal Bleeding, Pelvic and Perineal Injuries)	2 mo. (5.5%)*	2 mo. (5.5%)**
Radiology (especially Diagnostic, and to include, if possible, ultrasound diagnostic	3 mo. 8.3%)**	3 mo. 8.3%)**
Orthopedics (especially Fractures, Sprains, Dis- locations and Traction Procedures)	2 mo. (5.5%)**	2 mo. (5.5%)**
Neurology and Neurosurgery (especially Head Injuries, Coma, and Nerve Injuries, the management of like, Threatening injuries)	1 mo. (2.8%)**	1 mo. (2.8%)**
Psychiatry and Toxicology (especially Acute Neuroses, Acute Psychoses, Suicidal patients, and Poisonings)	1 mo. (2.8%)**	1 mo. (2.8%)**
Opthalmology and Otorhinolaryngology (especially Injuries, Foreign Bodies, Hemorrhage and Infections)	1 mo. (2.8%)**	1 mo. (2.8%)**
Anesthesia and P.A.R. (especially Airways, Fluids, Supportive Care, Pulmonary Physiology, Inhala- tion techniques and treatment	1 mo. (2.8%)**	1 mo. (2.8%)**
Emergency Services	8 mo. (25%)* & **	8 mo. (25%)**
Electives	4 mo. (11%)* & **	2 mo. (6%)**

---

* Internship
** Residency

5. Also included should be a series of didactic lectures through the entire three years to cover Emergency Department Administration and Hospital Administration and the basic aspects of the various medical specialties, as well as forensic medicine.
6. He should be a member of the Hospital's C.P.R. team.
7. At least two months of the first year must be spent in the Emergency Department, and two months in the second year.
8. On each rotation, the resident is to see the acutely ill patient and to follow him to the conclusion of treatment.
9. In the senior year of residency, he must participate in community emergency care councils and emergency planning.

VI. Goals
   A. It is anticipated that this recommended training program will accomplish the basic goal of training physicians qualified to deliver primary emergency health services. It is further anticipated that graduates of such a program will be eligible to take a certifying examination when an American Board for certification in this specialty is established.
   B. The training of Emergency Physicians should include research centered in the field of Emergency Care and its delivery.

Revised Draft
Unofficial—2/12/71

APPENDIX C

COMPREHENSIVE INJURY SCALE FOR RATING THE SEVERITY OF TISSUE DAMAGE*

ABBREVIATIONS AND QUANTITATIVE TERMINOLOGY USED IN COMPREHENSIVE INJURY SCALE

Terminology	Abbreviation	Quantitation Code
ENERGY DISSIPATED	ED	Little 1 Minor 2 Moderate 3 Major 4 Maximum 5
THREAT TO LIFE	TL	None 1 Minor 2 Moderate 3 Severe 4 Maximum 5
PERMANENT IMPAIRMENT	PI	20% or less 1 21%-40% 2 41%-60% 3 61%-90% 4 91%-100% 5
TREATMENT PERIOD	TP	2 weeks or less 1 2 to 8 weeks 2 8 to 26 weeks 3 26 to 52 weeks 4 52 weeks or more 5
INCIDENCE	IN	Unusual 1 Occasional 2 Common 3 Very Common 4 Most Frequent 5

---

* Reproduced with permission. *JAMA,* vol. 220, 1972, pp. 717-720.

COMPREHENSIVE INJURY SCALE
Internal Medicine—General Surgery

AIS	INJURY DESCRIPTION	ED	TL	PI	TP	IN
	CHEST					
1	Abrasion	1	1	1	1	5
1	Contusion	2	1	1	1	4
1	Laceration	1	1	1	1	4
4	Crush	4	4	3	3	2
	Fracture [open fracture: +1, AIS, ED, TL, TP; —1 IN]					
2	Sternum	4	2	2	3	2
2	Rib	3	1	1	2	4
4	Puncture (sucking wound)	4	4	3	3	1
	Injury involving					
5	Hemomediastinum	4	4	3	3	1
3	Hemothorax	3	3	2	2	3
4	Pneumomediastinum	4	4	2	2	2
3	Pneumothorax	3	3	2	2	3
5	Tracheo-bronchial system	5	5	4	4	1
	HEART AND GREAT VESSELS					
	Contusion					
3	Pericardium	3	3	1	2	3
	[+1 PI; —1 IN with pericarditis]					
4	Myocardium	4	3	3	2	1
	[+1 AIS, ED, TL PI, TP for severe]					
	Laceration					
4	Pericardium	3	3	2	2	2
	[+1 PI; —1 IN with pericarditis]					
5	Aorta	4	5	3	3	3
5	Coronary artery	4	5	4	3	1
5	Myocardium	4	4	3	3	2
5	Pulmonary vein	5	5	3	3	1
5	Pulmonary artery	5	5	3	3	1
5	Superior/inferior vena cavae	5	5	3	3	1
5	Heart/great vessels	5	5	5	4	1
5	Intracardiac (valve, septum)	5	5	5	4	1
	Puncture, Rupture					
5	Heart/great vessels	5	5	5	4	1
	ABDOMEN					
	Abrasion					
1	Abdominal wall	1	1	1	1	4
	Contusion					
1	Abdominal wall	2	1	1	2	4
3	Pancreas	4	3	2	3	1
	Laceration					
1	Abdominal wall	1	1	1	1	4
3	Stomach	3	3	3	3	2
	Liver					
4	Minor	3	3	2	2	3
5	Extensive/severe	4	4	3	3	2
4	Duodenum	3	3	3	3	2
4	Pancreas	4	4	4	3	2
	[+1 AIS, ED, TP; —1 IN if duodenum involvement]					
3	Mesentary	4	2	3	2	2
	[+1 AIS, TL, PI, TP; —1 IN if vascular involvement]					

AIS	INJURY DESCRIPTION	ED	TL	PI	TP	IN
5	Major vessels	5	5	4	3	2
	Muscle transection					
3	Abdominal wall	3	1	2	2	2
4	Pancreas	5	4	4	4	1
	Rupture					
2	Abdominal wall	3	1	1	3	2
	[+1 PI if herniated]					
3	Diaphragm [+1 PI if herniated]	4	3	2	3	2
4	Spleen	3	4	2	2	3
5	Liver	4	5	3	3	2
	Puncture					
4	Small bowel	4	3	2	2	1
	[+1 AIS, ED, TL, PI, TP for multiple]					
4	Large bowel	4	4	3	3	1
	Injury involving					
4	Biliary tract	4	4	4	3	2

COMPREHENSIVE INJURY SCALE

Neurological Surgery*

AIS	INJURY DESCRIPTION	ED	TL	PI	TP	IN
	EXTRAVRANIAL SCALP					
1	Abrasion	2	1	1	1	3
1	Contusion	2	1	1	1	2
	Laceration					
1	Minor	2	1	1	1	2
2	Extensive	3	1	1	2	1
2	Hematoma	2	1	1	1	2
	SKULL					
	Fracture					
2	Linear, no loss of consciousness	3	1	1	2	2
	[+1 TL for temporal]					
2	Basilar	3	3	1	2	1
	Closed, depressed					
3	no sinus or arterial injury	3	2	1	2	2
4	sinus or arterial injury with clot	3	5	3	4	1
4	Depresed, cerebral laceration	3	3	4	3	1
	[+1 TP & IN for frontal & occipital]					
	Cerebral Concussion, loss of consciousness					
2	<15 min	3	1	1	1	5
3	15 min-24 hrs	4	2	1	2	2
5	<24 hrs, associated					
	neurological signs	5	4	4	4	2
5	>hrs, intracerebarl clot	5	5	5	5	2
	Lesion, Cerebellum & Posterior Fossa					
4	Hematoma [+1 AIS, TL, PI, TP for intracerebellar]	4	4	3	4	1
	Contusion					
5	Medulla	5	5	4	5	2

---

* See also ORTHOPEDIC SURGERY SCALE for spinal cord injuries.

AIS	INJURY DESCRIPTION	ED	TL	PI	TP	IN
	SPINAL CORD**					
1	Cerivical spine injury complaint— no anatomical or radiological evidence ("whiplash")	2	1	1	1	4
	Cervical spine injury					
4	Partial paralysis	4	3	4	5	1
5	Total paralysis	4	5	5	5	2
	Dorsal spine injury					
4	Total paralysis	4	2	5	5	2
	[—1 AIS, PI for partial]					

** It should be noted that although nerve injuries, cranial and peripheral, do occur in varying degrees of severity, they often are connected with other more serious injuries, and, therefore, are implied in the ratings for these latter injuries.

COMPREHENSIVE INJURY SCALE

Obstetrics and Gynecology

AIS	INJURY DESCRIPTION	ED	TL	PI	TP	IN
	BREAST					
1	Abrasion	1	1	1	1	4
1	Contusion	1	1	1	1	4
	Laceration					
1	Minor	1	1	1	1	4
2	Extensive/severe	3	2	1	1	3
	PELVIS					
	Hematoma					
2	Below levator ani muscles	1	2	1	1	2
3	Above levator ani muscles	3	3	3	3	2
	VULVA, PERINEUM, VAGINA [—1 IN for VAGINA]					
1	Abrasion	1	1	1	1	2
1	Contusion	1	1	1	1	2
	Laceration					
1	Minor	1	1	1	1	2
3	Severe, no organ/peritoneal cavity involvement	3	2	1	1	2
	PERITONEUM					
	Laceration					
	Extensive/severe					
4	No bladder/rectum involvement	3	3	2	2	1
5	Bladder/rectum rupture	4	5	3	3	3
4	Hematoma—retroperitoneal	3	3	3	3	3
	UTERUS, OVARY					
	Avulsion					
4	No bladder/rectum involvement	5	4	5	3	1
5	Bladder/rectum rupture	5	5	5	4	1

COMPREHENSIVE INJURY SCALE
Ophthalmology

AIS	INJURY DESCRIPTION	ED	TL	PI	TP	IN
	Abrasion					
1	Lids	1	1	1	1	4
1	Conjunctiva	1	1	1	1	3
1	Cornea	1	1	1	1	3
	Contusion					
1	Lids	1	1	1	1	4
	Laceration					
1	Lids	1	1	2	2	3
1	Canaliculus	1	1	3	2	2
1	Conjunctiva	1	1	1	1	3
2	Cornea	1	1	3	2	2
2	Sclera	1	1	2	2	2
1	Retina	3	1	2	3	2
	Rupture					
2	Sclera	3	1	3	2	1
1	Choroid	3	1	3	2	1
	Hemorrhage					
1	Retina	3	1	2	2	2
1	Vitreous body	3	1	2	2	2
	Detachment					
1	Iris	3	1	2	2	2
2	Retina	3	1	3	4	2
	Edema					
1	Retina	3	1	2	2	2
	Foreign Body					
1	Cornea	1	1	2	1	2
2	Cataract	3	1	3	4	2
2	Paresis/Paralysis	3	1	2	2	2
	Avulsion					
2	Lids	3	1	3	4	2
3	Optic Nerve	4	1	4	4	1

COMPREHENSIVE INJURY SCALE

Orthopedic Surgery

AIS	INJURY DESCRIPTION	ED	TL	PI	TP	IN
	UPPER EXTREMITIES					
1	Abrasion	1	1	1	1	5
1	Contusion	1	1	1	1	5
	Laceration					
1	Minor	1	1	1	1	5
2	Extensive	1	1	1	2	5
3	Severe involving major nerves	3	2	3	5	1
3	Severe involving major vessels	3	4	1	2	1
	Sprain					
3	Major joint	2	1	1	2	4
1	Minor joint	2	1	1	1	3

AIS	INJURY DESCRIPTION	ED	TL	PI	TP	IN
	Crush					
4	Limb	4	3	4	5	1
3	Digit	4	2	3	4	2
	Fracture [open fracture: +1 ED, TL, TP; −1 IN]					
2	Scapula/clavicle	2	1	1	2	4
2	Humerus	3 (−1E1)	2	1	3	3
2	Elbow [multiple: +1 ED, TP, PI]	3	2	1	2 (−1Ch)	3
2	Radius/ulna [if both: +1 ED, PI, TP]	3	2	3	3	2
2	Carpus, metacarpus	3	1	2	3	2
1	Digit	3	1	2	2	3
3	Multiple segment or long bone	4	3	4	4	1
	Dislocation					
3	Shoulder	3	1	1	2	2
3	Elbow	3	1	1	3	2
3	Wrist	3	1	3	4	2
2	Carpus, metacarpus	3	1	3	4	2
1	Digit	3	1	2	2	3
	Amputation					
4	Above elbow	5	4	5	3	1
4	Below elbow	5	3	5	3	2
2	Digit [thumb: +1 PI]	4	2	2	2	2
	LOWER EXTREMITIES					
1	Abrasion	1	1	1	1	5
1	Contusion	1	1	1	1	5
	Laceration					
1	Minor	1	1	1	1	5
2	Extensive	2	3	2	2	1
3	Severe involving major nerves	3	2	3	5	1
3	Severe involving major vessels	3	4	1	2	1
	Sprain					
3	Major joint	2	1	1	1	3
1	Minor joint	2	1	1	1	2
	Crush					
4	Limb	5	4	3	5	1
3	Digit	5	3	2	4	2
	Fracture [open fracture, major bones: +1 ED, TL, TP; minor bones: +1 ED]					
2	Femoral neck	4 (−1E1)	3 (+1E1)	4	5	1
2	Femoral shaft	4	3 (−1Ch)	1	4	3
2	Patella	3	1	1	3	4
2	Tibia with or without Fibula	4	2 (−1Ch)	2	4 (−2Ch)	4
2	Fibula	2	1	1	2	2
2	Malleolus	3	1	2	3	3
	Foot					
2	Single	2	1	1	2	2
3	Multiple	5	2	2	4	2
3	Talus displaced	4	2	3	4	1

AIS	INJURY DESCRIPTION	ED	TL	PI	TP	IN
1	Digit	2	1	1	2	3
4	Multiple segment or long bone	5	4	4	5	2
	Dislocation					
3	Hip	4	2	4	5	2
3	Knee	4	3	3	4	1
			(—1Ch)			
3	Ligament tears	4	3	3	4	1
			(—1Ch)			
3	Ankle	3	1	2	3	3
2	Tarsus	4	2	3	3	1
1	Digit	2	1	1	2	3
	Amputation					
4	Above knee	5	5	5	3	1
4	Below knee	4	4	4	3	1
2	Digit	2	2	1	3	2
	PELVIS					
	Fracture involving sacrum					
2	Simple	4	2	1	2	3
3	Severe	5	3	2	3	2
3	Sacro-iliac fracture/dislocation	5	3	2	3	1
3	Symphysis pubis separation	5	3	2	3	1
	CERVICAL SPINE					
	Acute strain					
1	No neuro damage	2	1	1	1	4
2	Nerve root damage	3	1	3	3	2
5	Cord transection	5	5	5	5	1
3	Fracture, transverse or spinous process	3	2	1	3	1
	Fracture/dislocation					
3	No neuro damage	3	2	2	3	2
4	Nerve root damage	4	3	3	4	2
5	Cord transection	4	5	5	5	1
	THORACO-LUMBAR SPINE					
	Acute strain					
1	No neuro damage	3	1	1	3	4
2	Nerve root damage	3	1	3	3	2
5	Cord transection	5	2	3	3	1
4	Fracture, transverse or spinous process	4	2	3	3	2
	Fracture/dislocation					
2	No neuro damage	4	1	2	3	2
4	Nerve root damage	5	2	3	4	2
5	Cord transection	4	4	5	5	1

COMPREHENSIVE INJURY SCALE

Otolaryngology

AIS	INJURY DESCRIPTION	ED	TL	PI	TP	IN
	EAR					
	Abrasion)					
1	Contusion) Pinna	1	1	1	1	4
	Laceration)					
	Avulsion					

AIS	INJURY DESCRIPTION	ED	TL	PI	TP	IN
3	Pinna	2	1	3	2	2
	Fracture					
	Temporal bone with					
2	Deafness	4	2	3	1	2
4	Vertigo	5	4	3	3	2
				(+1E1)		
5	Hemorrhage	5	5	2	2	1
	Dislocation					
2	Ossicular chain	3	1	2	1	2
	Rupture					
2	Tympanic membrane	1	1	1	2	3
	Injury to					
1	Ear canal	1	1	1	1	3
	Inner ear with					
2	Deafness or vertigo [if both,					
	+1, AIS, PI]	3	1	3	3	1
				(+1E1)		
	*NOSE**					
	Fracture					
	Ethmoid					
2	Hemorrhage	2	4	1	2	2
2	Hypertelorism	3	4	2	2	2
2	Nasolacrimal or nasofrontal duct	3	2	2	2	1
3	Dural tear & CSF leak	3	4	2	2	2
	Sphenoid					
4	Hemorrhage	4	4	1	1	1
4	CSF leak	4	4	1	2	1

* See also PLASTIC SURGERY

AIS	INJURY DESCRIPTION	ED	TL	PI	TP	IN
	THROAT					
	Contusion					
1	Pharynx [+1 AIS,, TL for					
	hematoma]	1	1	1	1	2
2	Esophagus	2	1	1	1	1
	Laceration					
1	Pharynx [+ AIS, ED, TL, IN					
	for hemorrhage]	1	1	1	1	1
5	Esophagus	5	5	4	4	1
4	Larynx	2	3	3	2	2
4	Trachea	1	3	1	2	2
	Fracture					
4	Larynx	3	4	4	2	2
	Foreign body without blockage					
2	Esophagus	1	3	1	1	3
5	Larynx	2	5	1	1	2
	Obstruction					
5	Pharynx	2	4	1	1	1
4	Esophagus	4	4	3	1	3
5	Larynx	2	5	1	1	2
	Upper airway					
2	Moderate respiratory difficulty	2	2	1	2	3
5	Serious respiratory difficulty	3	5	3	3	2
	Hematoma					

AIS	INJURY DESCRIPTION	ED	TL	PI	TP	IN
4	Larynx	2	4	1	1	3
	Puncture					
1	Pharynx	2	1	1	1	2
	Crush					
3	Trachea	2	2	1	2	1
	Dislocation					
4	Cricothyroid	3	3	2	2	1
	Paralysis					
2	Larynx	2	1	2	2	2
	Avulsion					
5	Esophagus	4	5	4	3	1
5	Larynx	4	5	4	2	1
5	Trachea	3	5	4	3	1

COMPREHENSIVE INJURY SCALE

Plastic Surgery

AIS	INJURY DESCRIPTION	ED	TL	PI	TP	IN
	FACE					
1	Abrasion	1	1	1	1	2
1	Contusion	1	1	1	1	3
	Laceration					
1	Minor	2	1	1	1	5
2	Extensive	3	1	1	1	4
3	Nerves/vessels involvement	4	2	3	1	3
4	Severe hemorrhage	4	3	1	2	1
	Fracture [open fracture: +1 AIS, ED, TL, TP; —1, IN]					
2	Mandile [—1 PI for ramus]	3	1	2	3	3
2	Temporo-mandibular joint	3	1	1	3	2
2	Maxilla	4	1	1	3	3
2	Zygoma	4	1	1	2	4
3	Comminuted	4	1	3	3	2
3	Depressed	4	1	3	2	3
	Temporal bone					
4	Longitudinal	3	3	2	3	2
4	Transverse	4	4	3	4	1
4	Frontal bone	4	4	3	4	1
	*NOSE**					
2	Fracture [open fracture: +1 AIS, ED, TL, TP; —1 IN]	2	1	3	2	5
	*EYE***					
3	Fracture—orbit, blowout [open fracture: +1 AIS, ED, TL, TP; —1 IN]	4	3	3	3	3

---

* See also OTOLARYNGOLOGY SCALE
** See also OPHTHALMOLOGY SCALE

COMPREHENSIVE INJURY SCALE

Urology

AIS	INJURY DESCRIPTION	ED	TL	PI	TP	IN
	Contusion					
3	Kidney	2	2	1	2	5
3	Bladder	3	2	1	3	2
3	Urethra	1	1	1	1	3
2	Penis	1	1	1	1	3
1	Scrotum and contents	1	1	1	1	4
	Laceration					
4	Kidney	3	4	1	3	3
3	Urethra	3	2	2	3	2
3	Penis	3	2	1	1	3
1	Scrotum and contents	3	1	1	1	3
	Rupture					
4	Kidney	5	5	1	5	1
4	Renal pelvis	4	3	1	5	1
3	Bladder [+1 AIS, IN for intraperitoneal]	4	4	1	5	3
	Avulsion					
5	Kidney pedicle	5	5	1	5	1
3	Ureter	5	3	3	5	1
3	Urethra	5	3	4	5	1
4	Penis	5	2	5	5	1
4	Scrotum and contents	5	2	4	4	1
				(+1Ch)		

INDEX